ENHANCING FOOD SAFETY

THE ROLE OF THE
FOOD AND DRUG ADMINISTRATION

Committee on the Review of the Food and Drug Administration's Role in Ensuring Safe Food

Food and Nutrition Board

Board on Agriculture and Natural Resources

Robert B. Wallace and Maria Oria, *Editors*

INSTITUTE OF MEDICINE *AND*
NATIONAL RESEARCH COUNCIL
OF THE NATIONAL ACADEMIES

THE NATIONAL ACADEMIES PRESS
Washington, D.C.
www.nap.edu

THE NATIONAL ACADEMIES PRESS   500 Fifth Street, N.W.   Washington, DC 20001

NOTICE: The project that is the subject of this report was approved by the Governing Board of the National Research Council, whose members are drawn from the councils of the National Academy of Sciences, the National Academy of Engineering, and the Institute of Medicine. The members of the committee responsible for the report were chosen for their special competences and with regard for appropriate balance.

This study was supported by Contract No. HHSF2232008100201 between the National Academy of Sciences and the Food and Drug Administration of the U.S. Department of Health and Human Services. Any opinions, findings, conclusions, or recommendations expressed in this publication are those of the author(s) and do not necessarily reflect the view of the organizations or agencies that provided support for this project.

Library of Congress Cataloging-in-Publication Data

Institute of Medicine (U.S.). Committee on the Review of Food and Drug Administration's Role in Ensuring Safe Food.
  Enhancing food safety : the role of the Food and Drug Administration / Committee on the Review of Food and Drug Administration's Role in Ensuring Safe Food, Food and Nutrition Board, Board on Agriculture and Natural Resources ; Robert B. Wallace and Maria Oria, editors.
      p. ; cm.
  Includes bibliographical references.
  ISBN 978-0-309-15273-0 (pbk.) — ISBN 978-0-309-15274-7 (pdf)
  1. Food—Safety measures—Government policy—United States. 2. United States. Food and Drug Administration. 3. Food—Safety regulations—United States. I. Wallace, Robert B., 1942- II. Oria, Maria. III. Title.
  [DNLM: 1. United States. Food and Drug Administration. 2. Food Supply—United States. 3. Food Contamination—prevention & control—United States. 4. Health Policy—United States. 5. Resource Allocation—United States. 6. Risk Assessment—United States. 7. United States Government Agencies—United States. WA 695]
  RA601.I39 2010
  363.19'20973—dc22
                                          2010029845

Additional copies of this report are available from the National Academies Press, 500 Fifth Street, N.W., Lockbox 285, Washington, DC 20055; (800) 624-6242 or (202) 334-3313 (in the Washington metropolitan area); Internet, http://www.nap.edu.

For more information about the Institute of Medicine, visit the IOM home page at: **www.iom.edu.**

Printed in the United States of America

The serpent has been a symbol of long life, healing, and knowledge among almost all cultures and religions since the beginning of recorded history. The serpent adopted as a logotype by the Institute of Medicine is a relief carving from ancient Greece, now held by the Staatliche Museen in Berlin.

Suggested citation: IOM (Institute of Medicine) and NRC (National Research Council). 2010. *Enhancing Food Safety: The Role of the Food and Drug Administration.* Washington, DC: The National Academies Press.

THE NATIONAL ACADEMIES
Advisers to the Nation on Science, Engineering, and Medicine

The **National Academy of Sciences** is a private, nonprofit, self-perpetuating society of distinguished scholars engaged in scientific and engineering research, dedicated to the furtherance of science and technology and to their use for the general welfare. Upon the authority of the charter granted to it by the Congress in 1863, the Academy has a mandate that requires it to advise the federal government on scientific and technical matters. Dr. Ralph J. Cicerone is president of the National Academy of Sciences.

The **National Academy of Engineering** was established in 1964, under the charter of the National Academy of Sciences, as a parallel organization of outstanding engineers. It is autonomous in its administration and in the selection of its members, sharing with the National Academy of Sciences the responsibility for advising the federal government. The National Academy of Engineering also sponsors engineering programs aimed at meeting national needs, encourages education and research, and recognizes the superior achievements of engineers. Dr. Charles M. Vest is president of the National Academy of Engineering.

The **Institute of Medicine** was established in 1970 by the National Academy of Sciences to secure the services of eminent members of appropriate professions in the examination of policy matters pertaining to the health of the public. The Institute acts under the responsibility given to the National Academy of Sciences by its congressional charter to be an adviser to the federal government and, upon its own initiative, to identify issues of medical care, research, and education. Dr. Harvey V. Fineberg is president of the Institute of Medicine.

The **National Research Council** was organized by the National Academy of Sciences in 1916 to associate the broad community of science and technology with the Academy's purposes of furthering knowledge and advising the federal government. Functioning in accordance with general policies determined by the Academy, the Council has become the principal operating agency of both the National Academy of Sciences and the National Academy of Engineering in providing services to the government, the public, and the scientific and engineering communities. The Council is administered jointly by both Academies and the Institute of Medicine. Dr. Ralph J. Cicerone and Dr. Charles M. Vest are chair and vice chair, respectively, of the National Research Council.

www.national-academies.org

Study Staff

MARIA ORIA, Study Director
RUTHIE S. ARIETI, Research Associate
ALICE VOROSMARTI, Research Associate
GUI LIU, Senior Program Assistant
STEPHANIE GOODWIN, Fellow
LINDA D. MEYERS, Director, Food and Nutrition Board
ROBIN SCHOEN, Director, Board on Agriculture and Natural Resources

Reviewers

This report has been reviewed in draft form by individuals chosen for their diverse perspectives and technical expertise, in accordance with procedures approved by the National Research Council's Report Review Committee. The purpose of this independent review is to provide candid and critical comments that will assist the institution in making its published report as sound as possible and to ensure that the report meets institutional standards for objectivity, evidence, and responsiveness to the study charge. The review comments and draft manuscript remain confidential to protect the integrity of the deliberative process. We wish to thank the following individuals for their review of this report:

HENRY J. AARON, Senior Fellow, The Brookings Institution, Washington, DC

JOHN BAILAR, III, Professor Emeritus, University of Chicago, Washington, DC

KATHRYN J. BOOR, Professor, Food Science Department, Cornell University, Ithaca, New York

BONNIE BUNTAIN, Professor, Ecosystem and Public Health Department, University of Calgary, Alberta, Canada

J. JOSEPH CORBY, Executive Director, Association of Food and Drug Officials, York, Pennsylvania

LESTER M. CRAWFORD, JR., Senior Counsel, Policy Directions, Inc., Georgetown, South Carolina

CAROLINE SMITH DEWAAL, Director, Food Safety Program, Center for Science in the Public Interest, Washington, DC

Although the reviewers listed above have provided many constructive comments and suggestions, they were not asked to endorse the report's conclusions or recommendations, nor did they see the final draft of the report before its release. The review of this report was overseen by **Enriqueta C. Bond,** President Emeritus, Burroughs Wellcome Fund, and **Elena O. Nightingale,** Scholar-in-Residence, Institute of Medicine. Appointed by the National Research Council and Institute of Medicine, they were responsible for making certain that an independent examination of this report was carried out in accordance with institutional procedures and that all review comments were carefully considered. Responsibility for the final content of this report rests entirely with the authoring committee and the institution.

Contents

Part III:
Implementation of the New Food Safety System

Appendixes*

* Appendixes B–G are not printed in this book. They are available on the CD in the back of this book.

Preface

This Institute of Medicine/National Research Council report was written in response to a congressional request that the U.S. Food and Drug Administration (FDA) contract with the National Academies for a comprehensive study of gaps in public health protection provided by the food safety system in the United States. In particular, the study was to review the role of the FDA in ensuring the safety of the nation's food supply. The committee that conducted this study hopes that the recommendations in this report will help the FDA in achieving the very important goal of protecting the health of the American public.

Important functions of the FDA in regard to food safety are too numerous to be listed here. To name but a few, they range from resolving crises in the most expeditious and efficient manner; to predicting the next intentional food contamination episode, whether here or abroad; to communicating with and educating the public about food safety. The committee found it difficult to make recommendations for enhancing the FDA's role in ensuring food safety without also addressing the rest of the complex system of local, state, and federal government agencies that, together with the FDA, govern food production in the United States. One main tenet of the committee's recommendations is a call for a risk-based approach to allocating food safety resources and efforts. The committee suggests a number of enhancements at the FDA that would improve the efficiency of resource allocation and protection of the public health and could be initiated independently from other agencies. For other enhancements, however, improvement will not come without seamless cooperation with other agencies. For some recommendations, changes in federal law or structural reorganization are essential. In essence, the committee found that the time has come to modernize the nation's food safety system so it becomes a truly integrated national program.

In addition, although most of the recommendations offered are directed to the FDA, it is imperative to recognize that the FDA cannot guarantee food safety on its own, given the many other private and public parties involved in the nation's food supply chain. Hence, some of the recommendations also assume the responsibility of others, including food producers and distributors and consumers. Although the committee's deliberations were focused on improving the FDA's functions and operations, the success of its food safety enterprise cannot be realized without the involvement of other responsible parties, and the report refers to them when appropriate.

On behalf of the committee, I would like to express my great appreciation to the staff at the FDA's Office of Foods (formerly the Office of Food Protection) for the substantial time and effort they put into supporting our work. They were available to clarify the committee's task and to educate its members about the FDA's operations, challenges, and aspirations. In particular, this study could not have been conducted without the assistance of Dr. David Acheson, Ms. Kari Barret, and Dr. Chad Nelson, who tirelessly assisted the committee with answering numerous questions and requests for information, meetings, and conference calls. I would like to thank Michael Taylor, who served as an unpaid project consultant until June 2009, prior to his appointment as senior advisor to the FDA commissioner. On behalf of the committee, I sincerely thank the participants and speakers who contributed to the two workshops held to inform this study (see Appendix A) for addressing topics critical to the completion of the committee's work. Their presentations served as essential references and resources for the committee.

I would also like to gratefully acknowledge the time, effort, and skill that committee members invested in this process, with a spirit of continuous improvement and with the ultimate goal of assisting the FDA in accomplishing its food safety mission. Their diverse backgrounds and experience ensured that all aspects of this challenging topic were addressed and that all deliberations were carried out with respect and empathy. Finally, I thank the project staff and support staff of the National Academies for their tireless dedication to the production of this report.

Robert B. Wallace, *Chair*
Committee on the Review of the Food and Drug
Administration's Role in Ensuring Safe Food

Summary

Providing nutritious, abundant, and safe food requires the efforts of many partners that together make up today's complex and evolving food system.[1] Since 1906, the U.S. Food and Drug Administration (FDA) and its predecessor agencies have regulated foods, among other products. Today the agency has oversight of approximately 80 percent of the U.S. food supply.[2]

Although there have been prior efforts to identify needed improvements in food safety, recent multistate foodborne illness outbreaks have again highlighted a food safety system that is not always effective in protecting the public health. The FDA has been criticized as responding only reactively to food safety problems and neglecting its preventive functions. With these concerns in mind, in 2008 Congress requested that the FDA contract with the National Academies for a comprehensive study of gaps in the FDA's food safety system. While the responsibility for addressing these challenges

---

[1] Unless otherwise indicated, the term "food" refers to both food and animal feed.

[2] The U.S. Department of Agriculture's Food Safety and Inspection Service is primarily responsible for the safety of meat, poultry, and unshelled egg products. The FDA shares responsibility for the safety of alcoholic beverages with the Alcohol and Tobacco Trade Bureau of the Department of the Treasury. The FDA shares jurisdiction with state and local governments over food in interstate commerce. State and local governments have the main responsibility for food produced or sold within their borders. The major FDA offices with responsibility for food safety are the Office of the Commissioner, the Office of Foods, the Center for Food Safety and Applied Nutrition, the Center for Veterinary Medicine, the Office of Regulatory Affairs, and the National Center for Toxicological Research.

does not lie solely with the FDA, the focus of this report is on enhancing that agency's food programs, specifically those devoted to food safety.

STUDY APPROACH

To conduct this study, a 13-member committee with extensive experience in FDA food programs and policies, food law and regulations, risk analysis and communication, economics, epidemiology, monitoring and surveillance, food microbiology and toxicology, feed issues, and state food programs was convened. The committee gathered information through six meetings, statements in response to specific queries to the FDA, and public documents.

As requested (Box S-1), the committee reviewed the FDA's 2007 Food Protection Plan (FPP), a road map aligned with the agency's strategic plan, but it also worked to identify additional tools and capacities to improve food safety. Since the publication of the FPP, organizational and leadership changes in the federal government[3] have altered the U.S. food safety scene. In this new environment, the committee envisioned the FPP as a point of departure but focused its attention on providing the FDA with concrete guidance in various areas of concern, including the need to implement a risk-based food safety management system.

The committee left many of the details of the implementation of its recommendations to the FDA, especially since food safety is just one of the agency's many responsibilities. The committee considered cost and resource issues in a general sense by drawing on the experience of members who formerly held senior leadership positions at the FDA. Because essential information was not always accessible, however, the committee lacked the full evidence base needed to address these issues in detail.

CONCLUSIONS

This section presents the committee's main conclusions. It begins with a brief review of the FPP, which is evaluated throughout the report as appropriate. It then presents conclusions concerning the development and implementation of a stronger, more effective food safety system built on a risk-based approach to food safety management.

---

[3] For example, these include a change in administration, the formation of the White House Food Safety Working Group, and the FDA's establishment of a new Office of Foods with oversight and authority over the two FDA centers that regulate food—the Center for Food Safety and Applied Nutrition and the Center for Veterinary Medicine.

BOX S-1
Statement of Task

An ad hoc committee of the Institute of Medicine and the National Research Council will undertake a study to examine gaps in public health protection provided by the farm-to-table food safety system under the purview of the Food and Drug Administration (FDA) and identify opportunities to fill those gaps. The study will address the recommendations of the November 2007 FDA Food Protection Plan by evaluating the plan and identifying gaps and opportunities (recommendations) to fill the gaps. The committee's consensus report will include legislative, regulatory, and administrative recommendations and estimates of costs of such recommendations, as feasible.

Specifically, the committee will:

- Evaluate the FDA Plan in light of past reports directed at strengthening food safety including, but not limited to *Ensuring Safe Food from Production to Consumption* (IOM/NRC, 1998), *Scientific Criteria to Ensure Safe Food* (IOM/NRC, 2003), the 2007 FDA Science Board report, and relevant GAO reports;
- Identify strengths and weaknesses of the FDA Plan, factors that may limit its achievement, and needed revisions or additions; and
- Identify and recommend enhancements in FDA's tools and capacity that are needed to implement a comprehensive plan and assure a risk-based preventive system, including in the areas of new regulatory tools and statutory authority; research mandate; resources required for research, scientific and technical infrastructure, standard setting, inspection, and enforcement; integration of programs with other regulatory and public health agencies involved in food safety surveillance, research and regulation at federal, state and local levels; expansion of FDA's international presence and international regulatory information exchange; and changes in organizational and leadership structures on food safety within the Department of Health and Human Services.

The FPP

Strategic planning is an essential element of a food safety program and should precede the design and implementation of a risk-based approach to food safety management. At a broad level, strategic planning entails identifying public health goals (e.g., reducing the number of infections caused by specific foods), identifying tools for attaining those goals (e.g., research, education activities), and developing measures with which to evaluate success. The FDA's strategic plan for food safety management should explain its risk-based regulatory philosophy and the factors it will weigh in making decisions about the prioritization of efforts, allocation of resources, and selection of interventions. At a specific level, all of the risk-based activities discussed in the report (e.g., data collection) should be undertaken only after strategic planning.

The FPP (Appendix G) presents the FDA's general philosophy on food safety, focusing on three core elements: (1) prevention, (2) intervention, and (4) response. It also outlines the following four cross-cutting principles: (1) focus on risks over a product's life cycle, (2) target resources to achieve maximum risk reduction, (3) address both unintentional and deliberate contamination, and (4) use science and modern technology systems.

The committee concluded that while the FPP can serve as a platform for initiating a transformation at the FDA, it lacks sufficient detail on which to base policy decisions on prevention and risk. For example, it does not provide specific strategies to achieve the actions proposed. Moreover, terms such as "risk" and "risk-based approaches" are not adequately defined in the FPP; thus they do not clearly elucidate the FDA's philosophy and can be misunderstood. The committee concluded that the FPP needs to evolve and be supported by the type of strategic planning described in this report.

Adopting a Risk-Based Decision-Making Approach to Food Safety

In a food safety system, decisions about resource allocation need to be made consistently in order to maximize benefits and reduce risks while also considering costs. Food safety risk managers must consider a wide variety of concerns in their decision making, including the needs and values of diverse stakeholders, the controllability of various risks, the size and vulnerabilities of the populations affected, and economic factors. Although the balancing of diverse risks, benefits, and costs is challenging, the lack of a systematic, risk-based approach to facilitate decision making can cause problems ranging from a decrease in public trust to the occurrence of unintended consequences to society, the environment, and the marketplace. Moreover, to carry out all its food safety responsibilities and ensure continuity of everyday operations, the FDA needs to have sufficient staff working on food issues to ensure that routine functions continue even when a crisis occurs.

The committee examined concrete examples of the FDA's risk-based activities and identified gaps. Although the FDA is to be commended for embracing classic tools of risk assessment and management, it currently lacks a comprehensive, systematic vision for a risk-based food safety system. Many of the attributes necessary for such a system, including strategic planning, transparency, and formalized prioritization processes, are lacking in the agency's approach to food safety management. The FDA also has made only limited progress toward establishing performance metrics for measuring improvements in food safety.

Food safety is a shared responsibility of industry, retailers, consumers, and government agencies, and determining their roles is an important component of strategic planning. Regulators also must establish a systematic means of evaluating, selecting, and designing interventions to address high-priority risks. The FDA lacks a clear regulatory philosophy for assigning responsibility and a comprehensive strategy for choosing the level and intensity of interventions, as well as the extensive resources necessary to design and support a comprehensive risk-based food safety management system.

The risk-based approach recommended by the committee is summarized in Box S-2.

Creating a Data Surveillance and Research Infrastructure

Data form the foundation of a risk-based decision-making approach, and vast amounts of such data are being collected by the government, industry, and academia. However, the FDA has not adequately assessed its data needs and lacks a systematic means by which to collect, analyze, manage, and share data. Barriers to the availability and utilization of data to support a risk-based approach include a lack of data sharing, the absence of a comprehensive data infrastructure, and limited analytical expertise within the FDA.

The FDA's surveillance role is supported by its research capacity, which gives the agency an opportunity to fill data gaps and address uncertainties to help refine its risk-based decision making. The FDA's current food safety research program appears to be fragmented and poorly managed, lacking strategic planning and coordination of research that is conducted intramurally and at the five extramural research centers. Many basic questions, such as the size and scope of the FDA's research program and the appropriate balance between basic and applied research, need to be addressed before the program can be supportive of a risk-based approach. In particular, inadequate attention is given to research aimed at determining the efficacy and value of specific food safety management policies.

Integrating Federal, State, and Local Government Food Safety Programs

Food safety activities of state and local (including territorial and tribal) governments, including inspection, surveillance, and outbreak investigation, have long been important contributors to the U.S. food safety system.

BOX S-2
A Recommended Risk-Based Approach

Step 1: Strategic Planning
1. Identify public health objectives related to food safety in consultation with stakeholders.
2. Establish a risk management plan (general and specific strategic plans for meeting public health objectives and for considering and choosing policy interventions to achieve those objectives).
3. Establish metrics with which to measure performance in consultation with stakeholders.

Step 2: Public Health Risk Ranking (Ranking of Hazards)
1. Develop or select tools (models, measures, or other) for public health risk ranking in consultation with stakeholders.
2. Rank risks based on public health outcomes.
3. Report results to stakeholders and solicit feedback.

Step 3: Targeted Information Gathering on Risks and Consideration of Other Factors That May Influence Decision Making
1. Identify and consider additional criteria upon which risk-based decision making will be based (e.g., public acceptance, cost, controllability, environmental effects, market impacts) in consultation with stakeholders.
2. Conduct targeted information gathering. For each high-priority and/or uncertain risk, determine the need for collection of additional information and implement accordingly:
   a. additional data collection (research, surveillance, survey, baseline data); and
   b. risk assessment (qualitative, quantitative, semiquantitative).
3. Based on that additional information, identify priority risks for which intervention analysis is needed.

However, these activities are not fully integrated so that duplication is minimized. Integration will require harmonization so that all programs and functions related to food safety meet a minimum set of standards. The FDA has standards in place that, if broadened and implemented properly, could serve as the basis for this harmonization. As with the federal system, state and local efforts should be built on a risk-based approach.

Step 4: Analysis and Selection of Intervention(s)
1. Identify an appropriate level of protection for each high-priority risk, based on available data and in consultation with stakeholders.
2. Identify intervention options in consultation with stakeholders.
3. Identify the types of technical analysis, including but not limited to risk assessment, needed to evaluate the options; identify performance measures and the initial design of databases.
4. Gather the information necessary to conduct the technical analysis.
5. Choose intervention strategies for implementation using multicriteria decision analysis.
6. Report results to stakeholders, solicit feedback, and modify intervention strategies if needed.

Step 5: Design of an Intervention Plan
1. Develop a plan for implementing the selected interventions in consultation with stakeholders.
2. Allocate resources and implement interventions.

Step 6: Monitoring and Review
1. Collect and analyze data on evaluation measures selected during strategic planning.
2. Interpret data and evaluate whether interventions result in the desired intermediate outcomes.
3. Determine whether public health objectives are being met by using performance metrics developed in Step 1 (broad strategic planning).
4. Communicate results to stakeholders.
5. Review and refine the entire process in an iterative manner as necessary to accomplish both intermediate outcomes and public health objectives so as to achieve continuous improvement over time.

Enhancing the Efficiency of Inspections

For years, the inspectional capacity and efficiency of the FDA have been criticized as inadequate. Although mindful of potential gains from allocating more resources to the FDA's inspection system, the committee focused on increasing the system's efficiency. One barrier to improved efficiency is that the FDA's food programs lack direct authority over the work of inspectors, resulting in potential substantial delays in policy implementation in the field. Nor have inspection procedures been reviewed for efficiency or consistency with a risk-based approach. The committee concluded that exploring alternative models for the inspection of food facilities (e.g., delegating some inspection activities to state and local governments, accepting third-party auditing of food facilities) could lead to gains in efficiency.

Improving Food Safety and Risk Communication

Risk communication is integral to risk-based food safety management. The FDA should envision risk communication not only as consultation with stakeholders at various steps of the risk-based process, but also as a form of policy intervention to achieve objectives in its strategic plan. The FDA's risk-based food safety management system must incorporate effective risk communication and food safety education for consumers and those who could impact public health through their professions, such as public health officials. The FDA should continue to use the advice of the Risk Communication Advisory Committee; below the committee offers several other recommendations to enhance risk communication.

Modernizing Legislation to Enhance the U.S. Food Safety System

Since 1938, Congress has occasionally amended the Federal Food, Drug, and Cosmetic Act (FDCA) to enhance the FDA's power to fulfill its food safety mission. In some fundamental respects, however, the law under which the FDA must ensure the safety of 80 percent of the nation's food has remained unchanged since 1938—despite the dramatic changes in food production and distribution patterns that have taken place. Those food safety provisions of the FDCA that are broad delegations of power rather than specific grants of authority have led to the FDA's vulnerability to court challenges and, consequently, the agency's reluctance to take action. This deficiency in the food safety system needs to be remedied.

Achieving the Vision of an Efficient Risk-Based Food Safety System

The committee is confident that the risk-based approach recommended in this report would enhance the FDA's ability to ensure food safety now and in the future. Nonetheless, the committee recognizes that this approach will not work optimally under the current organizational structure of the food safety system. The committee is encouraged by the establishment of the Office of Foods in 2009, but it has not been persuaded that this single consolidation step will resolve the important problems related to the separation of responsibilities in the FDA's food programs.

Food safety in the United States is managed by many government agencies. The ability of the FDA, and the government in general, to succeed in ensuring food safety through the development of a risk-based food safety management system would be greatly enhanced if the recommendations in this report were implemented in the context of organizational changes, such as the integration of activities currently scattered among poorly coordinated agencies. There are many potential avenues of organizational reform and many serious barriers to overcome. Hence, the importance of in-depth analysis and planning of such changes cannot be overemphasized.

RECOMMENDATIONS

The committee's deliberations resulted in suggested directions for improving food safety management (Box S-3) and specific recommendations for overcoming deficiencies in the food safety system (Box S-4).

LOOKING FORWARD

Although food safety is the responsibility of everyone, from producers to consumers, the FDA and other regulatory agencies have an essential role. In many instances, the FDA must carry out this responsibility against a backdrop of multiple stakeholder interests, inadequate resources, and competing priorities. The committee hopes that this report provides the FDA and Congress with a course of action that will enable the agency to become more efficient and effective in carrying out its food safety mission in a rapidly changing world.

BOX S-3
Suggested Directions for Improving the
U.S. Food and Drug Administration's (FDA's)
Food Safety Management

- Apply the recommended risk-based approach to the management of all food hazards.
- Address the lack of resources (e.g., data infrastructure, human capacity) and organization for the implementation of a risk-based food safety management system.
- Identify metrics with which to measure the effectiveness of intervention strategies and the food safety system as a whole.
- Define the roles of the various parties sharing responsibility for food safety, and develop a roadmap with defined criteria for the level and intensity of policy interventions and plans to evaluate them.
- Develop a strategic plan to identify data needs for a risk-based approach, and establish mechanisms to coordinate, capture, and integrate the data. Remove barriers to the practical utilization of data to support a risk-based system, including problems with data sharing and gaps in analytical expertise within the FDA.
- Conduct strategic planning and coordination of the FDA's food safety research portfolio.
- Integrate food safety programs at the federal, state, and local levels, with the ultimate goal of utilizing all food surveillance, inspectional, and analytical systems as part of the national food safety program.
- Address the existence of barriers to improving the efficiency of inspections, such as the inefficiency of inspection procedures and the fact that the FDA's food programs do not have direct authority over the work of inspectors.
- Continue development of a single source of authoritative government information on food safety, safe food practices, foodborne illnesses and risks, and crisis communications.
- Create a centrally controlled plan for communicating with one voice with all affected parties during food safety crises.
- Modernize the legislative framework to give the FDA the necessary legal authority to perform its role in ensuring the safety of FDA-regulated foods.
- Implement organizational changes that would greatly enhance the ability of the FDA to succeed in ensuring food safety.

BOX S-4
Recommendations

Toward a Risk-Based Approach

Recommendation 3-1: The type of risk-based food safety approach outlined by the committee in Box S-2 should become the operational centerpiece of the U.S. Food and Drug Administration's (FDA's) food safety program. This approach should be embraced by all levels of management and should serve as the basis for food safety decision making, including prioritization of resources dedicated to all agency functions (e.g., inspections, promulgation of regulations, research). This approach should be applied to all domestically produced and imported foods and to all food-related hazards, whether due to unintentional or intentional (i.e., with intent to harm) contamination. The FDA should work with local, state, and national regulatory partners to facilitate the incorporation of these principles into their programs.

Recommendation 3-2: The FDA should develop a comprehensive strategic plan for development and implementation of a risk-based food safety management system. The agency should also develop internal operating guidelines for the conduct of risk ranking, risk assessment, risk prioritization, intervention analysis, and the development of metrics with which to evaluate the performance of the system. The strategic plan and guidelines should include descriptions of data, methodologies, technical analyses, and stakeholder engagement. Further, the strategic plan and all guidelines for the risk-based system should be fully supported by the scientific literature and subjected to peer review. When appropriate, the FDA should adopt guidelines already established by other federal agencies or international organizations.

Recommendation 3-3: The FDA, in collaboration with partners, should identify metrics with which to measure the effectiveness of the food safety system, as well as its interventions. The FDA should include these metrics, and plans for any related data collection, as part of strategic planning. The metrics should have a clearly defined link to public health outcomes.

Recommendation 3-4: The FDA should identify expertise needed to implement a risk-based approach. This includes training current

continued

BOX S-4 Continued

and/or hiring new personnel in the areas of strategic planning; management of data; development of biomathematical models and other tools for risk ranking, prioritization, intervention analysis, and evaluation; and risk communication.

Sharing the Responsibility

Recommendation 4-1: To ensure food safety, the FDA should develop a plan for defining the extent of and form for sharing responsibilities with the states, the private sector, third parties (e.g., independent auditors), and other countries' governments.

Recommendation 4-2: The FDA should develop a comprehensive strategy for choosing the level and intensity of policy interventions needed for different food safety risks. Criteria for choosing the level and intensity of policy interventions and a plan for evaluating the selected interventions should be developed with transparency, stakeholder participation, and clear lines of communication.

Creating a Data Surveillance Infrastructure

Recommendation 5-1: Data collection by the FDA should be driven by the recommended risk-based approach and should support risk-based decision making. It is critical that the FDA evaluate its food safety data needs and develop a strategic plan to meet those needs. The FDA should review existing data collection systems for foods to identify data gaps, eliminate systems of limited utility, and develop the necessary surveillance capabilities to support the risk-based approach. The FDA should formulate and implement a plan for developing, harmonizing, evaluating, and adopting data standards. The FDA should also establish a mechanism for coordinating, capturing, and integrating data, including modernization of its information technology systems. To coordinate, capture, and integrate data, the FDA could lead the implementation of a multiagency food safety epidemiology users group (see Chapter 5). The centralized risk-based analysis and data management center proposed in recommendation 11-3 in Chapter 11 could serve the functions of data storage and analysis in support of a risk-based approach. Mechanisms should also be instituted to build trust with industry and, in partnership, collect and analyze industry data.

Recommendation 5-2: The FDA should evaluate its personnel needs to carry out its roles in collecting, analyzing, managing, and communicating food safety data. The agency should establish an analytical unit with the resources and expertise (i.e., statisticians, epidemiologists, behavioral scientists, economists, microbiologists, risk analysts, biomathematical modelers, database managers, information technology personnel, risk managers, and others as needed) to support risk-based decision making.

Recommendation 5-3: The FDA should evaluate statutes and policies governing data sharing and develop plans to improve the collection and sharing of relevant data by all federal, state, and local food safety agencies. For example, in collaboration with other food safety agencies, the FDA should develop and implement technologies and procedures that will ensure confidentiality and facilitate data sharing. Congress should consider amending the law, to the extent that legal changes are needed, to allow sufficient data sharing among government agencies.

Creating a Research Infrastructure

Recommendation 6-1: The FDA should have a food safety research portfolio that supports the recommended risk-based approach. To this end, the agency's current food safety research portfolio should undergo a comprehensive review. Following this review and with consideration of the agency's broad strategic plan, the FDA should examine the relevance and allocation of its research resources by using public health risk ranking and prioritization. Future research should address the most pressing public health issues and directly support further characterization of risk and selection, implementation, and evaluation of interventions. In addition, research should be coordinated to prevent duplication of effort, especially for cases in which research efforts are better suited to the academic or medical sector.

Recommendation 6-2: Implementation of recommendation 6-1 requires reorganization of the FDA's research portfolio, including reallocation of resources from irrelevant or poorly performing initiatives; hiring of new staff in critical areas and, where appropriate, retraining of existing staff; and identification of future resource

continued

BOX S-4 Continued

needs to support risk-based food safety management. Although the committee recognizes the difficulty of transferring scientists from one research focus to another, the FDA should foster an environment of fluidity in which teams of scientists can be formed with ease to address different research initiatives as necessary.

Recommendation 6-3: Keeping in mind that the FDA will not be able to address all important research needs, the agency should continue to utilize alternative funding mechanisms (e.g., cooperative agreements, university-based centers, contracts) based on a competitive, peer-review process. These efforts could be expanded by establishing a competitive extramural research funding program.

Integrating Federal, State, and Local Food Safety Programs

Recommendation 7-1: The FDA should utilize the surveillance, inspection, and analytic systems and resources of state and local governments in a fully integrated food safety program. As a prerequisite to such integration, the FDA should work with the states and localities to harmonize their programs by providing adequate standards and overseeing their implementation, beginning with those states that meet such standards. Standardization and integration of state and local food safety programs should be conducted in an evolutionary fashion, with intermediate goals and associated performance measures. The White House Food Safety Working Group should make integration of federal and state food regulatory programs a priority and provide leadership to the already established Integrated Food Safety System Steering Committee. The agency should provide training, auditing, and oversight of state and local programs and should facilitate nationwide implementation of the recommended risk-based approach.

Enhancing the Efficiency of Inspections

Recommendation 8-1: The FDA should work toward an inspection system in which the frequency and intensity of inspection of each facility are based on risk, with minimum standards for the frequency and intensity of inspection of all facilities. To support the establishment of such a system, an outside panel should review the potential legal and cultural roadblocks to streamlining inspections and revise the *Investigations Operations Manual* so as to enhance efficiency and protection of the public health. As a prerequisite for a risk-based inspection system, the FDA should update its Good Manufacturing Practices, including those for medicated animal feed, now and hereafter as necessary.

Recommendation 8-2: As alternative regulatory models emerge, the FDA should evolve toward conducting fewer inspections, instead delegating inspections to the states and localities (including territories and tribes). The FDA should maintain a cadre of inspectors for several critical tasks, such as auditing inspections, providing specialty expertise, developing training and instructional materials for inspectors, identifying and evaluating new inspection techniques, and serving as a backup corps in situations of special need. In preparation for this move, the FDA should review and update curricula specific to general food inspections as well as to particular types of inspections (e.g., seafood Hazard Analysis and Critical Control Points). Agency employees with responsibility for auditing inspections by others should also be provided with specific training. An FDA-sponsored food safety certification program should be established whereby inspectors become certified as they meet agency standards. The agency should include in its budget a line item to fund state contracts and partnerships to help the states move toward and maintain full certification. Plans for implementation of the suggested changes should proceed in an evolutionary fashion, with intermediate goals and associated performance measures.

Recommendation 8-3: The FDA should fully consider the implications of accepting inspection data from an auditing program in which third-party auditors would inspect facilities for compliance with food safety regulatory requirements. If this approach is utilized, the FDA should set minimum standards for such auditors and audits, with oversight and implementation being assigned to an accreditation and standards body.

Improving Food Safety and Risk Communication

Recommendation 9-1: In its effort to integrate risk communication into the recommended risk-based food safety management system, the FDA should play a leadership role in coordinating the education of the food industry, the public, clinical health professionals, and public health officials at all government levels. The FDA could carry out its leadership role in educating industry personnel, health pro-

continued

BOX S-4 Continued

fessionals, and public health officials by seeking authority to mandate the setting of training standards, preparing training materials, certifying trainers, and providing technical support for the interpretation of policies and for the implementation of the risk-based approach.

Recommendation 9-2: In collaboration with other federal agencies, the FDA should continue efforts to develop a single source of authoritative information on food safety practices, foodborne illness and risks, and crisis communications. The FDA, with other federal agencies, should develop a coordinated plan for communicating in one voice with all affected parties during crises so that stakeholders receive timely, clear, and accurate information from a single recognizable source.

Recommendation 9-3: The FDA should improve its understanding of the knowledge and behavior of industry, health professions personnel, and consumers with respect to food safety, paying specific attention to knowledge about demographic groups that are particularly susceptible to food risks.

In making critical decisions about risk communication to implement recommendations 9-1, 9-2, and 9-3, the FDA should explore new mechanisms (e.g., tabletop discussions,[a] public forums, consultations) for expanding its use of strategic partnerships and collaborations.

Modernizing Legislation

Recommendation 10-1: Congress should consider amending the Federal Food, Drug, and Cosmetic Act to provide explicitly and in detail the authorities the FDA needs to fulfill its food safety mission. The following are the most critical areas in which Congress should enact amendments: mandatory reregistration of food facilities and FDA authority to suspend registrations for violations that threaten the public health, mandatory preventive controls for all food facilities, FDA authority to issue enforceable performance standards, mandatory adoption by the FDA of a risk-based approach to inspection frequency and intensity, expansion of the FDA's access to records, FDA authority to mandate recalls, and FDA authority to

---

[a] A tabletop discussion is a focused practice activity that places the participants in a simulated situation requiring them to function in the capacity that would be expected of them in a real event.

identify countries with inadequate food safety systems and to ban all imports from such countries.

Realizing the Vision of an Efficient Food Safety System

Recommendation 11-1: The committee recommends that the FDA's Office of Foods have complete authority over and responsibility for all field activities for FDA-regulated foods, including inspection, sampling, and testing of foods. Implementing this recommendation would resolve issues associated with the separation between the agency's enforcement functions and larger public health roles and responsibilities, and ensure a well-trained field workforce with specialized expertise in food safety and risk-based principles of food safety management.

Recommendation 11-2: There is a compelling need to elevate and unify the nation's food safety enterprise so that the FDA and relevant sister agencies can better ensure a safe food supply. The committee recognizes that organizational change to enhance the effectiveness and efficiency of the nation's food safety system as a whole is an evolutionary process that would require careful analysis, planning, and execution. With this in mind, the committee recommends that the federal government move toward the establishment of a single food safety agency to unify the efforts of all agencies and departments with major responsibility for the safety of the U.S. food supply.

Recommendation 11-3: Regardless of the evolution of the food safety system, an integrated, unimpeded, and centralized approach to risk-based analysis and data management is required to enhance the FDA's and the broader federal government's ability to ensure a safe food supply. To achieve this goal, and as a potential intermediate step toward the creation of a single food safety agency, the committee recommends the establishment of a centralized risk-based analysis and data management center. This center should be provided with the staff and supporting resources necessary to conduct rapid and sophisticated assessments of short- and long-term food safety risks and of policy interventions, and to ensure that the comprehensive data needs of the recommended risk-based food safety management system are met. This center should be as free from external political forces and influence as possible and accountable to the public health needs and mission of the regulatory agencies.

Part I

Setting the Stage for Understanding and Improving the U.S. Food and Drug Administration's Role in the Food Safety System

1

Introduction

The nation's food supply has evolved into a complex system involving more than $450 billion worth of food each year under the jurisdiction of the U.S. Food and Drug Administration (FDA), more than 156,008 FDA-regulated firms (FDA, 2010), and an additional 2,000 FDA-licensed feed mills (Behnke, 2009). Many parties are responsible for providing safe food, including suppliers, farmers, food handlers, processors, wholesalers and retailers, food service companies, consumers, third-party organizations, and government agencies in the United States and abroad. The path from production to consumption can involve only one step—from a farmer directly to a consumer at a farmer's market—or as many as six or even more steps—for example, from a farmer, to various processors, to a warehouse, to a transporter, to a grocer, to a consumer.

Paralleling the evolution of the food system is a similarly complex history of legislative actions that form the foundation for the current governance of the safety of the food supply in the United States. Since 1906, the Federal Food, Drug, and Cosmetic Act (FDCA) and amendments thereto have charged the FDA with oversight of this governance function (with the exception of meat, poultry, and egg products). This means the FDA has regulatory authority over approximately 80 percent of the U.S. food supply, encompassing products from fresh produce, to seafood, to packaged snack foods, to cereal, to pet food, to animal feed for food-producing animals. The major FDA entities with responsibility for food safety are the Office of the Commissioner, the Office of Foods, the Center for Food Safety and Applied Nutrition (CFSAN), the Center for Veterinary Medicine (CVM), the Office of Regulatory Affairs, and the National Center for Toxicological

Research. At the same time, the FDA is only one of many federal agencies that administer at least 30 laws related to food safety. The U.S. Department of Agriculture (USDA) is responsible for the safety of meat, poultry, and egg products, while state and local governments have jurisdiction over foods produced or sold within their borders. All of the significant agencies and departments that are responsible for various aspects of food safety are detailed in Chapter 2.

According to a recent public opinion poll, in general, confidence about the safety of the food supply appears to be lower now than it has been since 2001 (Gallup, 2010). The complexity of the system, combined with highly publicized recalls and outbreaks costing millions of dollars, the resulting impacts on the public health, and the piecemeal nature of the current system, has raised concern about the FDA's ability to ensure the safety of the nation's food supply. The purpose of this study is to identify gaps in the FDA's food safety system and recommend actions that can be taken to fill those gaps.

STUDY CONTEXT

Increasing Discussion and Controversies About the FDA's Ability to Ensure Safe Food

Many recent changes in the nation's food system have prompted increasing discussion of the FDA's ability to ensure safe food. The 1998 Institute of Medicine (IOM)/National Research Council (NRC) report *Ensuring Safe Food: From Production to Consumption* identifies some of these changes, such as the food safety implications of emerging pathogens, the trend toward the consumption of more fresh produce, the trend toward eating more meals away from home, and changing demographics, with a greater proportion of the population being immunocompromised or otherwise at increased risk of foodborne illness.[1] These developments must be understood in the context of a wide range of global and societal changes that greatly increase the complexity of the food safety system and the challenges faced by those responsible for implementing the system. These changes, detailed in Chapter 2, include changes in the food production landscape, climate change, evolving consumer perceptions and behaviors (e.g., the growing demand for fresh produce and for its availability year-round[2]), globalization and increased food importation, the role of labor–management

---

[1] A demographic change receiving particular attention today is the growth of the elderly population, which is at higher risk of foodborne illness. It is estimated that by 2015, 20 percent of the population will be over age 60, and the number at risk will increase accordingly (GAO, 2010).

[2] From 1992 to 2005, there was a 180 percent increase in consumption of leafy greens in the United States (GAO, 2008a).

relations and workplace safety, heightened concern about bioterrorism, increased levels of pollution in the environment, and the increasing role of international trade agreements. Food production is changing as well, with the number of firms involved with food having increased by roughly 28 percent since 2001 (GAO, 2008b).[3] The importation of food is also increasing; roughly $49 billion worth of food was imported to the United States in 2007 (GAO, 2008a).

A number of high-profile food-related outbreaks have occurred in recent years, including *E. coli* O157:H7 in spinach in 2006, melamine in pet food in 2007, *Salmonella* in produce and in peanut butter in 2008, and *E. coli* O157:H7 in cookie dough in 2009. In 1999, Mead and colleagues estimated that foodborne infections caused about 76 million illnesses, 325,000 hospitalizations, and 5,000 deaths each year in the United States (Mead et al., 1999). It should be emphasized that these data were reported in 1999, and the morbidity, mortality, and hospitalization estimates would likely be different today; new estimates are in preparation but were not available at the time of this writing. Nonetheless, data for 2008 from the U.S. Centers for Disease Control and Prevention (CDC) suggest that there has been no significant change in the incidence of foodborne infections by the major bacterial agents transmitted through food over the last several years (in some cases, disease may be acquired through other nonfood vehicles, such as reptiles). CDC therefore concludes that problems with bacterial contamination through food are not being resolved (CDC, 2009). According to CDC, the lack of recent progress toward national health objectives for food safety and the continual occurrence of large multistate outbreaks point to gaps in the food safety system. The most recent FoodNet surveillance data (CDC, 2010) show reductions in 2009 (compared with 2006–2008) in the incidence of some infections (shiga toxin-producing *E. coli* O157:H7 and *Shigella*) but not others (*Campylobacter*, *Listeria*, *Salmonella*). The data also show an increase in other infections from food-associated pathogens (*Listeria* and *Vibrio*).

During the last two decades, many organizations and individuals, including the IOM, have devoted effort to identifying needed improvements in food safety. Attention has been focused in particular on the FDA's food safety program. According to a number of reports (GAO, 2004a,b, 2005, 2008a,b; FDA Science Board, 2007), although the FDA is working to ensure safer food, problems with its capacities, functions, and processes persist. The IOM, the NRC, and other groups, including consumer organizations, have made recommendations for strengthening food protection, a few of which are listed here (see Appendix B for a detailed listing):

---

[3] Between 2001 and 2007, the number of domestic firms under the FDA's jurisdiction increased from about 51,000 to more than 65,500 (GAO, 2008b).

- The 1998 IOM/NRC report *Ensuring Safe Food: From Production to Consumption* concludes that the U.S. food system is fragmented and is facing unprecedented challenges from a global marketplace, a greater reliance on imports, shifting demographics, and changing societal practices. The report recommends modifying the federal statutory framework for food safety to eliminate fragmentation and enable the development and enforcement of science-based standards as well as creating a single food safety agency.
- The 2003 IOM/NRC report *Scientific Criteria for Ensuring Safe Food* (IOM/NRC, 2003) examines the scientific basis for criteria that underlie U.S. food safety regulations, presents a blueprint for how agencies responsible for regulating food safety should develop appropriate science-based criteria, and identifies the failure to adopt new technologies and enforce standards as barriers that impede regulatory action.
- The 2009 IOM report *HHS in the 21st Century* (IOM, 2009) highlights food safety regulatory activities as an area of weakness within the U.S. Department of Health and Human Services (HHS). Specifically, the report offers recommendations for uniting the food safety responsibilities of the two salient agencies (the FDA and USDA's Food Safety and Inspection Service) within HHS.
- Both consumer groups and industry have issued reports addressing food safety: the Center for Science in the Public Interest issued a white paper, *Building a Modern Food Safety System for FDA Regulated Foods* (DeWaal and Plunkett, 2007), while the Grocery Manufacturers Association (GMA) issued *Commitment to Consumers: The Four Pillars of Food Safety*, which focuses on prevention of foodborne illness (GMA, 2007).

An important factor influencing the FDA's ability to fulfill its mission is the resources available to the agency given that, in addition to food, it is required to regulate cosmetics, drugs, biologics, medical devices, and tobacco. Although the agency is responsible for the safety of more than 80 percent of the nation's food supply, its budget accounts for only 24 percent of expenditures on food safety (GAO, 2008b) (see Chapter 2). Moreover, after the events of September 11, 2001, the FDA was given additional responsibilities related to bioterrorism (GAO, 2008b), stretching its funds even thinner. For example, even though the number of domestic food establishments was increasing, the numbers of inspectors and inspections (both domestic and abroad) and the amount of funding allocated to food safety both decreased during the period 2003–2006 (FDA/CFSAN, 2008; GAO, 2008b).

In the face of its decreasing resources, the FDA must continue to make decisions about both appropriate short-term responses to a food crisis and longer-term prevention functions focused on continued improvements in the public health. While the need to respond to a crisis is clear, the agency has been criticized as responding only reactively to food problems, to the neglect of its preventive functions. In addition to the need to increase efficiency and prioritize its efforts, the FDA's success depends greatly on maintaining strong cooperative relationships with other partners in food safety (e.g., other federal departments and agencies; local, state, and foreign governments; industry). Although the division of responsibilities for food safety with respect to research, commodities, and public health surveillance among different agencies has been long criticized, no genuine attempt has been made to consider alternatives for the governance of food safety. Technological, scientific, environmental, and societal shifts have generated discrete actions, such as reorganizations within the food program at the FDA or amendments to the law, and the result has been the current piecemeal approach to food safety. The unprecedented speed and nature of such changes in the 21st century demand a different kind of response at this time—one that is comprehensive and systematic, giving the FDA and its partners a real opportunity to realize the vision of an integrated food safety system.

There have also been significant leadership and organizational changes in the FDA's operations and their context since this study was requested by Congress in 2008. In addition to a new administration, some of the most significant of these have been the establishment of the White House Food Safety Working Group (FSWG) to advise the administration on food safety matters; the establishment of a new Office of Foods within the FDA, with oversight and authority over CVM and CFSAN; the development of plans for a state–federal Integrated Food Safety System; and the hiring of additional high-level leaders and subject matter experts in food safety management.

The FDA's Food Protection Plan

In 2007, the FDA issued its Food Protection Plan (FPP) (FDA, 2007) (Appendix G), setting forth a general strategy for food safety and defense and identifying three core elements—prevention, intervention, and response (Box 1-1). In each of these areas, the plan describes key actions and needed legislative authority (Box 1-2). The approaches laid out in the plan include new regulatory authority for recalls, preventive controls for high-risk foods, and a shift to a risk-based system for inspections.

PURPOSE AND SCOPE OF THIS STUDY

In response to the heightened public health concerns outlined above, the Consolidated Appropriations Act of 2008 tasked the FDA to contract

---

BOX 1-1
Three Core Elements of Food Safety in the
U.S. Food and Drug Administration's Food Protection Plan

1. Prevent foodborne contamination:
- Promote increased corporate responsibility to prevent foodborne illnesses.
- Identify food vulnerabilities and assess risks.
- Expand the understanding and use of effective mitigation measures.

2. Intervene at critical points in the food supply chain:
- Focus inspections and sampling based on risk.
- Enhance risk-based surveillance.
- Improve the detection of food system "signals" that indicate contamination.

3. Respond rapidly to minimize harm:
- Improve immediate response.
- Improve risk communications to the public, industry, and other stakeholders.

---

with the National Academies for a comprehensive study of gaps in the public health protection offered by the food safety system in the United States.[4] Box 1-3 presents the statement of task for this study.

The FPP's overarching strategy for food protection encompasses and focuses on microbiological and chemical contaminants that can affect public health. The committee was tasked to evaluate the FDA's plan and to identify its strengths and weaknesses, determine whether it can be implemented effectively, and identify what additional resources (e.g., finances, equipment, personnel) the agency may need for this purpose. The committee was also tasked with evaluating the various additional legislative authorities the FDA has requested and determining whether these authorities are adequate to fulfill the agency's public health mission.

Clarification of the committee's task came from extensive dialogue with FDA food program leadership. Accordingly, the committee addressed microbiological contaminants, chemical contaminants, and intentional food contamination, including financially motivated contamination (as in the

---

[4] *Consolidated Appropriations Act of 2008*, HR2764, Public Law 110-161, Division A, Title VI.

BOX 1-2
**Additional Protections That Involve
Legislative Changes to the U.S. Food and Drug
Administration's (FDA's) Authority**

Prevent foodborne contamination:
- Allow the FDA to require preventive controls to prevent intentional adulteration by terrorists or criminals at points of high vulnerability in the food chain.
- Authorize the FDA to institute additional preventive controls for high-risk foods.
- Require food facilities to renew their FDA registrations every 2 years, and allow the FDA to modify the registration categories.

Intervene at critical points in the food supply chain:
- Authorize the FDA to accredit highly qualified third parties for voluntary food inspections.
- Require a new reinspection fee from facilities that fail to meet current Good Manufacturing Practices.
- Authorize the FDA to require electronic import certificates for shipments of designated high-risk products.
- Require a new food and animal feed export certification fee to improve the ability of U.S. firms to export their products.
- Provide parity between domestic and imported foods if FDA inspection access is delayed, limited, or denied.

Respond rapidly to minimize harm:
- Empower the FDA to issue a mandatory recall of food products when voluntary recalls are not effective.
- Give the FDA enhanced access to food records during emergencies.

recent case of melamine in pet foods) and contamination by terrorists. The committee excluded from its deliberations management of the safety of certain products (see Table 1-1). In particular, although the FDA's regulatory authority encompasses dietary supplements and food additives, the committee was asked to exclude them from its deliberations because their safety determination is not usually based on issues of contamination. Dietary supplements fall into a "gray area" of being a special category of food, and the determination of their safety is typically made by the industry. Manufacturers need not obtain FDA approval before producing or selling them. The

BOX 1-3
Statement of Task

An ad hoc committee of the Institute of Medicine and the National Research Council will undertake a study to examine gaps in public health protection provided by the farm-to-table food safety system under the purview of the Food and Drug Administration (FDA) and identify opportunities to fill those gaps. The study will address the recommendations of the November 2007 FDA Food Protection Plan by evaluating the plan and identifying gaps and opportunities (recommendations) to fill the gaps. The committee's consensus report will include legislative, regulatory, and administrative recommendations and estimates of costs of such recommendations, as feasible.

Specifically, the committee will:

- Evaluate the FDA Plan in light of past reports directed at strengthening food safety including, but not limited to *Ensuring Safe Food from Production to Consumption* (IOM/NRC, 1998), *Scientific Criteria to Ensure Safe Food* (IOM/NRC, 2003), the 2007 FDA Science Board report, and relevant GAO reports;
- Identify strengths and weaknesses of the FDA Plan, factors that may limit its achievement, and needed revisions or additions; and
- Identify and recommend enhancements in FDA's tools and capacity that are needed to implement a comprehensive plan and assure a risk-based preventive system, including in the areas of new regulatory tools and statutory authority; research mandate; resources required for research, scientific and technical infrastructure, standard setting, inspection, and enforcement; integration of programs with other regulatory and public health agencies involved in food safety surveillance, research and regulation at federal, state and local levels; expansion of FDA's international presence and international regulatory information exchange; and changes in organizational and leadership structures on food safety within the Department of Health and Human Services.

safety of dietary supplements is regulated under the Dietary Supplement Health and Education Act of 1994 (DSHEA). The committee excluded from the study a review of the process for notification or self-determination of generally recognized-as-safe ingredients. Food and color additives for both human food and animal feed are subject, respectively, to the 1958 Food

TABLE 1-1 Scope of This Study

Outside the Scope	Within the Scope
• Dietary supplements • Food and color additives • Issues specifically pertinent to genetically modified foods • Issues specifically pertinent to organic foods	• Microbiological contaminants in foods and feed • Chemical contaminants in foods and feed

Additives Amendment[5] and the 1960 Color Additives Amendments[6] to the 1938 FDCA, and they must be preapproved for safety before being added to food or feed. In the case of such additives, the burden of proof is on the manufacturer, who must provide evidence that the additive is safe for consumption. In 1992, the FDA concluded that, with regard to genetically modified foods, "The agency is not aware of any information showing that foods derived by these new methods differ from other foods in any meaningful or uniform way, and that, as a class, foods developed by the new techniques present any different or greater safety concern than foods developed by traditional plant breeding."[7] Therefore, these foods were not considered separately in this study. Likewise, the safety of organic foods was not considered separately.

In defining the scope of the study described in its statement of task, the committee was also guided by the FDA's jurisdiction in food safety. The FDCA, section 201, defines "food" as (1) articles used for food or drink by man or other animals, (2) chewing gum, and (3) articles used for components of any such article.[8] In accordance with this definition, the FPP includes food for both humans and animals. The latter encompasses both pet food and feed for "food-producing animals," a category that includes animals whose products will end up in the human food supply (including, for example, dairy cattle, beef cattle, swine, and chickens [FDA, 2007]). The committee consulted with the FDA on the precise scope of the study with respect to pet food and animal feed. This dialogue resulted in a decision to include in the study issues related to pet food and animal feed only as they might directly affect human health (e.g., because of drug or contaminant residues in pet food consumed or handled by humans or in human foods of

---

[5] *Food Additives Amendment of 1958*, Public Law 85-929, 72 Stat. 1784 (1958).

[6] *Color Additive Amendments of 1960*, Public Law 86-618, 74 Stat. 397 (1960).

[7] "Statement of policy—foods derived from new plant varieties" (FDA, 1992).

[8] *Federal Food, Drug, and Cosmetic Act*, Sec. 201, 21 U.S.C. §§ 321.

animal origin). In this report, the term "food" encompasses pet food and animal feed unless explicitly indicated otherwise.

METHODS

Committee Composition and Membership

The committee was assembled to include individuals with extensive knowledge of FDA programs, policies, and operations, as well as those with expertise in health policy, food law and regulations, risk analysis and communication, economics, epidemiology, monitoring and surveillance, food microbiology, and toxicology. Representation of state officials with food safety responsibilities was crucial because of the key role of state governments in keeping food safe. In addition, perspectives of the food industry and consumer interest groups were necessary as these sectors are responsible partners in food safety and would be affected by the implementation of the recommendations in this report. Expertise in animal feed was also sought because, as noted above, the safety of these products has the potential to affect human health, and feed safety is within the purview of the FDA.

Information Gathering, Meetings, and Workshops

The committee gathered information for this study from previous NRC and IOM reports, reports from authoritative groups, plans and initiatives from industry, FDA leadership and staff, numerous public sessions at committee meetings, teleconferences and written statements in response to specific queries, expert testimony before congressional committees, and the FDA website. The committee held three workshops to hear expert perspectives and obtain answers to its questions (see Appendix A for the workshop agendas). Participants from all relevant sectors attended the workshops, and the committee found their experience and insights invaluable to this study. They spoke on such topics as the FDA's organization and responsibilities; approaches to food safety prevention, inspection, and research; and perspectives on the FDA from industry and consumer stakeholders. Additionally, the committee held six closed meetings and numerous conference calls.

Study Approach

As noted above, the FPP is a road map founded in basic principles of prevention, intervention, and response. Since its publication and the congressional request for this study, leadership and organizational changes in the government have altered the U.S. food safety scene and affected the FDA's food programs. As discussed above, these include a change in administration, the formation of the White House FSWG, and the FDA's establishment of the new Office of Foods.

Although the FPP is widely regarded as a positive development, it is only a first step. Since its release, questions have been raised, for example, by the Government Accountability Office (GAO), about the specifics of its implementation—including a lack of clarity on its execution, efficient targeting of resources, budgetary constraints, and the timeline for implementation—as well as about the agency's statutory authority (GAO, 2008a,b). Without sufficient attention to these matters, there is concern that the plan cannot be appropriately implemented, and the likelihood of its success cannot be determined. Additional concern has been raised because of the failure to implement many past recommendations to the FDA.

In this new food safety environment and based on nature of the FPP, the committee concluded that to be useful, the FPP needs to evolve and be supported by more detailed strategic planning. Therefore, in its deliberations, the committee envisioned the FPP as a point of departure but focused its efforts on identifying additional tools and capacities that the FDA needs to improve food safety today and in the future.

In adhering to its statement of task, the committee reviewed the Food Protection Plan and formulated its recommendations in the context of an evaluation of the FDA's functions and operations. Thus, elements of the Food Protection Plan are considered in all chapters of this report, and they are also discussed in the context of the committee's recommendations. As an example, the FPP states that the FDA needs to "strengthen the establishment of a risk-based process to continuously evaluate which FDA-regulated products cause the greatest burden of foodborne disease." The committee recommends a stepwise process for achieving that objective. A synthesis of the committee's evaluation is presented in Chapter 4, which focuses on governing philosophy. The committee took this approach to its task to provide the FDA with a report that would be useful today and reflect all organizational and leadership changes within the agency since the FPP was written in 2007.

In identifying tools and capacities for an effective food safety system, the committee focused on investigating the FDA's food safety programs and operations as well as its progress toward the committee's view of such a system. The committee took great pains to provide recommendations that would maintain a balance between being too general and too prescriptive, and it formulated a number of concrete recommendations to guide the FDA in its food safety management mission, emphasizing the need for the agency to move toward a risk-based approach. Some of these concrete recommendations, for example, are aimed at overcoming current limitations in the acquisition and sharing of data (Chapters 5 and 11), in the FDA's research capacity and portfolio (Chapter 6), in risk communication and education (Chapter 9), and in legal authorities (Chapter 10). The committee believes that many details of the implementation of its recommendations (e.g., the factors to consider when assessing interventions) are within the purview of the FDA, especially since the agency's food safety program functions in the context of its overall responsibilities for food, which, for example, also include a nutrition program.

Recognizing that many enhancements can be realized without structural changes (through, for example, leadership commitment, staff retention, strategic planning), the committee initially deliberated its recommendations in the context of the current food safety management structure. As the study progressed and the committee's ideas matured, it became clear that there were many reasons to call for a single food agency, including the fact that a risk-based approach should encompass all foods and hazards. This is not a new idea, but it is one that is fraught with challenges that the committee recognizes. To overcome these challenges and to maintain public health as the ultimate goal, the committee formulated a stepwise process for achieving a single food safety system and ensuring maintenance of the day-to-day operations necessary to protect the public health. In formulating its own recommendations, the committee also took into account many recommendations made by other groups and individuals to enhance food safety, some of which the committee explicitly supports. (Appendix B presents a sampling of past recommendations from other sources.) The committee also specified what legislative changes would be required to implement its recommendations.

Finally, the committee was asked, if feasible, to provide cost estimates for implementing its recommendations. However, because essential supporting information was not always accessible and the committee faced time constraints, the evidence needed to address this question in detail was lacking. The committee did consider cost and resource issues in a general sense in all of its deliberations by drawing on the experience of members who formerly held senior leadership positions at the FDA.

ORGANIZATION OF THE REPORT

This report is divided into three parts. Part I sets the stage for understanding and improving the FDA's role in the food safety system. Chapter 2 assesses the current system with respect to how well it has fulfilled its public health mission in the face of the significant changes in the food enterprise discussed briefly above; it also contains a summary of organizational and functional challenges at the FDA. The committee used previous NRC and IOM reports, as well as reports by the agency itself, GAO, industry, and consumer organizations, to document these challenges.

Each chapter in Parts II and III is dedicated to explaining the committee's understanding of the essential functions of a food safety regulatory agency; these chapters also include the committee's recommendations. Part II presents the committee's vision of a food safety system defined by a risk-based decision-making approach. Chapter 3 details the attributes of such an approach and identifies the infrastructure needed for its implementation, such as personnel and analytical capacity. It also presents an account of the science needed to build a risk-based system, including data analysis and laboratory research. Chapter 4 outlines the types of governance models that might be appropriate for managing food safety and explains the importance of defining the responsibilities of the various parties involved in food safety (e.g., industry, state and local governments).

Part III describes what is necessary to implement the food safety system proposed in Part II. Chapters 5 and 6, respectively, address the creation of the necessary data surveillance and research infrastructures. Chapter 7 describes state and local food safety programs nationwide and calls for their harmonization and integration with the programs of the federal government to achieve a seamless food safety program. Chapter 8 addresses the issue of how to enhance the efficiency of food inspections. Chapter 9 examines the critical issue of communicating about food safety and risks with those who can impact public health through their food safety–related conduct at home (consumers) or at work (e.g., personnel in industry and the health professions). Chapter 10 is dedicated to legislative needs for an enhanced food safety system. Finally, Chapter 11 sets forth the organizational changes needed to achieve the committee's vision of an efficient risk-based food safety system.

Appendixes B–G can be found on the inserted CD. They include the agendas of all public meetings (Appendix A), recommendations of selected past reports (Appendix B), a brief description of food safety systems in the United States and other countries (Appendix C), two commissioned papers on food defense and food importation (Appendixes D and E, respectively, prepared at the committee's request by outside experts and used as background for the committee's deliberations), a sampling of selected FDA research (Appendix F), the FPP (Appendix G), a glossary and a list of acronyms and abbreviations (Appendixes H and I, respectively), and biographical sketches of the committee members (Appendix J).

REFERENCES

Behnke, K. 2009. *Feed Manufacturing and the Connection to Human Health*. Paper presented at the Institute of Medicine/National Research Council Committee on Review of the FDA's Role in Ensuring Safe Food Meeting, Washington, DC, March 25, 2009.

CDC (U.S. Centers for Disease Control and Prevention). 2009. Preliminary FoodNet data on the incidence of infection with pathogens commonly transmitted through food—10 states, 2008. *Morbidity and Mortality Weekly Report* 58(13):333–337.

CDC. 2010. Preliminary FoodNet data on the incidence of infection with pathogens transmitted commonly through food—10 states, 2009. *Morbidity and Mortality Weekly
Report* 59(14)418–422.

DeWaal, C. S., and D. Plunkett. 2007. *Building a Modern Food Safety System for FDA
Regulated Foods.* CSPI White Paper. Washington, DC: Center for Science in the Public
Interest.

FDA (U.S. Food and Drug Administration). 1992. Statement of policy—foods derived from
new plant varieties. *FDA Federal Register* 57(104):22984. http://www.fda.gov/Food/
GuidanceComplianceRegulatoryInformation/GuidanceDocuments/Biotechnology/
ucm096095.htm (accessed March 22, 2010).

FDA. 2007. *Food Protection Plan. An Integrated Strategy for Protecting the Nation's Food
Supply.* Rockville, MD: FDA.

FDA. 2010. *Food and Drug Administration FY 2011 Congressional Budget Request: Narrative by Activity–Foods Program FY2011.* http://www.fda.gov/downloads/AboutFDA/
ReportsManualsForms/Reports/BudgetReports/UCM205367.pdf (accessed June 2, 2010).

FDA Science Board. 2007. *FDA Science and Mission at Risk. Report of the Subcommittee on
Science and Technology.* Rockville, MD: FDA.

FDA/CFSAN (Center for Food Safety and Applied Nutrition). 2008. *Fiscal Year (FY) 2008 Enforcement Statistics Summary.* Edited by CFSAN/FDA. http://www.fda.gov/downloads/
ICECI/EnforcementActions/EnforcementStory/UCM129824.pdf (accessed May 7,
2010).

Gallup (The Gallup Organization). 2010. *Nutrition and Food.* http://www.gallup.com/
poll/6424/Nutrition-Food.aspx (accessed on May 12, 2010).

GAO (U.S. Government Accountability Office). 2004a. *Federal Food Safety and Security
System: Fundamental Restructuring Is Needed to Address Fragmentation and Overlap.*
Washington, DC: GAO.

GAO. 2004b. *Food Safety: USDA and FDA Need to Better Ensure Prompt and Complete
Recalls of Potentially Unsafe Food.* Washington, DC: GAO.

GAO. 2005. *Oversight of Food Safety Activities: Federal Agencies Should Pursue Opportunities to Reduce Overlap and Better Leverage Resources.* Washington, DC: GAO.

GAO. 2008a. *Federal Oversight of Food Safety: FDA Has Provided Few Details on the
Resources and Strategies Needed to Implement Its Food Protection Plan.* Washington,
DC: GAO.

GAO. 2008b. *Federal Oversight of Food Safety: FDA's Food Protection Plan Proposes Positive
First Steps, but Capacity to Carry Them Out Is Critical.* Washington, DC: GAO.

GAO. 2010. *Food Irradiation: FDA Could Improve Its Documentation and Communication
of Key Decisions on Food Irradiation Petitions.* Washington, DC: GAO.

GMA (Grocery Manufacturers Association). 2007. *A Commitment to Consumers to Ensure the
Safety of Imported Foods: Four Pillars of Public–Private Partnership.* Washington, DC:
GMA. http://www.gmabrands.com/publicpolicy/docs/FourPillarsLongFINAL17Sept07.pdf
(accessed March 22, 2010).

IOM (Institute of Medicine). 2009. *HHS in the 21st Century: Charting a New Course for a
Healthier America.* Washington, DC: The National Academies Press.

IOM/NRC (National Research Council). 1998. *Ensuring Safe Food: From Production to
Consumption.* Washington, DC: National Academy Press.

IOM/NRC. 2003. *Scientific Criteria to Ensure Safe Food.* Washington, DC: The National
Academies Press.

Mead, P. S., L. Slutsker, V. Dietz, L. F. McCaig, J. S. Bresee, C. Shapiro, P. M. Griffin, and
R. V. Tauxe. 1999. Food-related illness and death in the United States. *Emerging Infectious Diseases* 5:607–625.

2

The Food Safety System:
Context and Current Status

Since humans began farming, agriculture has evolved rapidly, with pervasive effects on society. An example is the industrialization of food production in the twentieth century, which, among other things, dramatically changed perceptions and behaviors related to food (Hennessy et al., 2003). While this revolution in food production resulted in great benefits to today's consumers and the ability to feed a growing population, it also resulted in unanticipated foodborne risks. Regulatory agencies responsible for food safety thus are challenged not only to respond to current issues, but also to articulate a vision of food safety that anticipates future risks. This chapter sets the stage for the more detailed assessments, findings, and recommendations that follow by reviewing some of the developments that have contributed to the context for food safety in the United States and by providing an overview of the current U.S. food safety system.

A CHANGING WORLD

The Institute of Medicine (IOM)/National Research Council (NRC) report *Ensuring Safe Food: From Production to Consumption* (IOM/NRC, 1998) identifies a number of developments with implications for food safety, including (1) emerging pathogens, (2) the trend toward the consumption of more fresh produce, (3) the trend toward eating more meals away from home, and (4) changing demographics, with a greater proportion of the population being immunocompromised or otherwise at increase risk of foodborne illness. These developments continue to be important today, but many others affecting food safety have occurred in the decade since that

35

report was published. Together, these developments contribute to the current context for food safety in the United States, which is characterized by a number of features that must inform any assessment of the food safety system. These include changes in the food production landscape, climate change, changing consumer perceptions and behaviors, globalization and increased food importation, the role of labor–management relations and workplace safety, heightened concern about bioterrorism, increased levels of pollution in the environment, and the signing of international trade agreements.

Changes in the Food Production Landscape

In addition to constant changes in food production and substantial growth in the number of food facilities (the number regulated by the U.S. Food and Drug Administration [FDA] grew by 10 percent between 2003 and 2007 [GAO, 2008a]), the food and agriculture sector has experienced widespread integration and consolidation in recent years. For example, the consolidation of supermarkets has changed the retail grocery landscape in the United States, leading to the dominance of the industry by a small number of large companies. Apart from consequences for the market share of small retailers, the greater dependence of manufacturers on this limited number of retailers for sales volume gives these companies significant leverage to bargain for lower prices and demand safety standards. The result has been an increased tendency to establish private standards, which has changed the enterprise of food safety (Henson and Humphrey, 2009).

For example, large retailers and customers established the Food Safety Leadership Council on Farm Produce Standards to develop standards for the growing and harvesting of fresh produce (FSLC, 2007). Another private effort was the Global Food Safety Initiative, created in 2000 to set common benchmarks for different national and industry food safety programs. Its standards, now used widely around the world, require that the food protection practices of manufacturers of food, including produce, meat, fish, poultry, and ready-to-eat products such as frozen pizza and microwave meals, be audited at regular intervals (GFSI, 2007). Farmers, shippers, and processors in the business of producing leafy greens may participate in the California Leafy Greens Marketing Agreement, a private mechanism operating with oversight from the California Department of Food and Agriculture that verifies whether growers are following certain food safety practices (LGMA, 2010). Adoption of these private standards could be seen as an enhancement of food safety; however, private standards can also impose unnecessary burdens if they are not scientifically justified. For example, private standards may result in unnecessarily higher food prices (DeWaal and Plunkett, 2007). Therefore, a close look at such standards is warranted. As an alternative, public standards can be instituted. For example, Tomato

Good Agricultural Practices for tomato farms and Tomato Best Management Practices for tomato packinghouses are the first mandatory produce safety programs in the United States (Florida Department of Agriculture and Consumer Services, 2007).

Climate Change

Climate change is doubly relevant to the food enterprise: not only may climate change affect food yields, but food production may contribute to climate change by releasing a substantial amount of greenhouse gases, such as carbon monoxide and nitrogen monoxide (Stern, 2007). Stern (2007), among others, has highlighted serious concerns regarding the effects of climate change on future food security, especially for populations in low-income countries that are already at risk of food insecurity.

Climate change can affect food systems directly, by affecting crop production (e.g., because of changes in rainfall or warmer or cooler temperatures), or indirectly, by changing markets, food prices, and the supply chain infrastructure—although the relative importance of climate change for food security and safety is expected to differ among regions (Gregory et al., 2005). A recent Food and Agriculture Organization paper, *Climate Change: Implications for Food Safety* (FAO, 2008), identifies the potential impacts of anticipated changes in climate on food safety and its control at all stages of the food chain. The specific food safety issues cited are increased range and incidence of common bacterial foodborne diseases, zoonotic diseases, mycotoxin contamination, biotoxins in fishery products, and environmental contaminants with significance for the food chain. To raise awareness and facilitate international cooperation, the paper also highlights the substantial uncertainty on the effects of climate change and the need for adequate attention to food safety to ensure effective management of the problem.

Changing Consumer Perceptions and Behaviors

With an increasingly global food market, consumer expectations and behaviors with regard to food have changed dramatically over the past hundred years. Consumers have grown to expect a wide variety of foods, including exotic and out-of-season foods. As a result, the consumption of fresh fruits and vegetables has increased (IOM/NRC, 1998) and is expected to continue to do so: per capita fruit consumption is predicted to grow in the United States by 5–8 percent by 2020, with a smaller increase predicted for vegetables (Lin, 2004). Additionally, consumers are spending more money on food away from home, which accounted for 48.5 percent of total food dollars, or approximately $565 billion, in 2008 (ERS, 2010).

At the same time, consumer perceptions and behaviors with respect to food safety have also changed significantly. Consumer knowledge about foodborne pathogens, high-risk foods, vulnerable populations, and safe food-handling practices has increased in recent years, although this knowledge is sometimes wrong or incomplete (FSIS, 2002). Recent foodborne illness outbreaks have further increased consumer awareness about food safety; in fact, a majority of consumers believe foodborne illnesses are a serious or very serious worry (FSIS, 2002; Hart Research Associates/Public Opinion Strategies, 2009). Further, recent polls indicate a lack of confidence in the ability of the FDA to protect consumers against food-related threats (Hart Research Associates/Public Opinion Strategies, 2009).

While food producers, processors, and retailers have the primary responsibility for the safety of the food they produce, food preparers also play an important role in preventing foodborne illness. Accordingly, several groups have developed educational messages aimed at teaching safe food-handling behaviors to consumers and other food preparers. The Clean, Separate, Cook, Chill approach, for example, is focused primarily on consumers in the home. However, this initiative has proven to be largely ineffective (Anderson et al., 2004). Several studies have found that, although self-reported use of safe food-handling practices has increased, consumers and other food preparers do not always follow these practices (Redmond and Griffith, 2003; Howells et al., 2008; Abbot et al., 2009). Further, the International Food Information Council Foundation found that many consumers fail to use some important food safety practices; for example, just 50 and 25 percent of consumers, respectively, use a different or freshly cleaned cutting board for each type of food and check the doneness of meat and poultry items with a food thermometer (IFICF, 2009). Several factors have been identified as affecting the adoption of safe food-handling practices, including attitudes, lack of motivation, sociodemographic factors, and cultural beliefs (Medeiros et al., 2004; Patil et al., 2005; Pilling et al., 2008). In addition, the media often promote poor food-handling practices during on-air cooking demonstrations and frequently give misinformation on the subject (Mathiasen et al., 2004). The decline of home economics classes in schools, coupled with the increasing trend to eat out, further contributes to the lack of food safety knowledge. In addition, few medical providers diagnose and report foodborne illness, and fewer yet discuss safe food-handling practices with their patients (Wong et al., 2004; Henao et al., 2005).

Globalization and Increased Food Importation

The expansion and liberalization of international trade in recent decades have resulted in an increase in food imports. By 2005, the volume of imported medical supplies and food had increased seven-fold over that in 1994, and this trend is expected to continue (Nucci et al., 2008). Among foods, the increase has been especially dramatic in the seafood sector, which the FDA oversees. From 1996 to 2006, the volume of FDA-regulated food imports increased almost four-fold, from 2.8 billion to 10 billion pounds (Nucci et al., 2008). About 230,730 facilities that deal with imported foods are registered with the FDA, including foreign manufacturers, packers, holders, and warehouses (FDA, 2010a). Consequently, there is a growing need for a robust regulatory system that can ensure the safety of food imports. This concern over the safety of imported foods is reflected in the number of congressional hearings on the subject in 2007 and 2008 (GPO, 2010).

Various countries are experimenting with models for regulating food imports (e.g., third-party certification, inspections at the border, country certifications; see Appendix E), but there is no consensus on the best regulatory models. In this environment, the United States is attempting to determine the best model to implement given available resources and the vast amount of imported foods to oversee. For example, in 2007, at the request of the White House, the Interagency Working Group on Import Safety was established. It included, among others, representatives of the Department of Health and Human Services (HHS), the parent agency of the FDA, and the Department of Agriculture (USDA). The working group developed a road map recommending both broad and specific actions that would enhance the safety of all food imports (Interagency Working Group on Import Safety, 2007).

The Role of Labor–Management Relations and Workplace Safety

The crucial role of food employees and employers in food safety cannot be overstated, particularly since food workers have been implicated in the spread of foodborne illness (Todd et al., 2007). When addressing food safety, therefore, it is important to consider the potential role of labor–management relations and workplace conditions. For example, if the labor force responsible for producing food on farms and in factories is inadequately trained or paid, is forced to work under unsafe or unsavory conditions, or is ignored by management when it attempts to express concerns, workers may respond by applying less care in the production, processing, or preparation of food, leading to increased risk for consumers. Some elements of this association may be direct since many human pathogens are easily transmitted to foods via contact with human vehicles, and worker sanitation and hygiene are critical factors in this process. Specifically, ensuring that workers have access to appropriate sanitary facilities, providing adequate sick leave, and making hand washing a critical control point are vital to controlling many hazards in the food supply. For example, if farm laborers in the field are not provided with adequate sanitary facilities, there will be increased opportunity for crop exposure to infectious agents. And if workers are not given sufficient training for their basic work activities, they are also less likely to be trained in minimizing risks for food products.

Regulation and oversight of all phases of the food supply chain by all levels of government can help enhance food safety by identifying situations in which work procedures need improvement or workers need training. Cooperation between the FDA and labor regulatory agencies such as the National Institute for Occupational Safety and Health and the Occupational Safety and Health Administration would appear to warrant exploration.

Heightened Concern About Bioterrorism

Although public health agencies have been concerned about the potential for intentional contamination of food in the past, this concern increased greatly after the events of September 11, 2001. The volume of food animals and commodities, the lack of physical security and robust surveillance systems for food products, and the rapid movement of food products over a broad geographic range and through many hands make the U.S. food supply highly vulnerable to intentional contamination (Kosal and Anderson, 2004). A major activity in response to this threat was the FDA's establishment, with USDA and the U.S. Department of Homeland Security (DHS), of a food defense partnership (i.e., sector organization) with all relevant federal, state, local, and industry counterparts (see Appendix D). Various other efforts followed the establishment of this partnership, increasing the responsibilities of all involved and of the FDA in particular. The FDA is engaged in food defense activities to implement new presidential directives and congressional legislation, as well as to educate and communicate with industry, its own staff, and state, local, and foreign counterparts about matters related to food defense. The issue of terrorism-related prioritization of efforts is highly problematic, however, because of the uncertainty concerning the likelihood and nature of an attack (information about which is generally classified). This uncertainty makes comparisons with other risks and justifications for resource allocation and prioritization difficult.

Increased Levels of Pollution in the Environment

An undesirable consequence of the industrialization of agriculture and manufacturing is the release of chemicals to the environment. Not all food pollutants come from industrial processes, however. For example, dioxins and furans are contaminants released unintentionally into the environment as a result of both preindustrial combustion processes (e.g., the combustion of forests or brush) and modern combustion processes (e.g., industrial burning, landfill fires, structural fires) (IOM/NRC, 2003). Whether exposure to these pollutants has increased over the years depends on the pollutant, and the data needed to assess trends are often lacking (IOM, 2007).

The bioaccumulation of pollutants in the food chain (e.g., methylmercury in seafood) has received a great deal of attention. The pollutants of concern may change over time as manufacturing processes evolve, but those that are persistent in the environment can be a chronic issue for public health and environmental agencies. The growing attention to the problem is due to both increased understanding of bioaccumulation and greater public concern about environmental pollutants in general, both domestically and internationally. The potential long-term effects of these pollutants, coupled with the difficulty of measuring multiple exposures and potential interactions, present a complex problem.

Although the U.S. Environmental Protection Agency (EPA), not the FDA, is the agency that regulates levels of pollutants in the environment, food commodities are subject to contamination via the environment. Much of the work on collecting and analyzing environmental and toxicological data on food pollutants has already been done by EPA, and EPA's risk assessments can often be used as the basis for food policy. A recent report, however, found that the national residue program is not accomplishing its mission of monitoring the food supply for harmful residues (USDA, 2010a).

The Signing of International Trade Agreements

In the wake of the establishment of the World Trade Organization (WTO) in 1995 and the signing of the Agreement on the Application of Sanitary and Phytosanitary Measures, countries are obliged to follow some basic rules in the application of food safety measures and plant and animal regulations. Countries can set their own standards for safety, but those standards must be based on science. The intent is to avoid protectionism on behalf of domestic producers of food and allow for free trade based on competitive principles. Although the obligations of this agreement were not fully understood at first by governments, it is increasingly viewed as a legal document with the same force as domestic law (Carnevale, 2009). In practical terms, this means that unscientific regulations that affect trade could be successfully challenged at WTO.

As an example, the United States and Canada brought to WTO the European Union's (EU's) ban on the importation of meat and meat products that had been treated with any of six hormones, which favored EU meat producers and blocked exports from the United States and Canada. The WTO Panel and Appellate Body concluded that the prohibition was not based on scientific evidence, and a settlement was reached (Lugard and

Smart, 2006). Policies of the United States have also been under scrutiny. A recent analysis suggests that foreign food producers may be at a disadvantage when they want to export to the United States because they need to comply with costly requirements under the Public Health Security and Bioterrorism Preparedness and Response Act of 2002, such as providing prior notice of shipment (GAO, 2004a; Boisen, 2007).[1] As the volume of imported foods continues to rise, such international agreements are becoming more important and must be considered in any discussion of enhancing food safety in the United States. (International trade agreements and their influence on food safety oversight and regulations are discussed in detail in Appendix E.)

LIMITS ON FOOD SAFETY

In examining how to improve a food safety system, one must acknowledge that foodborne illness cannot be completely eliminated. Many factors affect the degree of safety that is achievable, some related to the state of science and others to human factors, such as economic considerations and people's desire to enjoy certain foods whose safety cannot be ensured (e.g., raw milk). The degree of food safety that is attainable also depends on management and oversight practices, on costs versus benefits, and on such factors as regulatory limits, public perceptions, consumer education and responsibility, and public communication.

It is important to stress that responsibility for food safety falls on everyone, from farmers to consumers. However, the FDA is often held responsible for negative events related to food safety, given that ensuring food safety is part of the agency's core mission. This focus on the FDA's responsibilities has grown as such events have become more widespread, garnering increased media attention. Moreover, in recent years, reductions in the incidence of foodborne illness seen in the late 1990s appear to have leveled off (CDC, 2009), and for some pathogens the incidence has recently increased (CDC, 2010). Because many government agencies are responsible for food safety, it is not possible to attribute changes in the rate of foodborne illness to any particular agency. Still, the FDA's responses to these events have sometimes been less than optimal (Produce Safety Project, 2008).

One limit on the degree of food safety attainable is the fact that to achieve a complete absence of pathogens and other contaminants in food is an unrealistic goal (IOM/NRC, 2003). Although the concept of zero tolerance for a particular pathogen may appear justifiable, it is merely a

---

[1] *Public Health Security and Bioterrorism Preparedness and Response Act of 2002 (Bioterrorism Act)*, Public Law 107-188, 107th Cong., 2nd sess. (January 23, 2002), 306.

regulatory term with little scientific basis. As the IOM/NRC report *Scientific Criteria to Ensure Safe Food* states: "Scientists are often dismayed by the use of the term [zero tolerance] because they recognize the inability to ensure, in most situations, the complete absence of pathogens and contaminants and the limitations of any feasible sampling plan to check for their total absence" (IOM/NRC, 2003, p. 25). Moreover, most interventions to minimize food hazards have only limited effects in decreasing the prevalence of pathogens, and for some foods, such as those sold raw, few interventions are possible. Recognizing these realities, zero tolerances are viewed as an enforcement tool applied to the most problematic hazards with the goal of communicating that the highest level of public health protection is needed (DeWaal, 2009).

The creativity of those seeking to compromise food safety for profit, the evolution of bacteria to increased virulence, and the inevitability of human errors will continue to challenge regulators, producers, and consumers. As demonstrated by the recent incident in which several brands of pet food were contaminated with melamine, researchers struggle with the question of how to predict, mitigate, and prevent such relatively rare events. The predictability of such events must be taken into account when decisions are made about allocating resources to prevention versus rapid response.

OVERVIEW OF THE CURRENT FOOD SAFETY SYSTEM

Although the FDA's role in ensuring safe food needs to be reviewed in the context of the U.S. national food safety system, for brevity the discussion in this section is limited to information that pertains to the FDA and is needed as context for the reminder of this report. Previous reports have reviewed the food safety system in the United States (IOM/NRC, 1998; GAO, 2004a,b,c, 2008b; Becker and Porter, 2007), and the reader is referred to those reports for a more detailed description and historical context of the U.S. food safety system as a whole.

Organization

Table 2-1 lists the main federal agencies that have responsibility for food safety under at least 30 laws. Of these agencies, eight have primary responsibility for ensuring food safety: two under HHS—the FDA and the U.S. Centers for Disease Control and Prevention (CDC); four under USDA—the Food Safety and Inspection Service (FSIS), the Agricultural Marketing Service, the Agricultural Research Service, and the National Institute of Food and Agriculture; DHS; and EPA (GAO, 2004b,c, 2005, 2008a, 2009a).

State and local governments also have food and feed safety responsi-

TABLE 2-1 Food Safety Responsibilities by Federal Agency

Abbreviation	Name	Food Safety Responsibilities
CDC	U.S. Centers for Disease Control and Prevention	Prevents disease, disability, and death caused by a wide range of infectious diseases and does the following:
		• Investigates with local, state, and other federal officials sources of foodborne disease outbreaks.
		• Maintains a nationwide system of foodborne disease surveillance (designs and puts in place rapid electronic systems for reporting foodborne infections, works with other federal and state agencies to monitor rates of and trends in foodborne disease outbreaks, develops state-of-the-art techniques for rapid identification of foodborne pathogens at the state and local levels).
		• Develops and advocates for public health policies to prevent foodborne diseases.
		• Conducts research to help prevent foodborne disease.
		• Trains local and state food safety personnel.
DHS	U.S. Department of Homeland Security	Leverages resources within federal, state, and local governments, coordinating the transition of multiple agencies and programs into a single, integrated agency focused on protecting the American people and their homeland.
DHS/CBP	Customs and Border Protection	Works with federal regulatory agencies to ensure that all goods entering and exiting the United States do so according to U.S. laws and regulations.
DHS/OHA	Office of Health Affairs	• Serves as DHS's principal agent for all medical and health matters.
		• Leads veterinary and agro-defense activities, addressing animal and zoonotic diseases, as well as livestock, food, and water security issues.
DOJ	U.S. Department of Justice	• Prosecutes companies and individuals suspected of violating food safety laws.
		• Through the U.S. Marshals Service, seizes unsafe food products not yet in the marketplace, as ordered by courts.

TABLE 2-1 Continued

Abbreviation	Name	Food Safety Responsibilities
EPA	U.S. Environmental Protection Agency	Oversees drinking water and certain aspects of foods made from plants, seafood, meat, and poultry; establishes safe drinking water standards; regulates toxic substances and wastes to prevent their entry into the environment and food chain; assists states in monitoring the quality of drinking water and finding ways to prevent contamination of drinking water; and determines the safety of new pesticides, sets tolerance levels for pesticide residues in foods, and publishes directions on the safe use of pesticides.
EPA/OECA	Office of Enforcement and Compliance Assistance	Responsible for inspection/enforcement of pesticide regulations, including the misuse of pesticides.
EPA/OPPTS	Office of Prevention, Pesticides, and Toxic Substances	Responsible for risk assessment of pesticide residues in food, pesticide registration.
EPA/ORD	Office of Research and Development	Provides scientific support for pesticide-related public health issues.

continued

TABLE 2-1 Continued

Abbreviation	Name	Food Safety Responsibilities
FDA	U.S. Food and Drug Administration	Oversees all domestic and imported food sold in interstate commerce, including shell eggs, but not meat and poultry, bottled water, and wine beverages with less than 7 percent alcohol. Also enforces food safety laws governing domestic and imported food, except meat and poultry, by inspecting food production establishments and food warehouses and collecting and analyzing samples for physical, chemical, and microbial contamination; reviewing the safety of food and color additives before marketing; reviewing animal drugs for the safety of animals that receive them and humans who eat food produced from the animals; monitoring the safety of animal feed used for food-producing animals; developing model codes and ordinances, guidelines, and interpretations and working with states to implement them in regulating milk and shellfish and retail food establishments, such as restaurants and grocery stores (e.g., the model Food Code, a reference for retail outlets and nursing homes and other institutions on how to prepare food to prevent foodborne illness); establishing good food manufacturing practices and other production standards, such as plant sanitation and packaging requirements and Hazard Analysis and Critical Control Points (HACCP) programs; working with foreign governments to ensure the safety of certain imported food products; requesting manufacturers to recall unsafe food products and monitoring those recalls; taking appropriate enforcement actions; conducting research on food safety; and educating industry and consumers on safe food-handling practices. See Table 2-2 for detail on the responsibilities of the FDA centers and offices involved in food safety.
FTC/BCP	Federal Trade Commission/ Bureau of Consumer Protection	Protects consumers against unfair, deceptive, or fraudulent practices, including advertising claims for foods, drugs, dietary supplements, and other products promising health benefits.

TABLE 2-1 Continued

Abbreviation	Name	Food Safety Responsibilities
NOAA/NMFS	National Oceanic and Atmospheric Administration/ National Marine Fisheries Service (under the U.S. Department of Commerce [DoC])	Through its voluntary fee-for-service Seafood Inspection Program, inspects and certifies fishing vessels, seafood processing plants, and retail facilities for federal sanitation standards. Provides scientific oversight and system surveillance of the DoC inspection program and seafood HACCP training.
USDA	U.S. Department of Agriculture	Primarily responsible for meat, poultry, and egg products; see also below.
USDA/AMS	Agricultural Marketing Service	Provides standardization, grading, and market news services for five commodities: (1) dairy, (2) fruits and vegetables, (3) livestock and seed, (4) poultry, and (5) cotton and tobacco. Enforces such federal laws as the Perishable Agricultural Commodities Act and Country-of-Origin Labeling. AMS's National Organic Program develops, implements, and administers national production, handling, and labeling standards for organic agricultural products.
USDA/APHIS	Animal and Plant Health Inspection Service	Responsible for monitoring/surveillance of egg products, risk assessment and data collection for pesticides, and inspections, enforcement for the pesticide record-keeping program, including border quarantine activities to detect and eliminate animal health problems and exotic organisms that might harm U.S. agriculture, many of which also pose potential food safety threats.
USDA/ARS	Agricultural Research Service	Provides data for food products and contaminants (fruits and vegetables, dairy products, eggs/egg products, meat/poultry, seafood, grain/rice/related products, imported foods, animal drugs/feeds, and pesticide residues) to support risk assessment by the Food Safety and Inspection Service (FSIS), the Economic Research Service (ERS), the Office of Risk Assessment and Cost-Benefit Analysis (ORACBA), the FDA, and EPA; broad support of Land Grant Universities for research and education across all product areas; and education in the form of information to the National Agricultural Library (NAL) and educational workshops.

continued

TABLE 2-1 Continued

Abbreviation	Name	Food Safety Responsibilities
USDA/ERS	Economic Research Service	Provides risk assessment for meat and poultry and data collection to support the pesticide risk assessment process as well as technical assistance to identify education needs and to analyze the effectiveness of food safety education programs.
USDA/FSIS	Food Safety and Inspection Service	Oversees domestic and imported meat and poultry and related products, such as meat- or poultry-containing stews, pizzas, and frozen foods, as well as processed egg products (generally liquid, frozen, and dried pasteurized egg products). Also enforces food safety laws governing domestic and imported meat and poultry products by

- inspecting food animals for diseases before and after slaughter;
- inspecting meat and poultry slaughter and processing plants;
- with USDA's Agricultural Marketing Service, monitoring and inspecting processed egg products;
- collecting and analyzing samples of food products for microbial and chemical contaminants and infectious and toxic agents;
- establishing production standards for the use of food additives and other ingredients in preparing and packaging meat and poultry products, plant sanitation, thermal processing, and other processes;
- making sure all foreign meat and poultry processing plants exporting to the United States meet U.S. standards;
- seeking voluntary recalls of unsafe products by meat and poultry processors;
- sponsoring research on meat and poultry safety; and
- educating industry and consumers on safe food-handling practices.

As of April 2010, FSIS is responsible for mandatory inspection of catfish and catfish products.[a]

TABLE 2-1 Continued

Abbreviation	Name	Food Safety Responsibilities
USDA/GIPSA	Grain Inspection, Packers, and Stockyards Administration	Through its oversight activities, including monitoring programs, reviews, and investigations, fosters fair competition, provides payment protection, and guards against deceptive and fraudulent trade practices that affect the movement and price of meat animals and their products. Protects consumers and members of the livestock, meat, and poultry industries. Its Federal Grain Inspection Service facilitates the marketing of U.S. grain and related agricultural products by establishing standards for quality assessments, regulating handling practices, and managing a network of federal, state, and private laboratories that provide impartial, user fee–funded official inspection and weighing services.
USDA/NAL	National Agricultural Library/USDA/FDA Foodborne Illness Education Information Center	Collects information on human nutrition and food to support USDA programs. These programs encompass areas as diverse as human nutritional needs, food production, safety and inspection, distribution, economics, and consumer education. Because of USDA's responsibility for food safety and inspection, NAL comprehensively collects works addressing foodborne illness, food toxicology, and food inspection. In addition, in support of USDA's close relationship and regulatory role with the food industry, NAL collects information on the food industry and technology, including food irradiation and biotechnology.
USDA/NASS	National Agricultural Statistics Service	Performs data collection for risk assessment of pesticides.
USDA/NIFA[b]	National Institute of Food and Agriculture	Advances knowledge for agriculture, the environment, human health and well-being, and communities by supporting research, education, and extension programs in the Land Grant University System and other partner organizations. Does not perform actual research, education, and extension but helps fund them at the state and local levels and provides program leadership in these areas.
USDA/ ORACBA	Office of Risk Assessment and Cost-Benefit Analysis	Provides technical assistance to identify education needs and to analyze the effectiveness of food safety education programs.

continued

TABLE 2-1 Continued

Abbreviation	Name	Food Safety Responsibilities
US DOT/BATF	U.S. Department of the Treasury/ Bureau of Alcohol, Tobacco, and Firearms	Oversees alcoholic beverages except wine containing less than 7 percent alcohol, enforces food safety laws governing the production and distribution of alcoholic beverages, and investigates cases of adulterated alcoholic products, sometimes with help from the FDA.

^a *The Food, Conservation, and Energy Act of 2008,* 21 U.S.C. §§ 601 et seq., 2008 (also known as the 2008 Farm Bill).

^b The Cooperative State Research, Education, and Extension Service became the National Institute of Food and Agriculture on October 1, 2009.

SOURCE: IOM/NRC, 1998; DHS, 2004; GAO, 2005; Becker and Porter, 2007; AMS/USDA, 2009; FDA, 2009a; APHIS/USDA, 2010; FoodSafety.gov, 2010; USDA, 2010b.

bilities (see also Chapter 7). Forty-four states conduct inspections of food-manufacturing firms under contract to the FDA, and all 50 states have food safety and labeling programs. Additional responsibilities of state and local governments include the following:

- implementing food safety standards, such as Good Manufacturing Practices and Hazard Analysis and Critical Control Points (HACCP), for fish, seafood, milk, and other foods manufactured within state borders with the assistance of the FDA and other federal agencies;
- inspecting restaurants, grocery stores, and other retail food establishments, as well as dairy farms, milk-processing plants, grain mills, and food-manufacturing plants, within the state (the states collect and analyze many food product samples);
- using advisory and enforcement actions to protect the health of their citizens, including placing embargoes on (i.e., stopping the sale of) unsafe food products manufactured, transported, or distributed within state borders;
- providing safety training and education to food establishment personnel and industry as requested;
- preparing for and participating in food recall events and foodborne outbreak investigations independently or with the FDA and other federal agencies (this may include ordering recalls of contaminated foods within state borders and taking enforcement actions against firms within state borders);
- collecting representative samples according to established procedures and with a documented chain of custody (These samples are

then tested at state regulatory laboratories so they can be evaluated for compliance with food regulatory laws.);

- receiving, evaluating, and responding to consumer complaints relating to products manufactured, purchased, or consumed in their state;
- conducting epidemiological investigations of people who have become ill or injured (State, county, and local health officials serve the primary on-site epidemiological role in the United States and coordinate among one another and with CDC in situations of multistate outbreaks.);
- responding to natural disasters—earthquakes, floods, hurricanes— to assess the impact on food safety and take immediate action to prevent problems in affected areas; and
- issuing consumer health advisories or warnings through typical media and outreach channels.

The FDA's Responsibilities for Food Safety

The FDA's responsibilities for food safety are only part of its wide range of responsibilities. The agency has regulatory authority over more than $1 trillion in products sold annually—about 25 cents of every dollar spent by consumers (Fraser, 2009). The FDA is required to oversee the safety of all food products with the exception of meat, poultry, and some egg products. Additionally, the agency's food safety charge includes the safety of animal feed for both pets and food-producing animals (e.g., swine, dairy cattle). In addition to food, moreover, the FDA's jurisdiction extends to drugs, biologics, medical devices, and tobacco.[2] According to the agency's mission statement,

> 1) FDA is responsible for protecting public health by ensuring the safety, efficacy and security of human and veterinary drugs, biological products, medical devices, our nation's food supplies, cosmetics and products that produce radiation. 2) The FDA is also responsible for advancing the public health by helping to speed innovations that make medicine and foods more effective, safer, and more affordable; and helping the public get the accurate science-based information they need to use medicines and foods to improve their health. (FDA, 2009a)

The FDA has six program centers: (1) the Center for Biologics Evaluation and Research, (2) the Center for Drug Evaluation and Research, (3) the Center for Devices and Radiological Health, (4) the Center for Food Safety

---

[2] The FDA acquired jurisdiction over tobacco products in 2009.

and Applied Nutrition (CFSAN), (5) the Center for Tobacco Products, and (6) the Center for Veterinary Medicine (CVM). The FDA also has a number of cross-cutting offices that report directly to the FDA Commissioner, including the Office of Operations, the Office of Scientific and Medical Programs, the Office of Regulatory Affairs (ORA), the Office of International Programs, and the Office of Planning, Policy, and Preparedness. A recent addition has been the Office of Foods, which reports directly to the Commissioner (see Figure 2-1) (FDA, 2010b).

In response to the increasing volume of imported products, including foods, the agency recently embarked on the Beyond Our Borders initiative, establishing offices in foreign countries under the Office of International Programs. As of 2009, countries with one or more U.S. offices included Belgium, China, Costa Rica, India, and Mexico. Although the long-term roles of these offices are still in the planning stages, the Beyond Our Borders initiative is designed to build or further strengthen relationships, help in learning more about the industries in these countries, facilitate and leverage inspection resources, increase interactions with foreign manufacturers, and verify that products meet U.S. standards (FDA, 2009b).

The main FDA offices with responsibility for food safety are the Office of the Commissioner, the Office of Foods, CFSAN, CVM, ORA, and the National Center for Toxicological Research (NCTR) (see Table 2-2) (FDA, 2010c).

The regulatory authority for foods is derived primarily from the Federal Food, Drug, and Cosmetic Act (FDCA)[3] and its amendments. Recent amendments include the Infant Formula Act of 1980, the Nutrition Labeling and Education Act of 1990, the Public Health Security and Bioterrorism Preparedness and Response Act of 2002, and, more recently, the Food and Drug Administration Amendments Act of 2007 (Fraser, 2009). In some fundamental respects, the law under which the FDA must ensure the safety of 80 percent of the nation's food supply[4] remains unchanged since 1938, despite the dramatic changes in food production, processing, and distribution that have taken place since (as discussed earlier in this chapter). Bills currently under consideration in Congress would give the FDA new authorities and, if enacted, would result in significant changes in the way food safety is managed.[5]

---

[3] *Federal Food, Drug, and Cosmetic Act (FDCA)*, 21 U.S.C. §§ 301 et seq., 1938.

[4] The term "food," as defined in the FDCA, includes "all articles used for food or drink for man or other animals," and thus encompasses what is commonly known as animal feed. Throughout this chapter, therefore, as throughout the report generally (see Chapter 1), the word "food" includes animal feed unless otherwise noted.

[5] HR 2749, *Food Safety Enhancement Act of 2009*; S510 IS § 206: *FDA Food Safety Modernization Act 2009*.

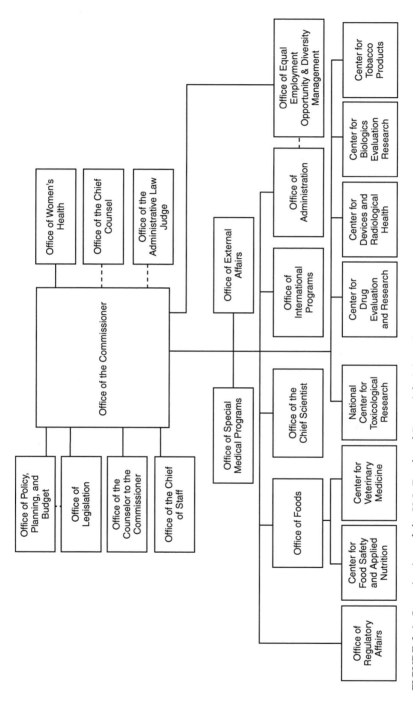

FIGURE 2-1 Organization of the U.S. Food and Drug Administration.
SOURCE: FDA, 2010b.

TABLE 2-2 U.S. Food and Drug Administration (FDA) Offices and Centers with Responsibility for Food Safety

Office	Responsibilities
Office of Foods	• Devises strategic and substantive agencywide domestic and imported food-related policies. • Develops and implements an agencywide visionary strategy for food protection and an approach to promoting and protecting public health with respect to foods (FDA, 2009c; Fraser, 2009).
Center for Food Safety and Applied Nutrition (CFSAN)	Focuses on foods and applied nutrition, but also has responsibility for regulating the safety of cosmetic products. Except for food and color additives, generally it does not have premarket approval authority (in contrast with the centers that deal with drugs and devices, which generally must preapprove products before they can be put on the market). The prevailing regulatory philosophy is that the manufacturer has the primary responsibility for putting a safe product on the market. According to CFSAN's mission statement, "CFSAN, in conjunction with the agency's field staff is responsible for promoting and protecting the public's health by ensuring that the nation's food supply is safe, sanitary, wholesome, honestly labeled, and cosmetic products are safe and properly labeled." Specific responsibilities include • safeguarding the nation's food supply by making sure products are safe, • conducting activities in conjunction with ORA and other groups within the agency, and • ensuring that food is free of contaminants (FDA, 2009c; Fraser, 2009).
Center for Veterinary Medicine (CVM)	Regulates foods used to feed animals, including pet food, as well as devices and drugs for animals, which must gain FDA premarket approval (except animal devices). According to CVM's mission statement, "It's a consumer-protection organization that fosters public and animal health by approving safe and effective products for animals and by enforcing other applicable provisions of the FDCA [Federal Food, Drug, and Cosmetic Act] and other authorities" (FDA, 2009c; Fraser, 2009).
Office of Regulatory Affairs (ORA)	With a headquarters location and field offices across the country, serves as the FDA's broad compliance and enforcement arm. ORA has responsibility to "protect consumers and enhance public health by maximizing compliance of FDA regulated products and minimizing risk associated with those products." In a presentation to the committee, the FDA clarified that within ORA, work to foster compliance is often done in partnership not only with the FDA centers but also with industry. During an outbreak, ORA field investigators work closely with the center that is impacted, conduct investigations, and decide on courses of action (FDA, 2009c; Fraser, 2009).
National Center for Toxicological Research (NCTR)	• Focuses on peer-reviewed research and provides expert advice and training to enable the FDA to make science-based decisions. • Focuses on critical biological events and toxicity (Fraser, 2009; NCTR, 2009).

Budget, Strategic Planning, and Performance Measures

Budget

Annual funding for the FDA is provided in the Agriculture, Rural Development, Food and Drug Administration, and Related Agencies appropriations bill and is handled by the corresponding appropriations subcommittees in the House and Senate. The total amount the agency can spend is composed of direct appropriations (budget authority) and other funds, mainly user fees. Occasionally, funds are earmarked for various activities or offices by Congress. Implementation of the budget for food programs involves a great deal of collaboration among the centers, ORA, and leadership of the FDA food programs.

Table 2-3 shows the FDA budgets for fiscal years (FYs) 2008, 2009, and 2010 and the President's FY 2011 budget as presented in February 2010. After many years of declining funds and personnel, resources for the agency's food programs have recently increased from 2007 levels (note that the food programs include food safety and nutrition funding).

Appropriations for the FDA's food safety program increased in FY 2009 by $141.5 million to a total of about $644 million, or a little less than 25 percent of the agency's overall budget. The distribution of FY 2009 $141.5M food safety budget increase was as follows: CFSAN received $32 million, ORA $90 million, and CVM $6.4 million.

The FDA's budget for food safety comes not only from its budget for food programs, but also from the budgets for the animal drug and feeds program and NCTR, as well as other budgets. In 2009, the FDA proposed an initiative called Protecting America's Food Supply[6] for which a budget increase of $259.3 million was requested for FY 2010, bringing the total budget for food safety to more than $1 billion (HHS, 2009). This increase was the highest among FDA programs for that year. The administration justified the budget request with reference to investments that would strengthen the safety and security of the food supply chain, including enhancements to the system needed as a result of recent food safety events, the dramatic growth in food imports, and changes in food processing and distribution practices. Among the priorities mentioned in the budget justification were the creation of a food safety system that would integrate federal and state programs, the development of preventive controls, increased frequency of domestic and foreign inspections, improved laboratory capacity and food surveillance, and enhanced information technology (IT) to support all food safety programs. The proposed 2011 budget increases the agency's

---

[6] See http://www.fda.gov/NewsEvents/Newsroom/PressAnnouncements/ucm152276.htm (accessed October 8, 2010).

TABLE 2-3 U.S. Food and Drug Administration (FDA) Budgets for Fiscal Years (FYs) 2008, 2009, 2010, and 2011 (in millions)

	FY 2008 (Enacted)	FY 2009 (Enacted)	FY 2010 (Appropriation)	2011 President's Budget
Total FDA	2,420	2,691	3,284	4,023
$	1,870	2,055	2,362	2,508
User fees	549	636	922	1,233
FTEs[a]	NA	11,413	12,335	13,677
Total Food Programs	577	644	784	1,042
Center	NA	210	237	337
Field	NA	434	547	705
User fees[b]	0.00	0.00	0.00	194
FTEs (center)	NA	854	981	1,186
FTEs (field)	NA	2,165	2,505	2,902
Total Animal Drugs and Feeds	115	133	156	175
Center	NA	90	102	113
Field	NA	43	53	62
User fees	14	20	23	24
FTEs (center)	NA	424	447	472
FTEs (field)	NA	238	278	319

NOTE: FTE = full-time equivalent; NA = not available.

[a] In general, the numbers of FTEs decreased from 1992 to 2007 and increased thereafter, in parallel with increases in the FDA's budget for food programs. (The FDA could not provide the number of food-dedicated FTEs at the Center for Veterinary Medicine because its staff is also responsible for products other than foods [e.g., approval of animal drugs]).

[b] Current law includes user fees for animal drug approval and export color certification (certification ensures that products meet regulatory requirements for exportation). Incorporated in the FY 2011 budget for the FDA's food programs is approximately $194 million in user fees, which has been proposed by Congress for registration of food facilities, reinspection, and food and feed export certification.

SOURCES: HHS, 2008, 2009, 2010.

funding for food safety by $318 million. Major activities mentioned to justify this increase include setting standards to integrate state and federal programs and enhancing analytical tools and laboratory capacity. Increased inspection is also proposed.

Strategic Planning and Performance Measures

Strategic planning involves fundamental decisions about the nature, mission, and goals of an organization. When a strategic plan is linked to performance measures, an approach that has been adopted by the federal government, it is also a tool to enhance accountability, which is especially important as the FDA uses public money to implement its plan. The Government Performance and Results Act of 1993 requires that all cabinet-level departments and independent agencies develop a strategic plan covering 6 years, with updates every 3 years.[7] Under this act, HHS is required to have a strategic plan, but not the FDA, which is a sub-cabinet-level department within HHS; however, all the operating divisions of HHS do in fact develop such a plan. As discussed further below, the FDA last developed a strategic plan in 2007.

An additional requirement of the 1993 act is an annual performance plan and a report on how well that plan was implemented during the previous year. During the Bush Administration, the performance plan and report for HHS were integrated with the annual budget submission to Congress. This year, the integrated FY 2010 performance plan and report for HHS were provided as an appendix to the budget request to Congress in compliance with HHS performance planning and reporting requirements (HHS, 2009). The Program Assessment Rating Tool was also introduced during the Bush Administration as a governmentwide evaluation tool, with strategic planning being one of the areas assessed (OMB, 2008). Chapter 3 of this report includes a list of performance measures that have been used by the FDA and are linked to long- and short-term objectives. The President's FY 2011 budget as presented in February 2010 introduces a significant number of new performance measures in the area of food. For example, a reduction in the number of days spent on subtyping priority pathogens in food is linked to the strategic objective of detecting safety problems earlier (HHS, 2010).

Reorganization at the FDA

CFSAN has undergone various reorganizations in an attempt to become more efficient and to adopt new ways of accomplishing its mission under new circumstances. For example, in 1992, as a result of concern expressed by FDA leadership about the ability of the agency's food programs to address emerging food safety issues, the FDA (1) conducted a management study of CFSAN'S programs and activities, (2) reorganized CFSAN and created organizational units to respond directly to certain new food technologies, and (3) established an advisory committee on issues related to food safety. The intent was to make the center more efficient in performing its scientific and regulatory activities and to enhance its ability to meet new challenges. The reorganization was aimed at integrating policy, regulatory, and scientific specialists into offices according to their areas of expertise.

---

[7] *Government Performance and Results Act of 1993 (GPRA)*, Public Law 103-62, 107 Stat. 285.

The FDA believed this new structure would increase managers' accountability for program results and streamline approvals (Suydam, 1996; Johnson et al., 2008). This reorganization was a major change for a center that had been organized by scientific discipline (i.e., toxicology, physical sciences, and nutrition) for the previous 20 years. According to the U.S. Government Accountability Office (GAO, 1992), concern arose at the time that the reorganization's dispersion of scientists could threaten the agency's science base and impede consistency.

Since 1992, other reorganizations have occurred at the FDA. Most notably, the agency was reorganized in 2007 in an effort to consolidate its structure, realign programs with similar or overlapping functions and operational activities, and improve communication and coordination.[8] To reduce the number of management layers, most research activities were merged into two primary offices and the compliance and enforcement functions into one office. The ultimate goal was to maintain a strong and flexible food safety system as new public health challenges continued to emerge. In 2007, the Office of Food Protection was established under the commissioner's oversight to develop an agencywide, visionary strategy for food protection and serve as a liaison to HHS on food protection issues. This office has now merged into the new Office of Foods, headed by a new deputy commissioner of foods and having responsibility and authority for all aspects of food policy under agency jurisdiction (see Box 2-1). Figure 2-1 (presented earlier) reflects these latest changes, plus the addition of the Office of Foods, in 2009 (FDA, 2009d).

Since the Obama Administration took office, the FDA has undergone further changes, which continue even as this report is being written. With a greater emphasis on food safety and public health and an increase in resources for 2010 (see above) (Hamburg and Sharfstein, 2009), the new administration is making substantive attempts to effect strategic changes, for example, through the creation of the White House Food Safety Working Group (FSWG).

RECENT ANALYSES OF
FOOD SAFETY MANAGEMENT AT THE FDA[9]

Over the years, the U.S. government has changed its food safety management approach to meet new challenges and adapt to changes in cir-

---

[8] Personal communication, Robert Brackett, Director and Vice President, National Center for Food Safety and Technology, Illinois Institute of Technology, Chicago, July 14, 2009.

[9] This section does not reflect the conclusions of the committee but instead summarizes the findings of various other reviews of the U.S. food safety system focusing on the FDA. (To complement this section, Appendix B contains numerous recommendations made over the last two decades for enhancing the FDA's management of food safety.)

BOX 2-1
Responsibilities of the Office of Foods

- Provides executive leadership and management to all U.S. Food and Drug Administration (FDA) food-related programs.
- Exercises, on behalf of the Commissioner, direct line authority over the Center for Food Safety and Applied Nutrition (CFSAN) and the Center for Veterinary Medicine (CVM).
- Exercises, on behalf of the commissioner, all food-related legal authorities that the Commissioner is empowered to exercise under the Federal Food, Drug, and Cosmetic Act, as amended; the Public Health Service Act; and other applicable laws.
- Directs efforts to integrate the programs of CFSAN, CVM, and the Office of Regulatory Affairs and thereby ensure the optimal use of all available FDA resources and tools to improve the safety, nutritional quality, and proper labeling of the food supply.
- Directs the development of integrated strategies, plans, policies, and budgets to build the FDA's food-related scientific and regulatory capacities and programs, including recruitment and training of key personnel and development of information systems.
- Represents the FDA on food-related matters in dealings with the Office of the Secretary of the U.S. Department of Health and Human Services, the Centers for Disease Control and Prevention, the U.S. Department of Agriculture, the White House, and other elements of the executive branch.
- Represents the FDA on food-related matters in dealings with Congress.
- Represents the FDA on food-related matters in dealings with foreign governments and international organizations.
- Directs FDA efforts to build an integrated national food safety system in collaboration with other federal agencies and state and local governments.
- Directs a program of public outreach and communication on food safety, nutrition, and other food-related issues to advance the FDA's public health and consumer protection goals.

SOURCE: FDA, 2009d.

---

cumstances and expectations, scientific advances, and new evidence-based understanding of effective management practices. For example, since the mid-1990s, greater emphasis has been placed on preventive programs, such as HACCP, and on industry responsibility. In 1997, after a series of serious foodborne outbreaks, President Clinton announced a request for $43.2 million to fund a nationwide early-warning system for foodborne illness, increase seafood safety inspections, and to expand food safety research, training, and education. In addition, the Secretary of Agriculture, the Secretary of HHS, and the Administrator of the EPA were directed to identify specific steps to improve the safety of the nation's food supply (FDA/USDA/EPA/CDC, 1997).

Several initiatives, including science-based HACCP regulatory programs for seafood (FDA/HHS, 1995), meat and poultry (FSIS, 1996), and juice (FDA/HHS, 2001), reflected an effort not only to place greater emphasis on prevention, but also to be more flexible in the governance of food safety by allowing manufacturers to identify their own preventive controls. (For a more detailed description of the progression of food safety philosophies over the years, see Chapter 1 of the IOM/NRC report *Scientific Criteria to Ensure Safe Food* [IOM/NRC, 2003]).

Reported Funding Discrepancies Based on Volume of Foods

According to GAO, the FDA is responsible for approximately 80 percent of the nation's food supply, yet the federal funds the agency receives do not reflect this level of responsibility (GAO, 2004c).[10] Whereas more than 75 percent of consumer expenditures on food are for FDA-regulated products, roughly 60 percent of food safety funding is allocated to USDA (GAO, 2004c). The reason for this disparity lies partly in the federal laws governing food safety, which require USDA/FSIS (the agency with responsibility for meat, poultry, and egg products) to conduct daily inspections of meat and poultry processing plants and carcass-by-carcass inspections of slaughtered animals (GAO, 2004c).

Fragmented Nature of the Food Safety System

The 30 laws that govern food safety activities were enacted over time between 1906 (the 1906 Pure Food and Drugs Act) and today (e.g., HR3580, the Food and Drug Administration Amendments Act of 2007), and they are based on the issues that were faced in each time period—there has been no overall strategic design to the food safety system. For example,

---

[10] In 2009, the budgets for food safety were $649 million for the FDA and $1,092 million for USDA's Food Safety and Inspection Service (www.fda.gov; www.usda.gov).

the FDA was created (in its first incarnation as the Bureau of Chemistry under USDA) to prohibit adulterated and misbranded food and drugs in interstate commerce. The FDCA of 1938, which established the current FDA, was passed in response to the 1937 Elixir Sulfanilamide disaster.[11]

According to a recent GAO report, this situation results in "fragmentation and overlap," as well as the lack of a strategic design to protect the public health. According to GAO, "What authorities agencies have to enforce food safety regulations, which agency has jurisdiction to regulate what food products, and how frequently they inspect food facilities is determined by the legislation that governs each agency, or by administrative agreement between the two agencies, without strategic design as to how to best protect public health" (GAO, 2004c, p. 4).

Gaps in the System

Although there is overlap in the U.S. food safety system in some areas (e.g., inspection of certain establishments), past reviews have identified some gaps that could result in threats to food safety. These gaps are most obvious in two areas—imported foods and on-farm food safety—and relate to both intentional and unintentional threats. For example, GAO has expressed concern about the food safety system because both the FDA and USDA lack statutory authority to "regulate all aspects of security at food-processing facilities" (GAO, 2004c, p. 16).

Imported Foods

As discussed earlier, a significant portion of the nation's food supply—and more than 75 percent of its seafood—comes from abroad; however, the FDA inspects less than 2 percent of imported foods (GAO, 2004c; FDA Science Board, 2007). GAO also found that while USDA saves money and time by mandating U.S.-equivalent food safety standards for countries supplying imports, the ability of the FDA to do the same needs strengthening (GAO, 2004c). The Interagency Working Group on Import Safety's 2007 *Action Plan for Import Safety* requests additional, expanded, or strengthened authorities for the FDA to require preventive controls for certain foods, measures to prevent the intentional contamination of foods, and certification or other assurance that a product under its jurisdiction complies with agency requirements (Interagency Working Group on Import Safety, 2007). The report specifically cites the FDA as the lead for its recommendations or requests for new authorities more frequently—28 times—than is the case

---

[11] See http://www.fda.gov/AboutFDA/WhatWeDo/History/ProductRegulation/Sulfanilamide Disaster/default.htm (accessed October 8, 2010).

for any other agency (Interagency Working Group on Import Safety, 2007). A 2009 GAO report recognizes that some steps have been taken to ensure the safety of imported foods but also highlights gaps in enforcement and collaboration among U.S. Customs and Border Protection, the FDA, and FSIS (GAO, 2009b). Appendix E contains a detailed discussion of the FDA's imported food program.

On-Farm Food Safety Policies

On-farm regulation has received increased attention recently as a result of outbreaks involving pathogen-contaminated fresh produce. The FDA relies almost completely on voluntary guidance documents and initiatives (for example, the Produce Safety Initiative) for on-farm regulation (Becker, 2009). Occasionally it will inspect farms, but almost exclusively during periods of crisis (FDA Science Board, 2007). Although the FDA had requested authority to regulate shell eggs, such measures were postponed because of industry concerns (Becker, 2009); the Egg Safety Rule, which regulates the production of shell eggs on the farm, was published only recently (FDA/HHS, 2009). A further barrier to the FDA's on-farm efforts lies in the FDCA, in which farms are specifically exempted from requirements for record keeping (Consumers Union, 2008) and registration. Both exemptions hinder traceability, and ending these exemptions is a recurrent recommendation of GAO and other groups to help protect the public health (DeWaal, 2003; Consumers Union, 2008).

Lack of Mandatory Recall Authority

Also lacking is authority for the FDA to order mandatory food recalls—aside from infant formulas (USDA also lacks this authority [Brougher and Becker, 2008; GAO, 2008b]). The need for this authority is controversial because some argue that in the majority of cases, food companies voluntarily recall products suspected of being contaminated (Degnan, 2006), and that the FDA already has legal authority to seize adulterated and misbranded products and to administratively detain articles of food for which it "has credible evidence or information indicating that such article presents a threat of serious adverse health consequences or death."[12] In addition, the FDA routinely uses the embargo authority of the states to remove and hold products off market until federal seizure actions can be implemented. In support of mandatory authority, however, others observe that detention procedures must be carried out through the courts and therefore are not expeditious; meanwhile, the food supply and public health are endangered

---

[12] FDCA 304(h)(1).

(GAO, 2004b, 2008b). Moreover, when manufacturers or producers issue a recall, neither the FDA nor USDA has mechanisms for tracking the recall's effectiveness or accounting for the recalled products. Nor does either agency mandate timelines for recalls (GAO, 2004b). A 2004 GAO report found that, in some cases, the time it took for the agency to verify a recall was longer than the shelf life of the recalled products (GAO, 2004b). Accordingly, both consumer groups and GAO have recommended that the FDA and USDA be given mandatory recall authority (GAO, 2004b, 2008b; Consumers Union, 2008), and in the FDA's Food Protection Plan (FPP), the agency itself requests this authority (FDA, 2007; GAO, 2008b).

The FDA's Use of Resources

Groups such as the Alliance for a Stronger FDA,[13] Consumers Union, and the IOM have for years called for increased funding for the FDA (IOM/NRC, 1998; Consumers Union, 2008). Yet while the FDA's funding and staffing levels have not kept pace with its increased workload, the agency has opportunities to improve the management of its resources (GAO, 2008a). For example, GAO has identified some overlap in the activities of USDA and the FDA, including inspection and enforcement, training, research, and rulemaking. By simply enforcing interagency agreements, the FDA could "leverage inspection resources and possibly avoid duplication of effort" (GAO, 2005, p. 33). The same report suggests that the FDA and USDA consider a joint inspection training program. These examples illustrate the potential for savings and better use of limited resources (GAO, 2005, 2008a).

Inspection

In 2004 and 2005, GAO identified the three main deficiencies in the FDA's inspection program as (1) duplication of effort, (2) insufficient inspection, and (3) a poor basis for determining which facilities to inspect (GAO, 2004c, 2005). According to GAO, in 2003 USDA and FDA inspection and enforcement activities included overlapping inspections of 1,451 domestic food-processing facilities that produce multi-ingredient foods. This overlap occurs because of the differences in the statutory responsibilities of the two agencies.

Insufficient inspection takes many forms. Facilities can go as long as 10 years without an inspection, and the rate of inspection has declined by 78 percent in the past 35 years (FDA Science Board, 2007). GAO reported in 2004 that the FDA had roughly 1,900 full-time equivalents (FTEs) who

---

[13] See http://www.strengthenfda.org/members.htm (accessed October 8, 2010).

inspected an estimated 57,000 facilities. In comparison, USDA had 9,170 inspectors for "daily oversight of approximately 6,464 meat, poultry, and egg product plants" (GAO, 2004c, p. 10). Further, these 1,900 FTEs were also responsible for inspecting other FDA-regulated products. In fact, the FDA was unable to tell the committee specifically how many FTEs were dedicated to food inspections (Givens, 2009). Without a sufficient number of inspectors and inspections, the agency cannot ensure the safety of the food supply (FDA Science Board, 2007). To illustrate the problem, the Peanut Corporation of America facility, at the root of a 2009 salmonella outbreak that sickened 700 people and contributed to 9 deaths, had last been inspected by the FDA in 2001, 8 years before the outbreak. Intermittent inspections had been conducted by the state of Georgia, but significant problems had not been detected, leading the recently appointed Advisor to the FDA Commissioner on Food to say during the outbreak that it was an example of "a basic breakdown" and to call for the agency to raise its standards (Schmidt, 2009).

Prior reports have expressed concern about insufficient inspection with respect to certain kinds of commodities—fresh produce and imported products—and certain kinds of facilities, such as farms (see On-Farm Food Safety Policies). When the FDA conducts fresh produce inspections—which declined in number to just 478 in FY 2007—it tests primarily for pesticide rather than microbial contamination (GAO, 2008c).

The 1998 IOM/NRC report *Ensuring Safe Food* notes that, although there is a computer system to track FDA- and USDA-regulated imported products and their inspection, "there is no way to determine whether the agencies are focusing their attention on the most important health risks" (IOM/NRC, 1998, p. 89). The FDA lacks control over detained imported shipments and does not punish those who violate the rules. Seafood is inspected minimally, although, as noted earlier, 75 percent of seafood consumed in the United States is imported, and shellfish alone is reported to have caused 21 percent of all foodborne illness from 1978 to 1992 (IOM/NRC, 1998; GAO, 2004c). This situation reflects an inherent flaw in FDA inspections: they are not risk-based in frequency or in facilities targeted (GAO, 2004c). Federal regulation, not risk, determines which facilities are inspected by which agency. For example, according to GAO, the frequency of inspection of a facility that produces ham and cheese sandwiches depends on the percentage of meat used rather than on risk (GAO, 2004c). The law, in this case, inhibits science-based decisions in food safety programs (IOM/NRC, 1998).

Research

Without an adequate research program, there is insufficient information with which to make science-based decisions (IOM/NRC, 1998). Indeed, a thorough scientific understanding of threats to the food supply would likely be more cost-effective for the FDA in the long term than simply adding more inspectors.

In 2007, the FDA Science Board completed a general review of the agency's research programs. The review concluded that these programs were in urgent need of enhancement. The Science Board's report stated that basic research programs and risk assessments would determine pressing risks to the food supply so that the agency's limited funds could be used for targeted research to address those risks (FDA Science Board, 2007). The agency maintains several research centers at academic institutions, but these, too, are poorly funded. When the Science Board examined CFSAN's critical research priorities, such as detection of foodborne viruses, many were found to be on target, but the agency does not always maintain staff with scientific expertise in those areas. It was suggested that some of these priorities could be shared with USDA (FDA Science Board, 2007). The FDA also lacks plans for critical research in other areas, such as produce safety (GAO, 2008c).

In 2007, a new center was formed to conduct research and serve as a source of scientific information to enhance food safety and defense. The Western Institute for Food Safety and Security is a program at the University of California, Davis, partnering with the California Department of Food and Agriculture, the California Department of Public Health, the FDA, and USDA. See Chapter 6 for further discussion of the FDA's research centers and their funding.

With limited funds and inadequate staff, the FDA relies on USDA to meet some of its research needs (FDA Science Board, 2007). Much of the data the FDA needs is expensive to acquire, however, and other agencies are not willing to make the investment (FDA Science Board, 2007). Data the FDA itself collects are not available to every researcher within the agency, and data obtained by other agencies often are not made available to the FDA (FDA Science Board, 2007; GAO, 2009a).

A review of CFSAN and CVM research programs was recently initiated by subcommittees of the FDA Science Board. As of this writing, only the CVM review had been completed. The report from that review highlights that since the 2007 review (FDA Science Board, 2009), CVM has made much progress in the research function, but the report also points to areas of weakness, such as regulatory science and the external consultative process for research planning.

Information Technology Infrastructure

Related to the above problems is the lack of an adequate IT infrastructure both within the FDA and between the FDA and related agencies responsible for food safety (see Chapter 5) (FDA Science Board, 2007). Although the FDA has made progress in addressing this deficiency by hiring new staff, forming internal IT governance boards, developing strong partnerships with other agencies, and updating management systems, in 2007 the Science Board found that the FDA's IT infrastructure could not support the agency's public health mission (FDA Science Board, 2007). Specific problems mentioned include (1) the quality of data, which are not standardized; (2) the integration of IT systems within centers; (3) inconsistent data collection across different centers and even within discrete agency program areas (GAO, 2009a); (4) antiquated hardware lacking security measures (FDA Science Board, 2007; GAO, 2009a); and (5) delays in sharing data (FDA Science Board, 2007). A 2008 report describing the FDA's plan to revitalize ORA proposes ways to deal with many of these IT issues. GAO supports such efforts but concludes that without initiating a strategic plan as is required by federal law, the agency may not be effective in carrying them out (Glavin, 2008; GAO, 2009a).

An example of how IT problems contribute to inefficiency is the significant duplication of effort among the agencies responsible for ensuring safe food discussed above. GAO has found that one reason this duplication occurs is that the agencies "do not have adequate mechanisms to track interagency food safety agreements" (GAO, 2005). An IT system should facilitate the FDA's public health mission by allowing data flow and being responsive to scientific innovation, but the agency's system does not meet these requirements (GAO, 2009a).

Lack of a Research and IT Strategic Plan

One key problem at the FDA has been the lack of an overarching strategic plan for research addressing the agency's food safety mission. Development of a new strategic plan is said to be under way (Musser, 2009). The FDA's efforts to enhance and modernize its programs are uncoordinated and inefficient and may lead to little or ineffectual improvement (GAO, 2009a). Without a clearly delineated mission statement, goals, and performance metrics, the agency cannot align itself with a direction, measure how well it fulfills its responsibilities, or determine the effectiveness of its programs (FDA Science Board, 2007; GAO, 2009a). The FDA needs to define its mission to meet its regulatory obligations and build its research, inspection, IT, and other programs to fulfill that mission. The Science Board report acknowledges both the lack of resources available to the FDA and the current initiatives to improve its programs, but it finds that without clear goals, the agency cannot know, for example, what expertise is needed as it recruits new staff, what laboratory capabilities are needed, or how to organize data in an efficient and productive way (FDA Science Board, 2007).

LOOKING FORWARD

The nation is undergoing many changes related not only to technology advances, but also to changes in the way business is conducted and the way its citizens interact with the rest of the world. Although ensuring food safety is the responsibility of everyone, the public will continue to view regulatory agencies as the ultimate repository of salient scientific knowledge, reliable advisors, and overseers of food safety activities in the private sector. The flaws in the existing food safety system have been well investigated, and recent changes in the approach to food safety offer cause for hope that the nation is ready to take the steps necessary to create an efficient and effective food safety system. The first signs of progress at the FDA were seen in the development and early stages of implementation of the FPP, a document that outlines basic principles of prevention, intervention, and response for food safety and defense of domestic and imported products (FDA, 2007). However, a 2008 GAO report states that, while the FPP proposes some positive first steps to enhance oversight of food safety, the plan lacks specific information about strategies and resources needed for its implementation (GAO, 2008b).

With a new FDA commissioner in place and the creation of the White House FSWG and the Office of Foods, many further positive changes are anticipated, and some of them are already well under way. In the following chapters, the committee encourages the FDA to continue with its recent initiatives and plans and to delineate a course of action that will enable it to become more efficient at carrying out its food safety responsibilities.

REFERENCES

Abbot, J. M., C. Byrd-Bredbenner, D. Schaffner, C. M. Bruhn, and L. Blalock. 2009. Comparison of food safety cognitions and self-reported food-handling behaviors with observed food safety behaviors of young adults. *European Journal of Clinical Nutrition* 63:572–579.

AMS/USDA (Agricultural Marketing Service/U.S. Department of Agriculture). 2009. *About AMS*. http://www.ams.usda.gov/AMSv1.0/ams.fetchTemplateData.do?template=TemplateD &navID=AboutAMS&topNav=AboutAMS&page=AboutAMS&acct=AMSPW (accessed May 13, 2010).

Anderson, J. B., T. A. Shuster, K. E. Hansen, A. S. Levy, and A. Volk. 2004. A camera's view of consumer food-handling behaviors. *Journal of the American Dietetic Association* 104(2):186–191.

APHIS/USDA (Animal and Plant Health Inspection Service/U.S. Department of Agriculture). 2010. *Animal Product Manual* (Second Edition). Washington, DC: APHIS/USDA. http://www.aphis.usda.gov/import_export/plants/manuals/ports/downloads/apm.pdf (accessed March 30, 2010).

Becker, G. S. 2009. *Food Safety on the Farm: Federal Programs and Selected Proposals.* Washington, DC: Congressional Research Service.

Becker, G. S., and D. V. Porter. 2007. *The Federal Food Safety System: A Primer.* Washington, DC: Congressional Research Service.

Boisen, C. S. 2007. Title III of the Bioterrorism Act: Sacrificing U.S. trade relations in the name of food security. *American University Law Review* 56(3):667–718.

Brougher, C., and G. S. Becker. 2008. *CRS Report for Congress: The USDA's Authority to Recall Meat and Poultry Products.* Washington, DC: Congressional Research Service.

Carnevale, C. 2009. *FDA and Import Food Safety: A Briefing Paper.* Paper presented at Institute of Medicine/National Research Council Committee on Review of the FDA's Role in Ensuring Safe Food Meeting, Washington, DC, October 15, 2009.

CDC (U.S. Centers for Disease Control and Prevention). 2009. Preliminary FoodNet data on the incidence of infection with pathogens commonly transmitted through food—10 states, 2008. *Morbidity and Mortality Weekly Report* 58(13):333–337.

CDC. 2010. Preliminary FoodNet Data on the incidence of infection with pathogens transmitted commonly through food—10 states, 2009. *Morbidity and Mortality Weekly Report* 59(14):418–422.

Consumers Union. 2008. *Increased Inspections Needed for Produce, Processing Plants to Protect Consumers from Unsafe Food.* http://www.consumersunion.org/pub/core_food_safety/005732.html (accessed January 28, 2010).

Degnan, F. H. 2006. *FDA's Creative Application of the Law: Not Merely a Collection of Words* (Second Edition). Washington, DC: Food and Drug Law Institute.

DeWaal, C. S. 2003. Safe food from a consumer perspective. *Food Control* 14(2):75–79.

DeWaal, C. S. 2009. *Zero Tolerance: Pros and Cons.* Paper Presented at the International Association for Food Protection 96th Annual Meeting, Grapevine, TX, July 15, 2009.

DeWaal, C. S., and D. Plunkett. 2007. *Building a Modern Food Safety System: For FDA Regulated Foods, CSPI White Paper.* Washington, DC: Center for Science in the Public Interest.

DHS (U.S. Department of Homeland Security). 2004. *Fact Sheet: Strengthening the Security of Our Nation's Food Supply.* http://www.dhs.gov/xnews/releases/press_release_0453.shtm (accessed March 25, 2010).

ERS (Economic Research Service). 2010. *Food CPI and Expenditures.* http://www.ers.usda.gov/Briefing/CPIFoodAndExpenditures/ (accessed January 28, 2010.

FAO (Food and Agriculture Organization of the United Nations). 2008. *Climate Change: Implications for Food Safety.* Rome, Italy: FAO. ftp://ftp.fao.org/docrep/fao/010/i0195e/i0195e00.pdf (accessed January 28, 2010).

FDA (U.S. Food and Drug Administration). 2007. *Food Protection Plan: An Integrated Strategy for Protecting the Nation's Food Supply.* Rockville, MD: FDA.

FDA. 2009a. *About FDA: What We Do.* http://www.fda.gov/AboutFDA/WhatWeDo/default.htm (accessed December 10, 2009).

FDA. 2009b. *FDA Beyond Our Borders.* http://www.fda.gov/ForConsumers/ConsumerUpdates/ucm103036.htm (accessed January 29, 2010).

FDA. 2009c. FDA. 2009. *FDA Staff Manual Guides, Organizations and Functions Volume I (1000–1300).* Rockville, MD: FDA. http://www.fda.gov/AboutFDA/ReportsManualsForms/StaffManualGuides/ucm136374.htm (accessed January 29, 2010).

FDA. 2009d. Office of the Commissioner reorganization; statement of organizations, functions, and delegations of authority: Action notice. *Federal Register* 74(158):41713–41734.

FDA. 2010a. *Food and Drug Administration FY 2011 Congressional Budget Request: Narrative by Activity—Foods Program FY2011*. http://www.fda.gov/downloads/AboutFDA/ReportsManualsForms/Reports/BudgetReports/UCM205367.pdf (accessed June 2, 2010).

FDA. 2010b. *About the FDA Organization Charts*. http://www.fda.gov/downloads/AboutFDA/CentersOffices/OrganizationCharts/UCM198460.pdf (accessed March 26, 2010).

FDA. 2010c. *Department of Health and Human Services Food and Drug Administration (FDA) Organization Charts Overview*. Rockville, MD: FDA. http://www.fda.gov/downloads/AboutFDA/CentersOffices/OrganizationCharts/UCM198460.pdf (accessed January 29, 2010).

FDA Science Board. 2007. *FDA Science and Mission at Risk. Report of the Subcommittee on Science and Technology*. Rockville, MD: FDA.

FDA Science Board. 2009. *Research Planning, Program and Facilities of the Center for Veterinary Medicine*. Report to the FDA Science Board. http://www.fda.gov/AdvisoryCommittees/CommitteesMeetingMaterials/ScienceBoardtotheFoodandDrugAdministration/ucm176816.htm (accessed March 22, 2010).

FDA/HHS (U.S. Department of Health and Human Services). 1995. Procedures for the safe and sanitary processing and importing of fish and fishery products. Final rule. *Federal Register* 60(242):65095.

FDA/HHS. 2001. Hazard Analysis and Critical Control Point (HAACP); Procedures for the safe and sanitary processing and importing of juice. Final rule, January 19, 2001. *Federal Register* 66(13):6137.

FDA/HHS. 2009. Prevention of salmonella enteritidis in shell eggs during production, storage, and transportation. Final rule. *Federal Register* 74(130):33030.

FDA/USDA/EPA/CDC (U.S. Department of Agriculture/U.S. Environmental Protection Agency/U.S. Centers for Disease Control and Prevention). 1997. *Food Safety from Farm to Table: A National Food Safety Initiative*. Report to the President. Washington, DC: FDA/USDA/EPC/CDC.

Florida Department of Agriculture and Consumer Services. 2007. *Tomato Best Practices Manual: DACS Tomato Best Practices Manual*. Tallahassee: Florida Department of Agriculture and Consumer Services. http://www.doacs.state.fl.us/fs/TomatoBestPractices.pdf (accessed March 30, 2010).

FoodSafety.gov. 2010. *Inspections and Compliance*. http://www.foodsafety.gov/compliance/index.html (accessed March 25, 2010).

Fraser, L. M. 2009. *FDA's Regulatory Authority and Division of Responsibility for Food Safety*. Paper presented at Institute of Medicine/National Research Council Committee on Review of the FDA's Role in Ensuring Safe Food Meeting, Washington, DC, March 24, 2009.

FSIS (Food Safety and Inspection Service). 1996. *The Final Rule on Pathogen Reduction and Hazard Analysis and Critical Control Point (HACCP) Systems*. Washington, DC: FSIS. http://www.fsis.usda.gov/OA/background/finalrul.htm (accessed January 29, 2010).

FSIS. 2002. *Changes in Consumer Knowledge, Behavior, and Confidence Since the 1996 PR/HACCP. Final Rule*. Pr/HACCP Rule Evaluation Report. www.fsis.usda.gov/oa/research/HACCPImpacts.pdf (accessed May 12, 2010).

FSLC (Food Safety Leadership Council). 2007. *On-Farm Produce Standards*. http://www.perishablepundit.com/DailyPundit/PunditImages/FSLC-On-FarmStandards-11-2007.pdf (accessed January 28, 2010).

GAO (U.S. Government Accountability Office). 1992. *Food Safety and Quality: Uniform, Risk-Based Inspection System Needed to Ensure Safe Food Supply*. Washington, DC: GAO.

GAO. 2004a. *Food Safety: FDA's Imported Seafood Safety Program Shows Some Progress, but Further Improvements Are Needed*. Washington, DC: GAO.

GAO. 2004b. *Food Safety: USDA and FDA Need to Better Ensure Prompt and Complete Recalls of Potentially Unsafe Food.* Washington, DC: GAO.

GAO. 2004c. *Federal Food Safety and Security System: Fundamental Restructuring Is Needed to Address Fragmentation and Overlap.* Washington, DC: GAO.

GAO. 2005. *Oversight of Food Safety Activities: Federal Agencies Should Pursue Opportunities to Reduce Overlap and Better Leverage Resources.* Washington, DC: GAO.

GAO. 2008a. *Federal Oversight of Food Safety: FDA has Provided Few Details on the Resources and Strategies Needed to Implement Its Food Protection Plan.* Washington, DC: GAO.

GAO. 2008b. *Federal Oversight of Food Safety: FDA's Food Protection Plan Proposes Positive First Steps, but Capacity to Carry Them Out Is Critical.* Washington, DC: GAO.

GAO. 2008c. *Food Safety: Improvements Needed in FDA Oversight of Fresh Produce.* Washington, DC: GAO.

GAO. 2009a. *Information Technology: FDA Needs to Establish Key Plans and Processes for Guiding Systems Modernization Efforts.* Washington, DC: GAO.

GAO. 2009b. *Agencies Need to Address Gaps in Enforcement and Collaboration to Enhance Safety of Imported Food.* Washington, DC: GAO.

GFSI (Global Food Safety Initiative). 2007. *The Global Food Safety Initiative: GFSI Guidance Document* (5th Edition). Paris, France: GFSI. http://www.ciesnet.com/pfiles/programmes/foodsafety/GFSI_Guidance_Document_5th%20Edition%20_September%202007.pdf (accessed January 28, 2010).

Givens, J. M. 2009. *Review of FDA's Role in Ensuring Safe Food (FDA's Approach to Risk Based Inspections—A Field Perspective).* Paper presented at Institute of Medicine/National Research Council Committee on Review of the FDA's Role in Ensuring Safe Food Meeting, Washington, DC, March 24, 2009.

Glavin, M. 2008. *Revitalizing ORA: Protecting the Public Health Together in a Changing World—A Report to the Commissioner.* Rockville, MD: FDA.

GPO (Government Printing Office). 2010. *Search Databases "House Hearings (Calendar Year 2007/2008); Senate Hearings (Calendar Year 2007/2008)" + "Food Safety."* http://frwebgate.access.gpo.gov/cgi-bin/multidb.cgi (accessed January 28, 2010).

Gregory, P. J., J. S. I. Ingram, and M. Brklacich. 2005. Climate change and food security. *Philosophical Transactions of the Royal Society B: Biological Sciences* 360(1463):2139–2148.

Hamburg, M. A., and J. M. Sharfstein. 2009. The FDA as a public health agency. *New England Journal of Medicine* 360:2493–2495.

Hart Research Associates/Public Opinion Strategies. 2009. *Americans' Attitudes on Food Safety.* Washington, DC: Hart Research Associates and Public Opinion Strategies.

Henao, O., E. Scallan, J. Choùdhuri, J. Nelson, D. Norton, K. Edge, P. Ryan, M. Tobin-D'angelo, S. Hanna, T. Jones, F. Angulo, and the EIP FoodNet Working Group. 2005. *Proportion of Visits to Health Care Providers Resulting in Request of Stool Samples: Data from the National Ambulatory Medical Care Survey (NAMCS) and the Foodborne Diseases Active Surveillance Network (FoodNet) Population Survey.* http://www.cdc.gov/enterics/publications/118-IDSA2005_Henao.pdf (accessed March 9, 2010).

Hennessy, D. A., J. Roosen, and H. H. Jensen. 2003. Systemic failure in the provision of safe food. *Food Policy* 28(1):77–96.

Henson, S., and J. Humphrey. 2009. *The Impacts of Private Food Safety Standards on Food Chain and on Public Standard-Setting Processes.* Paper presented at Report to the Codex Alimentarius Commission, 32nd Session, June 29–July 4, 2009.

HHS (U.S. Department of Health and Human Services). 2008. *FY 2009 President's Budget for HHS.* http://www.hhs.gov/asrt/ob/docbudget/budgetfy09.html (accessed March 25, 2010).

HHS. 2009. *FY 2010 President's Budget for HHS.* http://www.hhs.gov/asrt/ob/docbudget/budgetfy10.html (accessed March 25, 2010).

HHS. 2010. *FY 2011 President's Budget for HHS.* http://www.hhs.gov/asrt/ob/docbudget/index.html (accessed March 25, 2010).

Howells, A. D., K. R. Roberts, C. W. Shanklin, V. K. Pilling, L. A. Brannon, and B. B. Barrett. 2008. Restaurant employees' perceptions of barriers to three food safety practices. *Journal of the American Dietetic Association* 108(8):1345–1349.

IFICF (International Food Information Council Foundation). 2009. *2009 Food & Health Survey.* Washington, DC: IFICF. http://www.foodinsight.org/Resources/Detail.aspx?topic=2009_Food_Health_Survey_Consumer_Attitudes_toward_Food_Nutrition_and_Health (accessed May 24, 2010).

Interagency Working Group on Import Safety. 2007. *Action Plan for Import Safety. A Roadmap for Continual Improvement.* http://www.importsafety.gov/report/actionplan.pdf (accessed March 25, 2010).

IOM (Institute of Medicine). 2007. *Seafood Choices: Balancing Benefits and Risks.* Washington, DC: The National Academies Press.

IOM/NRC (Institute of Medicine/National Research Council). 1998. *Ensuring Safe Food: From Production to Consumption.* Washington, DC: National Academy Press.

IOM/NRC. 2003. *Scientific Criteria to Ensure Safe Food.* Washington, DC: The National Academies Press.

Johnson, J. A., D. V. Porter, S. Thaul, and E. D. Williams. 2008. *The Food and Drug Administration: Budget and Statutory History, FY1980–FY2007.* Washington, DC: Congressional Research Service.

Kosal, M. E., and D. E. Anderson. 2004. An unaddressed issue of agricultural terrorism: A case study on feed security. *Journal of Animal Science* 82 (11):3394–3400.

LGMA (California Leafy Green Products Handler Marketing Agreement). 2010. *About LGMA.* http://www.caleafygreens.ca.gov/ (accessed January 28, 2010).

Lin, B-H. 2004. *Fruit and Vegetable Consumption: Looking Ahead to 2020. USDA/ERS.* http://www.ers.usda.gov/publications/aib792/aib792-7/ (accessed January 28, 2010).

Lugard, M., and M. Smart. 2006. The role of science in international trade law. *Regulatory Toxicology and Pharmacology* 44(1):69–74.

Mathiasen, L. A., B. J. Chapman, B. J. Lacroix, and D.A. Powell. 2004. Spot the mistake: Television cooking shows as a source of food safety information. *Food Protection Trends* 24(5):328–334.

Medeiros, L. C., V. N. Hillers, G. Chen, V. Bergmann, P. Kendall, and M. Schroeder. 2004. Design and development of food safety knowledge and attitude scales for consumer food safety education. *Journal of the American Dietetic Association* 104(11):1671–1677.

Musser, S. 2009. *Food Safety Research at FDA.* Paper presented at Institute of Medicine/National Research Council Committee on Review of the FDA's Role in Ensuring Safe Food Meeting, Washington, DC, March 24, 2009.

NCTR (National Center for Toxicological Research). 2009. *NCTR Strategic Plan: 2009–2013.* Jefferson, AK: NCTR.

Nucci, M. L., J. E. Dellava, C. L. Cuite, and W. K. Hallman. 2008. *The US Food Import System: Issues, Processes, and Proposals.* New Brunswick: New Jersey Agricultural Experiment Station, Rutgers, the State University of New Jersey.

OMB (Office of Management and Budget). 2008. *Assessing Program Performance.* http://www.whitehouse.gov/omb/rewrite/part/index.html (accessed January 29, 2010).

Patil, S. R., S. Cates, and R. Morales. 2005. Consumer food safety knowledge, practices, and demographic differences: Findings from a meta-analysis. *Journal of Food Protection* 68(9):1884–1894.

Pilling, V. K., L. A. Brannon, C. W. Shanklin, A. D. Howells, and K. R. Roberts. 2008. Identifying specific beliefs to target to improve restaurant employees' intentions for performing three important food safety behaviors. *Journal of the American Dietetic Association* 108(6):991–997.

Produce Safety Project. 2008. *Breakdown: Lessons to Be Learned from the 2008 Salmonella Saintpaul Outbreak.* http://www.producesafetyproject.org (accessed January 28, 2010).

Redmond, E. C., and C. J. Griffith. 2003. Consumer food handling in the home: A review of food safety studies. *Journal of Food Protection* 66:130–161.

Schmidt, J. 2009. Broken links in food-safety chain hid peanut plants' risks. *USA Today,* April 28, 2009. http://www.usatoday.com/money/industries/food/2009-04-26-peanuts-salmonella-food-safety_N.htm (accessed January 29, 2010).

Stern, N. 2007. *The Economics of Climate Change: The Stern Review.* Cambridge, UK: Cambridge University Press.

Suydam, L. 1996. *Congressional Testimony Before the House Committee on Government Reform and Oversight, Subcommittee on Human Resources and Intergovernmental Relations, June 22, 1996.* http://www.hhs.gov/asl/testify/t960622a.html (accessed March 30, 2010).

Todd, E. C. D., J. D. Greig, C. A. Bartleson, and B. S. Michaels. 2007. Outbreaks where food workers have been implicated in the spread of foodborne disease. Part 3. Factors contributing to outbreaks and description of outbreak categories. *Journal of Food Protection* 70:2199–2217.

USDA (U.S. Department of Agriculture). 2010a. *FSIS National Residue Program for Cattle.* http://www.usda.gov/oig/webdocs/24601-08-KC.pdf (accessed on May 12, 2010).

USDA. 2010b. *Laws and Regulations.* http://www.usda.gov/wps/portal/!ut/p/_s.7_0_A/7_0_1OB?navtype=SU&navid=LAWS_REGS (accessed March 25, 2010).

Wong, S., R. Marcus, M. Hawkins, S. Shallow, K. G. McCombs, E. Swanson, B. Anderson, B. Shiferaw, R. Garman, K. Noonan, and T. Van Gilder. 2004. Physicians as food-safety educators: A practices and perceptions survey. *Clinical Infectious Diseases* 38(Suppl. 3):S212–S218.

Part II

Toward a Stronger and
More Effective Food Safety System

3

Adopting a Risk-Based Decision-Making Approach to Food Safety

As described in Chapter 2, the responsibilities of the U.S. Food and Drug Administration's (FDA's) new Office of Foods include providing executive leadership and management to all FDA food-related programs; directing the development of integrated strategies, plans, policies, and budgets to build the FDA's food-related scientific and regulatory capacities and programs, including the recruitment and training of key personnel and the development of information systems (FDA, 2009); and exercising direct line authority over the Center for Food Safety and Applied Nutrition (CFSAN) and the Center for Veterinary Medicine (CVM). Its responsibilities include both short-term decision making in direct response to a food crisis and longer-term initiatives focused on sustained, continued improvement in food safety and public health. The former responsibility requires rapid decision making in cooperation with multiple regulatory partners, while the latter requires long-term strategic planning aimed at proactive activities that are based on data and risk-based prediction and prioritization. For example, the FDA's responsibility during a foodborne illness outbreak would focus on identification of the source of contamination (product trace-back), initiation of regulatory action, and product recall. More proactive activities might involve conducting research to address crucial unknowns, undertaking formalized quantitative risk assessment, identifying candidate mitigation strategies to prevent repeat incidents, and ensuring the implementation of those strategies. Critical to both long- and short-term initiatives are improvements in cooperation with partners (see Chapters 4 and 7); efficient data collection, sharing, and analysis (Chapter 5); and communication with the public (Chapter 9).

Clearly, short- and long-term responsibilities coexist as the FDA seeks to both manage and prevent foodborne illness. As noted earlier, the FDA has often been criticized as responding reactively to food problems. Sometimes, this type of action is necessary; the FDA has no choice but to react when a problem manifests itself. However, greater proactive efforts by the FDA would enhance food safety. This chapter presents a conceptual approach for the prioritization of activities and allocation of resources to support both short- and long-term FDA responsibilities for food safety. Accordingly, the chapter lays out the foundation for a proactive, risk-based food safety system. Succeeding chapters describe elements of such a system that are dependent on the success of the approach presented here. For instance, application of a risk-based approach at all levels of regulation is a prerequisite for harmonization of federal, state, and local food safety programs (Chapter 7). Similarly, effective cooperation and communication with diverse stakeholders will require that all levels of the FDA embrace a proactive, risk-based approach to food safety management and facilitate its implementation (Chapter 9).

The committee did not conduct a comprehensive review of the details of all the risk-based activities of the FDA, such as the models utilized or factors considered in making individual decisions. The committee was provided with general information with regard to the FDA's risk-based activities and describes its understanding of those activities in this chapter. In this discussion, the committee uses concrete examples of those activities and identifies gaps with respect to the extent to which they adhere to the attributes and steps of the recommended approach. Although the committee concluded that those activities would have been enhanced by the use of a more extensive risk-based approach, in this and subsequent chapters the committee also recognizes that the FDA will face challenges in this regard. The committee identified challenges and courses of action to overcome them, for example, in hiring the appropriate personnel and coordinating data collection and sharing (Chapter 5), reorganizing the agency's food safety research portfolio (Chapter 6), integrating FDA programs with those of state and local governments (Chapter 7), carrying out risk communication and education (Chapter 9), and addressing organizational problems (Chapter 11).

There is consensus that food safety programs and any approach to food safety reform must be both science- and risk-based. This view was first articulated in the 1998 Institute of Medicine (IOM)/National Research Council (NRC) report *Ensuring Safe Food: From Production to Consumption* (IOM/NRC, 1998) and is also addressed by other reports of the IOM/NRC (IOM/NRC, 2003), the U.S. Government Accountability Office (GAO) (GAO, 2004a,b,c, 2005, 2007, 2008, 2009a,b), consumer groups (Consumers Union, 2008; Tucker-Foreman, 2009), and Congress (Becker,

2008, 2009; Brougher and Becker, 2008). These reports have emphasized the importance of using the best available science to understand foodborne illness, including the identification of causative agents (chemicals, toxins, and microbes) and transmission pathways and the development of appropriate surveillance systems. As the science base has developed, attention over the last decade has increasingly turned to its application within a risk-based framework, with the ultimate goal of improving public health. The term "risk-based" implies the existence of an underlying science base; however, it goes a step beyond to encompass use of the tools of risk and decision analysis to create systems that optimize the ability to prevent and control foodborne illness and improve public health. This chapter focuses on how this type of risk-based system might be constructed and implemented to enable the FDA to deal more effectively with food safety problems.

Ensuring Safe Food provides a rough description of the components necessary for the implementation of a risk-based system:

> . . . [It] require[s] identification of the greatest public health needs through surveillance and risk analysis. The state of knowledge and technology defines what is achievable through the application of current science. Public resources can have the greatest favorable effect on public health if they are allocated in accordance with the combined analysis of risk assessment and technical feasibility. . . . Thus, both the relative risks and benefits must be considered in allocating resources. (IOM/NRC, 1998, p. 93)

Other documents have furthered the concept of risk-based food safety management. For example, a 2002 discussion paper issued by Resources for the Future[1] states:

> If the primary objective of the food safety system is to reduce the burden of disease, success requires risk-based resource allocation. The food safety system must make the best possible use of its resources to reduce the disease burden. This means focusing government effort on the greatest risks and the greatest opportunities to reduce risk, wherever they may arise. It means adopting the interventions—presumably some combination of research, regulation, and education that will yield the greatest reduction in illness. (Taylor, 2002, p. 7)

These previous documents go beyond the scope of traditional technical risk assessment by introducing such terms as "risk-based resource allocation" and "relative risk and benefit." In its deliberations, the committee recognized the need to address risk analysis in the broader context of regu-

---

[1] See http://www.rff.org/rff/Documents/RFF-IB-02-02.pdf (accessed January 25, 2010).

latory decision-making processes and risk governance (see, for example, IRGC, 2005, 2009) to manage food safety.

The challenges and best practices for integrating science to support effective risk management decisions are widely recognized, as summarized by a recent NRC study (NRC, 2009a):

> The most effective decision support efforts are organized around six principles: begin with users' needs; give priority to processes over products; link information producers and users; build connections across disciplines and organizations; seek institutional stability; and design processes for learning. Following these principles improves the likelihood of achieving the three main objectives of decision support: increased usefulness of information, improved relationships between knowledge producers and users, and better decisions. (NRC, 2009a, p. 67)

In short, in a society with limited resources, decisions about allocation need to be made in a consistent manner and with the goal of maximizing benefits and reducing risks while considering associated costs. In the area of food safety, a process is needed for allocating resources based on public health data and information. Risk managers must consider a wide variety of factors in their decision-making process, including the needs and values of a diverse set of stakeholders, which may diverge even with respect to public health. These factors might include economic considerations, the controllability of risk, and the population affected. The committee recognizes that such multidimensional comparisons are a highly challenging endeavor. However, the lack of such a systematic approach to risk-based decision making causes problems, from a decrease in public trust to unintended consequences in the marketplace, the environment, and society. In addition, the lack of such an approach may make a regulatory agency more vulnerable to political influences. The need to formally acknowledge the complexity of such decision making and then establish a transparent and systematic way to carry out the decision-making process is the subject of the next section. In addition, in Chapter 4, the committee elaborates further on the issue of how to select interventions. It should be noted that, while the committee concluded that providing the FDA with a stepwise process as a tool for making decisions is appropriate, the development of the FDA's philosophy, including specific criteria and their weight, is a management decision beyond scope of this study. Thus in Chapter 4 (recommendation 4-2), the committees recommends that the FDA develop its philosophical approach by defining a strategy that delineates factors to consider (e.g., economic factors, public perception, environmental factors) and their weight.

A RISK-BASED APPROACH TO FOOD SAFETY MANAGEMENT

Definitions

Many groups have defined risk and risk characterization. For example, the World Health Organization's (WHO's) International Program on Chemical Safety defines risk as "the probability of an adverse effect in an organism, system, or (sub)population caused under specified circumstances by exposure to an agent" (IPCS, 2004). Others have expanded this definition to include the fact that this probability can be expressed quantitatively or qualitatively and that risk characterization includes a discussion of the significant scientific uncertainties in this information. Further, the committee agreed upon the following working definition for a risk-based approach: "a systematic means by which to facilitate decision making to reduce public health risk in light of limited resources and additional factors that may be considered." The committee identified the following as key attributes of a risk-based food safety system: (1) is proactive based on a strategic management plan; (2) is data driven; (3) is grounded in the principles of risk analysis; (4) employs analytical methods to rank risks based on public health impact; (5) incorporates deliberation with key food safety stakeholders; (6) considers factors such as consumer perception, public acceptance, market impacts, and environmental impacts in decision making when appropriate; (7) employs analytical methods to prioritize the allocation of limited resources to manage risk most effectively; (8) employs measures to evaluate the efficacy of the risk management program on a continuous basis; and (9) performs all of these functions in a systematic and transparent manner with the involvement of stakeholders. These attributes are further described in Box 3-1.

A Conceptual Approach to Risk-Based Food Safety Management

The risk-based system envisioned by the committee will entail analysis and prioritization at several distinct levels:

- the formulation of a strategic plan that identifies outcomes/goals of the risk-based system,
- broad-based risk ranking to identify the most important risks based exclusively on public health considerations,
- the identification of additional data/information needs upon which prioritization of resources may be based,
- the choice of intervention strategies and allocation of regulatory resources, and
- the evaluation of outcomes.

BOX 3-1
Attributes of a Risk-Based Food Safety System

A risk-based system is proactive and based on a strategic management plan. Notwithstanding the need to respond to unforeseeable crises, risk activities should be planned in advance, an exercise that should include various stakeholders and be based on the knowledge gained from past experience with a vision of predicting food contamination problems. Managing a crisis in the short term and implementing a well-developed strategic plan for managing food safety in the long term are equally important; attention to unanticipated outbreaks should not detract from implementation of the strategic plan.

A risk-based system is data driven. Although expert opinion is a valuable asset when there are uncertainties or data must be interpreted, a risk-based system should be grounded in science. That is, the collection, analysis, and interpretation of quality data, as well as data management, are essential tasks for the implementation of a risk-based system.

A risk-based system is grounded in the principles of risk analysis. A risk-based system should be grounded in risk analysis, with risk assessment, risk communication, and risk management as the essential basis for establishing a sound public health protection capability. If implemented appropriately, the system ideally provides a transparent, data-driven means by which to determine the extent of public health protection achieved as a result of different risk management actions, and therefore it provides a decision-making tool. This concept has worldwide support and has been applied for several decades by regulatory and public health agencies.

A risk-based system employs analytical methods to rank risks based on public health impact. A risk-based system systematically ranks risks even if those risks differ in complexity and uncertainty. The development of analytical methods (models) that can assign numerical values to the various risks based on public health impact is the foundation of this activity.

A risk-based system employs analytical methods to prioritize the allocation of limited resources to manage risk most effectively. The evaluation of intervention strategies is an essential element of risk management. Risk managers must consider multiple characteristics or attributes of different risks and integrate these data for the purpose of prioritizing and making effective use of resources. In this manner, decisions are made by considering the food system as a whole, that is, with a systems-based approach. Important decision analysis tools that may be used in this process are feasibility, cost-effectiveness, and cost–benefit analyses. A major element of this activity is a clear statement of regulatory philosophy and the use of a road map showing how decisions will be made regarding the mix of private responsibility, government incentives, and government regulation that will be used to manage different risks.

A risk-based system considers other factors, such as consumer perception, cost, controllability, public acceptance, environmental effects, and market impacts, in decision making when appropriate. Risk mitigation strategies and public policy decision making are influenced by factors other than public health risk. These considerations should be formally communicated to stakeholders.

A risk-based system employs measures to evaluate the efficacy of the risk management program on a continuous basis. An essential step in a risk-based system is evaluation of the efficacy of the system itself with respect to public health and other factors selected by decision makers. Evaluation of programs, always a daunting process, requires the identification of indicators by which to link interventions to public health outcomes. To collect and integrate food safety data so that attribution models can be built is a critical first step in this process.

A risk-based system performs all of these functions in a systematic and transparent manner with the involvement of stakeholders. Risk managers should develop a process for implementing a two-way communication approach whereby stakeholders have an opportunity to engage in the risk-based decision-making process. This approach should include input and access to discussions regarding the basis for decision making, as well as information about the uncertainties and variability of the underlying data. Likewise, a risk-based approach requires disclosure of all sources of information, comprehensive analysis, and transparency regarding the considerations taken into account in the decision-making process. In addition, independent peer review is fundamental to all scientific undertakings and critical for risk-based decision-making processes.

Figure 3-1 depicts the cycle of risk prioritization and regulatory (intervention) activities that constitutes the basis of a risk-based food safety system. As the figure shows, the system encompasses six basic steps. These steps are outlined below and then discussed in detail, recognizing that they could be ordered differently and are likely to be taken iteratively.

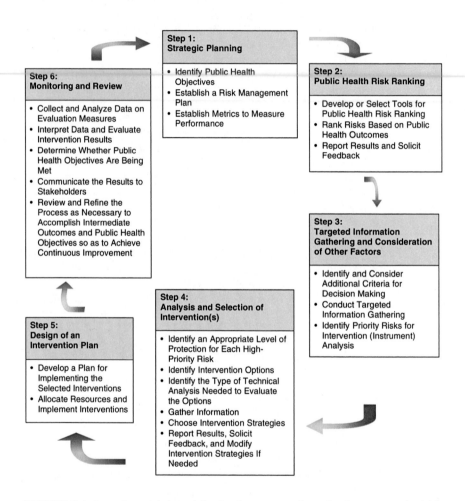

FIGURE 3-1 Steps in a risk-based food safety system (iterative between and within boxes).

Step 1: Strategic Planning

1. Identify public health objectives related to food safety in consultation[2] with stakeholders.
2. Establish a risk management plan (general and specific strategic plans for meeting public health objectives and for considering and choosing policy interventions to achieve those objectives).
3. Establish metrics with which to measure performance in consultation with stakeholders.

Step 2: Public Health Risk Ranking (Ranking of Hazards)

1. Develop or select tools (models, measures, or other) for public health risk ranking in consultation with stakeholders.
2. Rank risks based on public health outcomes.
3. Report results to stakeholders and solicit feedback.

Step 3: Targeted Information Gathering on Risks and Consideration of Other Factors That May Influence Decision Making

1. Identify and consider additional criteria upon which risk-based decision making will be based (e.g., public acceptance, cost, controllability, environmental effects, market impacts) in consultation with stakeholders.
2. Conduct targeted information gathering. For each high-priority and/or uncertain risk, determine the need for collection of additional information and implement accordingly:
    a. additional data collection (research, surveillance, survey, baseline data), and
    b. risk assessment (qualitative, quantitative, semiquantitative).
3. Based on that additional information, identify priority risks for which intervention analysis is needed.

Step 4: Analysis and Selection of Intervention(s)

1. Identify an appropriate level of protection for each high-priority risk, based on available data and in consultation with stakeholders.
2. Identify intervention options in consultation with stakeholders.
3. Identify the types of technical analysis, including but not limited

---

[2] In this context, the term "consultation" means "discussions with other interested individuals or groups to obtain advice."

to risk assessment, needed to evaluate the options; identify performance measures and the initial design of databases.

4. Gather the information necessary to conduct the technical analysis.
5. Choose intervention strategies for implementation using multi-criteria decision analysis.
6. Report results to stakeholders, solicit feedback, and modify intervention strategies if needed.

Step 5: Design of an Intervention Plan

1. Develop a plan for implementing the selected interventions in consultation with stakeholders.
2. Allocate resources and implement interventions.

Step 6: Monitoring and Review

1. Collect and analyze data on evaluation measures selected during strategic planning.
2. Interpret data and evaluate whether the interventions result in the desired intermediate outcomes.
3. Determine whether public health objectives are being met by using performance metrics developed in Step 1 (broad strategic planning).
4. Communicate the results to stakeholders.
5. Review and refine the entire process in an iterative manner as necessary to accomplish both intermediate outcomes and public health objectives so as to achieve continuous improvement over time.

Further Description of the Proposed Approach to Risk-Based Food Safety Management

Step 1: Strategic Planning

Strategic planning, conducted at several different levels, is an essential element of a successful food safety program. The highest level of strategic planning involves the identification of long-term and broadly stated goals for protecting public health from the threats associated with food contaminants, sometimes referred to as public health objectives. Perhaps the best example of such goals is those proposed for Healthy People (Box 3-2). These goals are considered national in scope and concern the entire food safety system, including components of the system not under FDA jurisdiction. In strategic planning, however, the FDA would also likely include agency-specific intermediate objectives, which might lead only indirectly to

---

BOX 3-2
Food Safety Goals Proposed for Healthy People 2020

Objectives Retained as Is from Healthy People 2010

FS HP2020–1: Reduce severe allergic reactions to food among adults with a food allergy diagnosis.

FS HP2020–2: (Developmental) Improve food-employee food preparation practices that directly relate to foodborne illnesses in retail food establishments.

Objectives Retained but Modified from Healthy People 2010

FS HP2020–3: Reduce infections caused by key pathogens commonly transmitted through food.

FS HP2020–4: Reduce infections associated with foodborne outbreaks due to pathogens commonly transmitted through food.

FS HP2020–5: Prevent an increase in the proportion of nontyphoidal *Salmonella* and *Campylobacter jejuni* isolates from humans that are resistant to antimicrobial drugs.

FS HP2020–6: Increase the proportion of consumers who follow key food safety practices.

Objectives New to Healthy People 2020

FS HP2020–7: Reduce the number of outbreak-associated infections caused by food commodity group.

FS HP2020–8: Reduce contamination of meat and poultry products by foodborne pathogens.

FS HP2020–9: (Developmental) Increase the number of States that have prohibited sale or distribution of unpasteurized dairy products (as defined by FDA, unpasteurized liquid milk and cheeses aged <60 days).

SOURCE: http://www.healthypeople.gov/hp2020/Objectives/TopicArea. aspx?id=22&TopicArea=Food+Safety (accessed October 8, 2010).

---

improvements in public health. Examples of these sorts of objectives might be improved efficiency of inspections or reorganization of the FDA research function. While accomplishing these objectives might not lead directly to improvements in public health, achieving efficiencies that would ultimately enable improvements in public health would represent measurable movement toward increased safety of the U.S. food supply.

Identification of the specific means by which the goals are to be achieved—for instance, defining the regulatory structures and the nature and size of the human and technical resources required—is another important component of strategic planning. The strategic planning phase is also when the agency further delineates how scientific research, inspection, and enforcement activities are to be prioritized and deployed. Budgetary issues are central to long-term strategic planning as well. Another important component of strategic planning is describing the metrics that will be used to measure the success of the strategic plan's implementation, that is, how the program will be evaluated with respect to its success in achieving the stated public health objectives. The issue of measuring success is an important and potentially troublesome one, as will be discussed later in this chapter.

In addition to broadly stated public health objectives, each specific agency function, such as research, inspection, and policy, needs its own strategic plan. Other more narrowly focused strategic planning requirements also arise frequently in conjunction with specific food safety issues. Sometimes these issues can be anticipated, but often they cannot. Therefore, an important aspect of a risk-based food safety management strategy is having the necessary structure and resources in place so the agency can respond rapidly to such emergent situations. Planning for emergencies must therefore be part of the strategic planning process.

The committee believes that all of the risk-based activities discussed in this chapter (e.g., risk assessment, collection of data, research, intervention analysis) should be undertaken only after sufficient strategic planning has been completed. Further, the results of strategic planning should be shared with all constituents involved in each path to decisions. Therefore, risk communication must be carried out during the earliest planning stage. In fact, provisions for the stakeholder contributions expected at all levels of food safety management should be outlined as part of the strategic planning process, to include defining the various stakeholders, the nature of the consultations that will take place with them, the methods to be employed to obtain their feedback and with what frequency, and the process by which the agency will respond to that feedback.

The committee is aware that a balance must be achieved between the time spent in planning and that spent on other, more narrowly focused risk management efforts, but it is convinced that inadequate attention to planning (and an ill-planned initiation of technical analysis) is fatal to an effective risk-based food safety program. Strategic planning is necessary to identify the most efficient path to achieve food safety objectives.

Step 2: Public Health Risk Ranking (Ranking of Hazards)

The first step in support of the strategic plan is to identify which risks constitute the greatest threat to public health and hence should be a priority for future analysis. This step is accomplished using tools of public health risk ranking, which itself is a type of risk assessment. Public health risk ranking is a formalized process that involves comparing the relative risk of multiple hazards, including foods, with the purpose of aiding in the establishment of risk management priorities, the allocation of resources, and the identification of critical data and research needs (CAST, 2006; Havelaar et al., 2006; Mangen et al., 2009). At this initial phase of the risk-ranking process, the emphasis is on identifying and comparing hazards and foods with the greatest impact on public health, without consideration of other factors that might also play a role in decision making.

A number of public health risk-ranking models have been produced over the last decade. They differ in their degree of complexity, level of quantification, and approach to model construction. The simplest approach to risk ranking involves the use of personal judgment to create a "risk versus severity" table or matrix to assign rankings. At the other extreme of the spectrum is the joint FDA (CFSAN)–U.S. Department of Agriculture (USDA, Food Safety and Inspection Service [FSIS]) *Listeria monocytogenes* in Ready-to-Eat Foods Risk Ranking (CFSAN/FSIS, 2003), which ranks foods based on their listeriosis risk and encompasses all the components of a full quantitative risk assessment. Somewhere in the middle are many simpler, semiquantitative public health risk-ranking tools, some of which are summarized in Table 3-1.

Each public health risk-ranking model has been designed with a specific purpose in mind, which then informs its design, scope, and degree of rigor. The general approach involves consideration of the body of scientific evidence on attributes (e.g., potential for amplification of the hazard in the food) that define the risk(s) posed by the various agent–food combinations. These attributes (or criteria) are described qualitatively or semiquantitatively and together are the basis for the risk ranking. Each criterion or attribute is defined by one or more input variables that are described using relevant data sources, usually a combination of personal judgment and scientific evidence. Some of the commonly used criteria are (1) burden of illness (epidemiological attribution), (2) illness severity, (3) population susceptibility, (4) likelihood of contamination, (5) potential for agent amplification, and (6) breadth of exposure. The inputs are combined using a mathematical algorithm that assigns a "rank" based on the values or weights given to each input variable. Although risk ranking can be done at a macro level (such as the entirety of risk associated with a specific food or hazard), it is most often applied to specific hazard–commodity pairs.

A useful way to differentiate risk-ranking approaches is by the features of the data sources used in model construction. In the surveillance-based or "top-down" approach, the level of risk associated with specific foods, hazards, or their combinations is based on information gathered

TABLE 3-1 Semiquantitative Food Safety Risk-Ranking Methods

Method	Brief Description	Metrics and Design	Originator(s)
Foodborne Illness Risk-Ranking Model[a]	A science-based tool for prioritization of resources in food safety. Consists of three modules: (1) disease incidence, (2) valuation of health outcomes, and (3) attribution.	Ranks on five measures of social burden. Analytical design with user-friendly interface.	Food Safety Research Consortium (U.S.).
iRISK	Semiquantitatively compares risks of hazard–commodity pairs. Allows for comparison of microbial and chemical hazards. Closest to the standard risk assessment paradigm. Considers (1) exposure assessment (populations, consumption), (2) hazard characterization (dose-response), (3) process information (effect on prevalence and level of contaminant through stages in continuum), and (4) public health metric pseudo-disability adjusted life years (pDALY).	pDALY calculation for comparative ranking purposes. Analytical platform with web-based user interface.	Institute of Food Technologists, Risk Sciences International, and the Food and Drug Administration (U.S.).
Risk Ranger[b]	Determines relative risks from different product–pathogen–processing combinations. Based on 11 questions posed to the user, which deal with (1) susceptibility and severity, (2) probability of exposure, and (3) probability of the food containing an infectious dose.	Excel-based mathematical model converts answers to numerical values; values combined to produce a risk-ranking score scaled logarithmically between 0 and 100.	Australian Food Safety Center of Excellence.
Food Safety Universe Database	Systematic ranking of food safety risks in three dimensions: food, hazard, and location in chain. Establishes two "axes" upon which are determined (1) probability (consumption, contamination, exposure) and (2) impact (P[illness], severity, difficulty of limiting impact).	Risk score calculated multiplicatively as a product of six subscores.	Ontario Ministry of Agriculture and Food.

[a] See http://www.thefsrc.org/firrm.htm (accessed October 8, 2010).
[b] See http://www.foodsafetycentre.com.au/riskranger.php (accessed October 8, 2010).

from epidemiological systems such as disease reporting and outbreak data-bases. It can be argued that these are the best sources of information for public health–based risk ranking because they reflect illness at the point of consumption (NRC, 2009b). However, good epidemiologically based foodborne illness attribution data are not available at this time for the vast majority of hazard–food combinations under FDA jurisdiction, and in most instances do not exist for chronic chemical exposures associated with foods. Another concern with this approach is that it represents disease risk only at the "point of consumption," which is the net sum of contamination occurring at the preharvest, processing, and final preparation stages (NRC, 2009b). This does not necessarily translate directly to an understanding of the possible source of contamination in the supply chain, including a source at the point of processing, which is the location of the large majority of the FDA's current activity. The overall role of foodborne illness attribution in a risk-based food safety management system is discussed further at the end of this chapter.

The alternative or "bottom-up" approach to public health risk ranking adheres roughly to the standard microbial risk assessment paradigm and follows the agent through the food chain to produce a prediction of risk to human health relative to other agents and/or foods. This approach is based on research data supplemented by expert judgment, and therefore can be resource-intensive and subjective. It frequently presupposes an understanding of the behavior of microorganisms in complex and changing environments, complexities that may be very difficult to model. It could be argued that some combination of both approaches (bottom-up and top-down) would be better than either one alone.

Many considerations arise in designing a public health risk-ranking model, including model structure, degree of resolution (categorization of foods and agents broadly or narrowly), choice of key risk attributes and their defining criteria, data sources, and weighting approach. Nonetheless, a good risk-ranking model should be fit-for-purpose and be scientifically credible, balanced, transparent, easy to use, and flexible. As such it must provide both the information and the framework necessary to facilitate public health risk ranking in a systematic manner.

As is the case for strategic planning, public health risk ranking can be applied to decision making at various levels. At the uppermost level, identification of the highest-priority risks can be used to support decisions about the balance of resources dedicated to different agency functions. For example, for risk X, what proportion of the agency's resources should go to research relative to inspection versus risk communication? Or within the inspection function, what proportion of resources should be dedicated to commodity A versus commodity B based on their relative risk ranking? At a lower level, predictive (bottom-up) risk-ranking models with a high degree of resolution can even function as preliminary risk assessments to determine the need for additional data collection or to predict the efficacy of competing mitigation approaches. In short, public health risk ranking supports the other functions of a risk-based food safety management system in the spirit of the iterative nature of the system.

Step 3: Targeted Information Gathering on Risks and Consideration of Other Factors That May Influence Decision Making

The committee recognizes that even a risk-ranking process based exclusively on public health aspects and grounded in scientific knowledge requires weighing competing values and objectives. Risk decision making takes place in a broader social context. In its mission to protect the safety of the public food supply, the FDA must usually consider such additional factors as (1) the feasibility of mitigation; (2) economic constraints (both costs and economic consequences); (3) additional public health and welfare concerns of consumers, farmers, the food processing industry, and other stakeholders; and (4) the environmental impacts of proposed mitigation measures. Therefore, it is critical during the information-gathering stage to identify which factors will be considered in the decision-making process.

Risk prioritization, an emerging approach in the food safety arena, uses the combined tools of risk assessment and decision analysis to determine the importance of one risk relative to another. Unlike risk ranking, which the committee has defined as a type of risk assessment exercise, risk prioritization is inherently a risk management tool. In particular, multiple criteria decision analysis (MCDA) shows promise for supporting complex decision making. MCDA allows for the systematic structuring of a decision problem from the perspective of multiple dimensions (not just public health). Implemented as an element of structured decision support (NRC, 2009a), it can assist in decision making by integrating value judgments as well as objective, quantitative measurements within a transparent and systematic framework.

Structured decision making incorporating MCDA consists of three basic phases (compare NRC, 2009a, p. 57). In the first phase, called problem structuring, the agency defines the decision problem with input from key stakeholders. This activity includes (1) bounding the problem and identifying the question to be addressed and the factors to be included or excluded from consideration, (2) identifying the values and objectives of the decision-making process, (3) identifying the specific criteria with which potential actions are to be compared, (4) identifying the attributes with which the performance of a given alternative will be measured, and (5) identifying the potential actions to be compared in the analysis. Examples of criteria that may be used are public health improvements, health risk reductions, economic impact, consumer perception, social sensitivity, and environmental effects. In the next phase, called preference modeling, analysts work with all parties to evaluate and represent agency and stakeholder preferences relative to each criterion and to develop an aggregated model that combines preferences across criteria for the purposes of comparing alternative actions (interventions) and assessing trade-offs among the alternatives. Finally, after the ranking of alternatives, sensitivity analysis is performed to identify the most influential criteria and attributes and to evaluate the influence of different preference judgments, an activity that may lead to a change in the ranking of the alternatives (Belton and Stewart, 2002). Recent examples of MCDA approaches applied to food safety include those of Ruzante and colleagues (Henson et al., 2007; Fazil et al., 2008; Ruzante et al., 2009). Ultimately, the outcome of Step 3 is to rerank or reprioritize competing risks.

In some cases, risk prioritization will result in the identification of substantial uncertainties that could well impact the decision-making process. For example, what are the major stakeholder concerns, and how important are they? Are candidate mitigation strategies available, and if so, what is known about their effectiveness? Is the degree of contamination in a product actually known? Is the infectivity/toxicity of a candidate hazard in a population of interest understood? In instances where unknowns are critical to informed decision making, Step 3 helps inform resource allocation with respect to surveillance, research, or further risk assessment efforts. This is not to say that decision making should be placed on hold until every piece of missing information is gathered. When there are sufficient uncertainties that might well impact the choice of a control strategy, however, it is prudent to invest in the collection of information that will improve the ability to make an informed, science-based decision. Alternatively, a risk-ranking/prioritization model (Steps 2 and 3 of the risk-based system) could be designed that would take into account the degree of certainty about public health impact or the need to prioritize based on the potential to cause a particularly serious disease (e.g., bovine spongiform encephalopathy).

Step 4: Analysis and Selection of Intervention(s)

The next step in a risk-based approach is to identify and select interventions (or instruments) for the highest-priority risks. In economic and policy analysis, the term "instrument" is used to describe the means a government has at its disposal to achieve public policy outcomes—to govern. Instrument types that are often used include laws, economic incentives, self-regulation, standards, contracts, and information and education, all of which establish relationships between the state and its citizens (Treasury Board of Canada Secretariat, 2007). However, the term "instrument" can be interpreted in many different contexts (e.g., the medical discipline), so to avoid potential misinterpretations, the committee chose to use the term "intervention" instead. For the purposes of this report, the term "intervention" should not be equated exclusively with legislation, but with any means by which policy objectives are pursued. This broad definition includes forms of government action in addition to legislation and encompasses a spectrum from no intervention through reliance on industry self-regulation, use of information and education strategies, coregulation, establishment of incentive-based structures, direct regulation, or a combination of actions (see Chapter 4).

Choosing interventions based on decision analysis is a process that involves multiple tasks. The first is to establish an acceptable level of risk (appropriate level of protection) for each high-priority risk, consistent with the broad goals for protecting public health identified in Step 1 (strategic planning). This task should, of course, be carried out in consultation with stakeholders. Next, it is necessary to identify interventions that could be used—alone or together with other interventions—to address each risk. Candidate interventions can be identified or designed through consultation with stakeholders and based on the scientific analyses performed in Step 3. In point of fact, many candidate interventions will already have been identified in Steps 1, 2, and 3 of the risk-based system during the gathering of information about the risks and the discussion of potential mitigation strategies. Because the objective of the risk-based approach is to allocate limited resources to maximize benefits and minimize risks, decisions about interventions should include an analysis of the value of public health outcomes and uncertainties as well as of the costs and risks of the intervention. This analysis should be undertaken with the understanding that for some interventions (e.g., a new regulatory approach to food inspections), the impact on public health and the cost will be realized only in the long term, and therefore the timing of the analysis is an important consideration. It is important at this stage to consider systematically the full spectrum of interventions (Treasury Board of Canada Secretariat, 2007) to ensure that the alternatives are not prejudged (see also Hammond et al., 1999).

Candidate interventions should then be evaluated by using analytical tools (e.g., risk assessment) that can help identify the types of additional information that might be needed to evaluate the alternatives and the data required. Based on this information and analysis, intervention strategies should be selected and assessed using formal MCDA approaches as described under Step 3. The MCDA approach does not need to be highly sophisticated, but it does need to provide a road map to ensure that the same factors and trade-offs are considered across intervention alternatives for different risk situations. A template (Treasury Board of Canada Secretariat, 2007) can help ensure that more salient aspects of a particular alternative do not dominate the overall choice among interventions (see

Chapter 4). Documenting intervention choices is essential to achieving transparent decision processes.

Step 5: Design of an Intervention Plan

The fifth step in a risk-based system is to design and implement the selected intervention(s) in consultation with stakeholders. Each intervention will have unique implementation needs, so the details of this step will vary based on the selected intervention and the risk being addressed. For example, this step may involve writing regulations, setting standards, overseeing self-regulation, or designing educational programs and tools, as might be the case for labeling. This step also requires the definition of interim measures (intermediate outcomes) with which to monitor the progress of the intervention's implementation; these measures, however, should not be a substitute for the ultimate performance measures identified in Step 1 (strategic planning), that is, the measurement of progress in meeting public health objectives. This step also involves systematically choosing the types of resources to be used in carrying out different intervention plans, for example, the mix of federal and state resources. The role of each partner (e.g., federal, state, and local governments; industry) in implementing the intervention needs to be discussed with partners and delineated in the plan.

Step 6: Monitoring and Review

Integral to any management system is continued monitoring of the system outcomes. In addition to common goals of greater accountability and improvements in performance-based decision making (Cavalluzzo and Ittner, 2004), performance measurement and monitoring can be used for evaluation, control, budgeting, learning, motivation or promotion, and recognition of achievement (Behn, 2003). The committee cautions that, while there is evidence that performance measurement can improve government performance (Bevan and Hood, 2006), it can also be ineffective or even harmful, producing gaming and other unintended consequences (Bird et al., 2005; Johnsen, 2005). For example, the Government Performance and Results Act (GPRA) has been criticized for focusing public managers more on procedural compliance than on performance (Lynn, 1998).

As each intervention is undertaken, it is essential to map appropriate predetermined goals (set during Step 1), such as public health objectives and intermediate objectives, to the actual outcomes of an intervention. Direct metrics of public health might include cases of illness, hospitalizations, deaths, measurements of disease burden (e.g., disability-adjusted life years), or economic costs (e.g., cost of illness). Intermediate metrics are those that, for example, measure contamination at a point between farm and table. As part of the strategic planning in Step 1, the agency should define one or more agencywide goals, ideally linked with national public health objectives and relating to national reductions in the incidence of key pathogens and their associated diseases or the presence of chemical contaminants. This should be seen as a means of measuring the overall outcome of the risk-based system, providing the agency with a way of assessing whether the selected approach to risk management is effective.

Needless to say, the identification and design of appropriate metrics must be consistent with the data collection system and the means by which the data are interpreted (see also Chapter 5). Foodborne illness attribution data can be particularly relevant in this regard. A prime example of an effort to link human health outcomes with regulatory controls is the creation of the Foodborne Diseases Active Surveillance Network (FoodNet) program in the late 1990s. FoodNet was initiated by the U.S. Centers for Disease Control and Prevention in collaboration with USDA and the FDA, and was intended to assess the effectiveness of the 1996 Hazard Analysis and Critical Control Points (HACCP)/Pathogen Reduction regulations (Scallan, 2007). While FoodNet has produced valuable information (e.g., improved foodborne illness estimates, standardization of methods, identification of risk factors for pathogen-specific illnesses), it does not meet the need for information for effective monitoring of the success of the HACCP/Pathogen Reduction regulations. The overall role of foodborne illness attribution in a risk-based food safety management system is discussed further at the end of this chapter.

The committee discussed and recognized the challenges associated with measuring the success of policy interventions, which have also been cited by others (Havelaar et al., 2006; Charlebois and Yost, 2008). For example, whereas intermediate variables (e.g., pathogen testing in food at the time of processing) may be relatively easier to correlate with the adoption of an intervention, such correlation is, in general, much more difficult for a public health outcome (e.g., measured by FoodNet or national public health trends), even in cases where a link has high face validity (e.g., an intervention that decreases food contamination would be expected to improve public health). In many instances, other factors that are not necessarily controllable confound the identification of such correlations. Although intermediate measures are useful, direct measures of public health impact are essential for truly evaluating the effectiveness of food safety interventions in the long term. Hence, again, the need for accurate and comprehensive foodborne illness attribution data is clear.

Ideally, the monitoring and review step should be performed not by the group planning the intervention but by a different group with expertise in designing the collection, analysis, interpretation, and communication of appropriate data and results to stakeholders (Chapter 5). As discussed in Chapter 11, this monitoring role could be assumed by an independent, centralized risk-based analysis and data management center. As with other aspects of a risk-based system, this process must be transparent and involve stakeholders meaningfully.

Finally, the entirety of the risk-based approach (Steps 1 through 6) should be seen as an iterative process, with a strong focus on continuous public health improvement. The monitoring and review process should be subject to rigorous quality assurance standards, with periodic quality reviews not only when goals are not being met, but also when goals are being consistently met, which may suggest the need for new standards or new measurement tools.

MOVING TOWARD THE DEVELOPMENT OF A COMPREHENSIVE RISK-BASED APPROACH TO FOOD SAFETY MANAGEMENT

The risk-based system described above is consistent with the principle of evidence-based public health, which has been defined as "the development, implementation, and evaluation of effective programs and policies in public health through application of principles of scientific reasoning, including systematic uses of data and information systems" (Brownson et al., 2003, p. 4). The evidence-based approach includes key characteristics of (1) interventions being based on the best possible science, (2) reliance on multidisciplinary problem solving, (3) systematic program planning, (4) sound evaluation of program efficacy, and (5) information dissemination. The committee advocates application of the evidence-based approach to food safety management.

The risk- and evidence-based food safety management approach described above is meant to be comprehensive in that the general steps are applicable to virtually all FDA food-related decision making. Certainly, the approach is relevant to broad-based prioritization, as might be the case for strategic planning of how best to use agency resources associated with specific functions (e.g., research, inspection, communication, surveillance). However, it is also applicable to decision making within any one unit of the agency, as might be the case for prioritization of the use of resources dedicated to the risk assessment function (e.g., which risk assessments to perform). It is fully applicable as well to specific decision making, such as deciding which of several competing risk reduction strategies to choose for implementation. The committee therefore sees the risk-based approach as providing the underlying structure for all of the FDA's food safety decisions.

The steps outlined above are not meant to be conducted in a fixed order; rather, the system as a whole should be envisioned as fluid. Furthermore, as noted above, the overall approach, like risk analysis, is intended to be iterative. For example, broad-based public health risk ranking (Step 2) might be applied at the general commodity level (produce versus fish) and considering all agents to identify those of greatest public health concern. This activity would be followed by prioritization and reranking (Step 3) on the basis of additional factors that might affect the decision to intervene. Once high-priority hazards and/or commodities had been identified, the agency might return to Step 2 to place the riskiest specific products and their hazards in a high-risk general commodity category, followed by prioritization (Step 3). Following prioritization would be analysis and selection of intervention(s) (Step 4), during which frequent iteration would occur between Steps 4 and 6 in an effort to establish appropriate levels of protection, identify and evaluate candidate intervention strategies, and collect the information necessary to support the choice of intervention(s), which might or might not include the need for a full quantitative risk assessment. Once the intervention plan had been implemented and monitored (Steps 5 and 6), there would be a need for periodic reevaluation using risk ranking and prioritization (back to Steps 2 and 3) to ensure that resources would continue to be allocated appropriately.

Indeed, given the diversity and inherent dynamics of food safety issues, it is impossible to account for all potential eventualities in advance. As noted earlier, therefore, the risk-based system must be sufficiently flexible to respond to rapidly emerging food safety issues, and it must be reactive enough to facilitate its use in emergency situations, such as the management of foodborne illness outbreaks. Activities within each step, such as data collection, analysis, and modeling, will depend on the type of hazard. During an outbreak, for example, decisions must be made quickly and possibly with an incomplete collection of data. For this reason, it is essential that strategic planning performed in emergency situations be largely standardized so that immediate decisions are based on lessons learned and the likely availability of needed data. As another example, government tools for overseeing the safety of imported foods necessarily differ from those available to ensure the safety of domestically produced food. (Appendix E contains background information on various tools that are used to oversee imported foods here and in other countries.) As discussed in Chapter 4, the lack of jurisdiction over the production of food in other countries is an important differentiating factor for governance purposes. In fact, for imported foods, the data available to make decisions based on risk may be very different from those available for domestic foods, and the analysis will need to take into consideration such factors as the FDA's knowledge of the foreign country's food safety system. Still, decision making about prioritizing inspections, allowing importation of a product into the United States, or responding to an emergency situation should be based on the same attributes listed in Box 3-1 and should follow the same basic risk-based approach. At a different level, flexibility needs to be integrated to allow for the "human element"; for example, an inspector should not be prevented from pursuing a hunch that something might be wrong.

RELATIONSHIP BETWEEN RISK ANALYSIS AND THE RISK-BASED FOOD SAFETY SYSTEM

To date, the term "risk-based" has been interpreted largely in the context of the basic elements of risk analysis. However, there has been some discussion for about a decade regarding the need to expand the meaning of the term. For example, a 2001 discussion paper issued by Resources for the Future[3] (Taylor and Hoffman, 2001) suggests that the role of risk analysis be broadened:

> There are, however, much broader roles for risk analysis at the level of system design and management. . . . They include: (1) guiding the allocation of inspection and enforcement resources, and (2) setting priorities for risk reduction initiatives. These are roles for risk analysis that can significantly enhance the effectiveness of the food safety system in reducing risk. (Taylor and Hoffman, 2001, p. 5)

The risk-based food safety management system presented here takes the concepts of risk analysis to an operational level by creating a process that uses analytical methodology to evaluate risk, and then facilitates decision making in light of the myriad factors that need to be considered in the risk management process. This sort of approach is not unlike that of HACCP, which provides the foundation for food safety control at the processing level of the food chain. Like HACCP, this conceptual approach to a risk-based food safety management program provides a road map that clearly defines the course of the process and the types of inputs that need to be considered along the way. This road map is a key component of the transparency of the system, with a focus not just on what has been done, but also on how the system will operate in the future. As envisioned by the committee, such a framework is comprehensive (providing a uniform means of assessing and comparing risk across the food safety system) and transparent (incorporating a clear understanding of how one goes from data to decisions); these and other key attributes of the risk-based system were noted earlier in Box 3-1.

---

[3] See http://www.rff.org/documents/RFF-DP-01-24.pdf (accessed January 26, 2010).

THE ROLE OF RISK ANALYSIS IN THE FDA'S CURRENT FOOD SAFETY MANAGEMENT PROGRAM

The FDA has been engaged in risk-based efforts in food safety management for more than a decade now. This section provides a brief synopsis of the committee's understanding of those efforts, based on a public workshop held March 24, 2009, in Washington, DC, and on follow-up questions and interviews with CFSAN and CVM staff as well as background analysis by the committee. Although the committee has not attempted an in-depth evaluation of the FDA efforts, it has identified some gaps in these efforts. The committee notes that creation of the Office of Foods in 2009 with direct line of authority over CFSAN and CVM will likely impact both the functioning of these units and the ultimate implementation of a risk-based food safety approach.

Risk-Based Activities of CFSAN

Although CFSAN has a long history of conducting safety assessments for food additives and risk assessments for chemicals, it was not until 1999 that the center conducted more complex quantitative risk assessments for pathogens. In 2002, a CFSAN risk analysis working group produced an internal report *Initiation and Conduct of All Major Risk Assessments Within a Risk Analysis Framework,* which is based on the principles of risk analysis and describes how to prioritize and conduct risk assessments.[4] Several offices within CFSAN have a role in developing and coordinating risk-based initiatives[5]:

- The Risk Assessment Coordination Team (RACT) in the Office of Food Defense, Communication, and Emergency Response coordinates and manages risk profiles and assessments that require representation from different offices within CFSAN, and sometimes outside of CFSAN or even outside of the FDA. The RACT oversees "virtual" teams that are formed to conduct a project. It also serves as a liaison to appropriate entities—federal, state, and local government; industry; consumer groups; and academia—in the planning of food safety risk analysis activities and related research, and it provides direction for the conduct and coordination of risk analysis activities related to food.
- In the Office of Food Safety, the Chemical Hazards Assessment Team conducts safety/risk assessments of industrial chemicals, both

[4] Personal communication, Chad Nelson, Office of Foods, FDA, September 3, 2009.
[5] Personal communication, Marianne Miliotis, Deputy Director, Office of Applied Research and Safety Assessment, CFSAN, FDA, April 21, 2009.

elemental and organic, including naturally occurring contaminants and allergens.

- The Economics Team in the Office of Regulations, Policy, and Social Sciences conducts analyses that are integrated with risk assessments, including economic impact analyses of decisions and cost–benefit analyses.
- The Division of Field Programs and Guidance in the Office of Compliance coordinates and provides oversight for risk-related initiatives that impact field work planning.
- Other offices at CFSAN that perform food safety assessments are the Office of Food Additive Safety and the Office of Nutrition, Labeling, and Dietary Supplements.

Risk-Based Activities of CVM

CVM also uses tools of risk ranking and risk assessment in its regulatory process (Hartogensis, 2009). CVM representatives stated that their risk management strategy is to prioritize activities aimed at reducing or mitigating risks according to the ranking of the risks and the limits of their authority and resources. However, CVM has not produced a document that delineates a standardized process for conducting risk assessments (or rankings) for potential contaminants in feed or specific guidelines for risk ranking or prioritization (Hartogensis, 2009). Only a few specific examples of CVM's risk-based activities were provided to the committee. Specifically, the Office of New Drug Evaluation, which reviews information on approvals to manufacture and market animal drugs, is also responsible for evaluating human health impacts that might result from the consumption of drug residues present in the tissues of food animals. To date, the committee is uncertain about the mechanism by which this evaluation is performed. In 2003, a group consisting of CVM officials, along with representatives from the Office of the Commissioner and state regulatory officials, announced the implementation of the Animal Feed Safety System (AFSS). This system represented the first step toward making the agency's animal feed safety program more comprehensive and risk based. To date, five public meetings to gather stakeholder input have been conducted, and this group is apparently developing a framework document describing the major processes, guidance, regulations, and policy issues entailed in addressing feed safety. As of this writing, however, the significance of the AFSS as applied to risk-based food safety management is unclear (Hartogensis, 2009).

Risk Analysis Products

Over the years, CFSAN and CVM have produced a variety of products related to risk analysis, including safety assessments, risk profiles, qualitative and quantitative risk assessments, and risk–benefit analyses. Perhaps the most comprehensive effort in this regard is the joint FDA (CFSAN)–USDA (FSIS) *L. monocytogenes* risk-ranking (assessment) model development mentioned earlier. Although the second iteration of this model was completed in 2003 (CFSAN/FSIS, 2003), action plan items are still being developed and implemented (CFSAN, 2008). Another notable risk assessment activity included evaluation of *Vibrio parahaemolyticus* risks associated with oyster consumption (FDA, 2005). In addition, the agency provides a high level of support to international organizations, such as the Food and Agriculture Organization/WHO and the Codex Alimentarius Commission, which have produced their own risk assessments. The FDA has also used others' risk assessments in formulating regulations, such as the Shell Egg Rule, for which USDA's "Risk Assessments for *Salmonella Enteritidis* in Shell Eggs and *Salmonella* spp. in Egg Products" was used. Similarly, the U.S. Environmental Protection Agency's risk assessments have been applied by the FDA for management of chemical contaminants in the food supply.

A complete review of all food safety risk analysis activities with which the FDA has been involved is beyond the scope of this report. However, three new approaches described by FDA representatives during the public workshop held March 24, 2009, are worth discussing.

Public Health Risk Ranking

Under an FDA cooperative agreement, the Institute of Food Technologists convened a panel of experts to develop a risk-ranking prototype designed to analyze data on hazards (both chemical and biological) in food and return an estimate of the resulting health burden at a population level. Termed the iRisk model, this is a bottom-up or predictive modeling approach to risk ranking that requires the application of data and expert judgment to assemble sufficient information with which to predict the ecology of the hazards in the food supply. These results are combined with food intake data and information on hazard virulence or toxicity to produce a prediction of the relative level of risk to human health of the particular hazard–food pair. The model produces a semiquantitative characterization of the disease burden, which can be used for comparison (ranking) purposes and can facilitate evaluation of the impacts of hazard control measures. The model was further developed by Risk Sciences International, a consulting company, into a web-accessible tool. RTI International is currently populating the iRisk model with data for proof-of-concept testing; Risk Sciences International is revising the model to improve its performance with respect to a variety of features (Wagner, 2009).

Risk-Based Inspection

Much like FSIS, the FDA has been developing models to assist in the allocation of inspectional resources, sometimes referred to as "risk-based inspection" (Engeljohn, 2009; Maczka, 2009). For example, CFSAN's Division of Field Programs and Guidance, which is responsible for developing tools to assist the Office of Regulatory Affairs (ORA) in resource management, has been working on the identification of high-risk food categories to support the targeting of field inspections and sample collection resources as applied to domestic food products and manufacturers. This effort began in 2002 as a simple document based on expert opinion from CFSAN technical experts. By 2008, a risk-based domestic priorities list had been developed for ranking particular product–hazard combinations and facilities (Wagner, 2009). The model appears to utilize such information as the occurrence of multiple hazards, the potential for fatal illness outbreaks, consumption by all segments of the population, and conditions under which the hazard is likely to occur. For ranking purposes, risk is considered a function of the likelihood of a hazard in a product and the severity of the health effect.

CFSAN also performed a risk-ranking exercise on food manufacturers based on their association with Class I recalls,[6] outbreaks, or serious adverse events during 2004, 2005, and 2006. The statistical analysis resulted in a scoring algorithm that was applied to each of the individual food firms. For fiscal year (FY) 2010, the FDA intends to design an updated version of the 2009 algorithm that will be overlaid with compliance history information for specific facilities. In the future, criteria such as the financial viability of the firms and their legal status may also be included as ranking criteria (Givens, 2009; Wagner, 2009).

ORA has reported prioritizing its inspectional resources for FY 2009 based on three categories: category 1, high-risk firm inspections; category 2, inspected plants with compliance issues; and category 3, low-risk industry blitzes. Likewise, CVM is in the process of changing its allocation of inspectional resources so that the resources are allocated in alignment with more objective ranking criteria for the various areas of each program (Hartogensis, 2009). The CVM efforts, which appear to be focused on medicated feeds, are still being developed in conjunction with AFSS; the committee was provided with only limited details.

---

[6] A Class I recall denotes a situation in which there is a reasonable probability that the use of or exposure to a violative product will cause serious adverse health consequences or death.

Risk-Based Management of Imported Foods

The FDA recently embarked on the development of a risk-based approach to managing the safety of food imports, which culminated in the release of the Predictive Risk-Based Evaluation for Dynamic Import Compliance Targeting (PREDICT) model (see also Appendix E). PREDICT is an import screening tool that is intended to automate decisions currently made by import entry reviewers by utilizing intelligence information from numerous sources so as to direct resources to products presenting the greatest risks to public health in a streamlined manner. Criteria such as information about recalls, registration of low-acid canned food processes, agreements with other countries, monitoring of products, and information on certification of facilities and from import certificates are used to calculate a risk score upon which decisions about a food import shipment are based. After a pilot study in June 2007 that the FDA judged to be successful, the agency estimated that PREDICT would be widely implemented by September 2009 (Solomon, 2009).

Food Safety Performance Measures

The Healthy People food safety goals could theoretically serve as the basis for the identification of specific performance measures. However, these goals now use such words as "reduce" and "improve," which cannot serve as metrics per se. Other targets and indicators for measuring the performance of the federal food safety system have been recently described. For example, the U.S. Department of Health and Human Services (HHS) has identified some food safety–related outcome indicators in its strategic plan (see Box 3-3). Elements of the 2004 FDA Program Assessment Rating Tool (PART) report and progress on implementation of the Food Protection Plan also can be used to identify some performance measures. PART was introduced in 2002 to standardize the measurement of performance in federal agencies, with the intent of linking performance to budgets (Gueorguieva et al., 2009) (see also Chapter 2). Presented by the Office of Management and Budget as a tool for implementing the GPRA, PART assesses GPRA performance strategies and goals, albeit to a limited extent. The GPRA requires that agencies demonstrate accountability and the effectiveness of programs to Congress and the public by establishing performance measures. PART has been described as applying a different level of analysis than the GPRA, conflicting with the GPRA regarding what to measure and how to measure it (GAO, 2005) and having serious limitations and questionable reliability (Radin, 2006; Gueorguieva et al., 2009). More specific to the FDA's food protection efforts, the agency's 2010 budget justification for implementation of the Food Protection Plan (FPP) includes several long-term objec-

---

BOX 3-3
Food Safety–Related Outcome Indicators Listed Under "Other Outcome Indicators," U.S. Department of Health and Human Services' Strategic Plan (2009)

1. Reduce the incidence of infection with key foodborne pathogens: *Campylobacter* species. 2010 12.3 cases/100,000 by December 2011.
2. Reduce the incidence of infection with key foodborne pathogens: *Escherichia coli* O157:H7. 2010 1.0 cases/100,000 by December 2011.
3. Reduce the incidence of infection with key foodborne pathogens: *Listeria monocytogenes.* 2010 0.24 cases/100,000 by December 2011.
4. Reduce the incidence of infection with key foodborne pathogens: *Salmonella* species. 2010 6.8 cases/100,000 by December 2011.

---

tives and associated measures (see Box 3-4). Overall, these objectives and measures focus on numbers of outputs, voluntary outcomes, and indirect measures of capacity to achieve public health, and hence they might be considered potentially useful metrics of performance. Recent progress reports on the implementation of the FPP also describe a wide variety of outputs (e.g., numbers of public meetings and workshops, technical guidance and rules issued, foreign offices established, memorandums of understanding, cooperative and interagency agreements).

COMPARISON OF THE CURRENT FDA APPROACH TO RISK MANAGEMENT AGAINST THE VISION AND ATTRIBUTES OF A TRUE RISK-BASED DECISION-MAKING APPROACH TO FOOD SAFETY MANAGEMENT

Based on the information presented in public meetings and conversations with FDA staff and other publicly available information, the committee concluded that the agency currently is not practicing some aspects of a systematic risk-based food safety management approach with the attributes identified in Box 3-1. The agency has embraced the tool of risk assessment, and it should be commended for doing so. The development of the risk-ranking/assessment model for *L. monocytogenes* mentioned above is a notable example of a comprehensive risk assessment produced in cooperation with another food safety agency and with stakeholder involvement.

BOX 3-4
Objectives Listed in the U.S. Food and Drug Administration's (FDA's) 2010 Congressional Budget Justification for Food

Long-Term Objective: Increase access to safe and nutritious new food products.
   Measure 213301: Complete review and action on the safety evaluation of direct and indirect food and color additive petitions, including petitions for food contact substances, within 360 days of receipt. (Output)

Long-Term Objective: Prevent safety problems by modernizing science-based standards and tools to ensure high-quality manufacturing, processing, and distribution.
   Measure 214101: Number of state, local, and tribal regulatory agencies in the U.S. and its Territories enrolled in the draft Voluntary National Retail Food Regulatory Program Standards. (Outcome)
   Measure 214102: Percentage of the enrolled jurisdictions which meet 2 or more of the Standards. (Outcome)

Long-Term Objective: Provide consumers with clear and timely information to protect them from foodborne illness and promote better nutrition.
   Measure 212401: Increase by 40 percent the percentage of American consumers who correctly identify that trans fat increases the risk of heart disease. (Outcome)
   Measure 212402: Increase by 10 percent the percentage of American consumers who correctly identify that saturated fat increases the risk of heart disease. (Outcome)

It appears that in general, the agency's microbial risk assessments have been performed in accordance with well-recognized standards (FAO/WHO, 2006; NRC/IOM, 2009).

However, the production of risk assessments and profiles alone does not constitute a risk-based food safety management system. The FDA does not employ the stepwise process outlined above, and it does not appear to have any strategic vision for a risk-based system. The fact that risk-based ranking and inspection models are under development and in various stages of implementation is commendable, but the use of these tools does not imply that a comprehensive risk-based approach is being pursued.

Measure 212403: Improve by 10 percent the percentage of American consumers who correctly identify that omega-3 fat is a possible factor in reducing the risk of heart disease. (Outcome)

Long-Term Objective: Detect safety problems earlier and better target interventions to prevent harm to consumers.
Measure 214201: Number of prior notice import security reviews. (Output)
Measure 214202: Number of import food field exams. (Output)
Measure 214203: Number of Filer Evaluations. (Output)
Measure 214204: Number of examinations of FDA refused entries. (Output)
Measure 214205: Number of high-risk food inspections. (Output)
Measure 214206: Maintain accreditation for Office of Regulatory Affairs labs. (Outcome)
Measure 214303: Convert data from new Electronic Laboratory Exchange Network (eLEXNET) participating laboratories via automated exchange or convert data from existing manual data streams to automated data exchange. (Outcome)
Measure 214305: Increase laboratory surge capacity in the event of terrorist attack on the food supply (radiological and chemical samples/week). (Outcome)

NOTE: "Output" and "Outcome" designations appear in the Budget Justification.

The absence of a strategic vision to embrace and implement a risk-based food safety management system is apparent at almost every level. Despite many counterexamples, the relative lack of strategic planning and incorporation of appropriate metrics for evaluating the efficacy of food safety control strategies illustrates the point well. For example, although the latest PART report[7] for the FDA, produced in 2003, resulted in a performance rating of "moderately effective," the report does not mention any direct public health

---

[7] See http://www.whitehouse.gov/omb/expectmore/detail/10001057.2003.htm (accessed October 8, 2010)

measures for food safety. Of the ten long-term performance goals[8] adopted by the FDA in 2003, the report includes only one that pertains directly to food safety: "increase laboratory surge capacity in the event of a terrorist attack on the food supply." In this case, it is unclear from the report how the specific targets (i.e., radiation and chemical contamination) for surge capacity were identified. In a similar manner, the recent FPP reports do not appear to map progress to metrics, and the 2010 FDA Congressional Budget Justification for the FPP does not appear to map directly to the plan's eight goals. Perhaps most notable, the FDA's 2010 Congressional Budget Justification for Food (Box 3-4) identifies objectives that are not necessarily consistent with the food safety goals proposed for Healthy People 2020 (Box 3-2), and specific metrics for the agency to use in measuring performance in food safety are not identified, with the exception of the few food safety outcome measures stated in the 2009 HHS Strategic Plan (Box 3-3). Briefly, it is not clear that efforts to identify performance measures for food safety or public health are linked to strategic goals as recommended by this committee.

Also, the measures identified in the FPP, the HHS Strategic Plan, and Healthy People 2020 fall short of suggested standards for performance indicators and systems (see, for example, the recommendations in Bird et al., 2005). GAO reports and other assessments suggest that performance indicators have been underutilized to improve agencies' decision making in the last decade (Cavalluzzo and Ittner, 2004; GAO, 2009a; Taylor, 2009). Among the obstacles to effective use of performance measurement are ambiguous goals and objectives, a lack of commitment to performance measurement on the part of top management, and inadequate measurement and analysis systems (Cavalluzzo and Ittner, 2004; Johnsen, 2005; Taylor, 2009). Overall, the committee found that the FDA and HHS have made limited progress toward establishing and applying performance measures, particularly those related to public health outcomes, as part of a risk-based food safety system.

Most of the other attributes of a risk-based food safety management system (e.g., public health risk ranking, prioritization for resource allocation, transparency in risk management, effective and frequent communication with stakeholders) are all but absent from the FDA's current approach to food safety. For example, well-articulated management objectives were not delineated when the iRisk model was presented to the committee. Likewise, the committee was not provided with additional details on the PREDICT model, which should undergo extensive peer review before being deployed

---

[8] Examples of such nonfood safety–related long-term goals laid out in PART include that the FDA shall "[i]ncrease by 40 percent the percentage of American consumers who correctly identify that trans fat increases the risk of heart disease" and "[r]educe the average time for marketing approval for safe and effective new devices."

in the field. Of interest, it was apparent during the workshop held on March 24, 2009, that stakeholders were unaware of many of the FDA's more recent risk-ranking/prioritization efforts, including its plans for a risk-based inspection system or the development of PREDICT as a risk-based tool to manage food imports (Bell, 2009; Gombas, 2009; Scott, 2009). Consistent with a recent report (USDA, 2010), the committee concluded that improvement of the agency's risk-based approach is also needed in the area of preventing risk from chemical contaminants.

The area of risk communication also remains a challenge. In general, the committee found a lack of transparency in the FDA's food safety activities and insufficient communication with stakeholders. Examples include insufficient description of risk-based initiatives and use of peer-review. Although the FDA's Risk Communication Advisory Committee (RCAC) was recently created to advise the agency on communication strategies and programs, and the FDA has created an internal Communication Committee to coordinate its communication activities, prioritizing and evaluating risk communication efforts remain a challenge (Chapter 9). During its August 2009 meeting, the RCAC discussed the FDA's research on consumer knowledge of food recalls and plans for monitoring the effectiveness of communication during recalls. An integrated risk-based management system should enable the FDA to target, design, and evaluate its risk communication more effectively (Morgan et al., 1992).

IMPLEMENTATION OF A RISK-BASED
FOOD SAFETY MANAGEMENT SYSTEM

Implementation of a risk-based food safety management system will be successful only if the necessary resources are dedicated to the effort. It should be clear from the preceding discussion that this will be a substantial undertaking. Virtually all of the recommendations in this report can and perhaps should be adopted with the stated purpose of supporting a risk-based approach to food safety management. Nonetheless, the committee has identified a few areas that it considers particularly critical to the successful implementation of a risk-based system, which are discussed below.

Personnel and Analytical Tools

There is a tendency on the part of government agencies, including the FDA, to assume that scientists are interchangeable: that individuals trained to conduct bench experiments in microbiology, for example, can easily be shifted to performing risk assessment or crisis management. It is essential that new scientific staff be acquired to provide the core competencies necessary to create a new, risk-based approach for the agency. The committee recognizes the difficulty of finding individuals trained in the breadth and depth of food safety problems who are also proficient in epidemiology, mathematical modeling, economics, or other disciplines necessary to support a risk-based approach. Academic institutions do not typically configure their programs with the necessary training to prepare students to be a part of a risk management team. Accordingly, it may be necessary to initiate agencywide recruitment and training efforts to train professionals in the skills necessary to support a risk-based approach. A good example of this sort of initiative is the new FDA Commissioner's Fellowship Program.

Further, the body of FDA scientists must be able to support both management of crises at the time they occur and prevention of future crises. To ensure that all of the FDA's responsibilities are met, resources need to be allocated for both routine operations and prevention of long-term food safety problems. While, as recommended here, a risk-based approach is institutionalized over time, the FDA should continue to attend to more immediate issues. The committee found disturbing various testimony confirming that during an emergency, work is redirected, and the FDA's focus on prevention and long-term efforts receives lower priority. To alleviate this situation and to advance the FDA toward a risk-based regulatory approach, experts will need to be hired in the areas recommended by the committee.

To carry out all its food safety responsibilities and specifically to ensure continuation of everyday operations, then, the FDA's food programs must include sufficient staff working on food issues to ensure that routine functions will continue even when a crisis emerges. A logical way to address this need is to form functional teams that would work in defined areas identified during the strategic planning process. Many of these teams could support efforts to manage the identified risk-based priorities with a focus on prevention. For example, there could be a Research Team, whose major function would be to support the high-priority research necessary to support the risk-based mission. Likewise, a Surveillance Team would be responsible for interacting with other federal agencies and state and local jurisdictions and for managing centralized epidemiological databases supporting modeling efforts. Similarly, there might be a Risk Assessment Team, a Risk Communication Team, and a Risk Management Team. Recognizing the need for continuous support of the crisis management function, it could be appropriate to have a separate team dedicated to this function. However, crises must not be allowed to preempt a substantial part of the effort allocated to essential noncrisis activities.

Alternatives to the development of agency competency to build and operate a risk-based food safety system are discussed in Chapter 11. One option is to create a centralized risk-based analysis and data management center, which would provide a multiagency and multidisciplinary core of expertise in risk analysis for all agencies with responsibilities for food safety.

This center would mirror the European model, in which such expertise is often housed in quasigovernmental research institutes (such as the National Institute for Public Health and the Environment in the Netherlands) that assist in data collection and provide independent analyses of incoming data for policy makers. Such a center would not subsume an agency's prerogative to develop food safety policy, and there would remain a need for analytic capacity at the top level of agencies, such as the FDA, with responsibility for food safety. However, the center's creation would eliminate the need for each agency involved in food safety to develop its own comprehensive expertise in risk analysis independently. As discussed in Chapter 11, a longer-term alternative would be the creation of a unified national food safety agency, which, as part of an overall consolidation of food safety activities (possibly though an intermediate office of food protection) would integrate the risk-based efforts of the multiple agencies currently involved in food safety.

Closely related to the personnel issue is the need for targeted research activities to permit the development of the information infrastructure required to support risk-based food safety management (see Chapter 5). At a basic level, the software needs for these activities are daunting, as most risk-modeling tools are not off-the-shelf software but highly customized. The FDA, alone or in collaboration with other agencies, must commit the resources required for the applied research needed to develop and test software and computer systems that are integral to infrastructure development. Again, the agency may want to support the creation of a risk-based analysis and data management center that would provide these services across all agencies involved in food safety.

Foodborne Disease Attribution Data and Models

The IOM/NRC report *Scientific Criteria to Ensure Safe Food* states that "science-based food safety criteria must be clearly linked to the public health problem they are designed to address. To accomplish this, a cause/effect relationship needs to be established between contaminants in foods and human disease, that is, to allocate the burden of foodborne disease among foods and food groups" (IOM/NRC, 2003, p. 250). This statement forms the basis of what is now referred to as foodborne disease attribution, defined as "the capacity to attribute cases of foodborne disease to the food vehicle or other source responsible for illness" (Batz et al., 2005, p. 993; EFSA, 2008, p. 5). While the concept is valuable, the committee recognizes the lack of truly reliable attribution data and the somewhat limited scope of this definition. A description of the current sources of foodborne disease attribution data as well as approaches to foodborne disease attribution and their advantages and limitations as reported by a recent NRC committee are summarized in Box 3-5 and Table 3-2, respectively. It is clear that substantially more

BOX 3-5
Sources of Foodborne Disease Attribution Data

Data on foodborne disease attribution generally come from three major sources: (1) outbreak reports, (2) case control studies, and (3) source tracking.

Outbreak Reports: Outbreak investigations have traditionally served as the primary means of identifying food sources for pathogens. When outbreaks are carefully investigated, such data can be extremely valuable. In the United States, however, almost all outbreak investigations are conducted by local health departments, which tend to be overworked and to lack either the laboratory or epidemiologic resources to identify a source. There are significant biases involved in the choice of which outbreaks get investigated (generally those that are large or involve an "interesting" pathogen), and the percentage of outbreaks reported and investigated ranges widely both among and within states. Outbreaks may also not be representative of routine foodborne disease cases: they generally represent a significant breakdown in food practices rather than the endemic pattern of transmission of pathogenic microorganisms. There are issues with timeliness as well: the U.S. Centers for Disease Control and Prevention tends to compile data from outbreak reports only on a sporadic basis, which often results in multiple-year gaps between reporting of national summary data. The United Kingdom has tended to rely on outbreak data in its food attribution/food safety efforts; however, its data collection is more standardized than that of the United States, without the wide variability in reporting from local health department to local health department (Batz et al., 2005).

Case Control Studies: When FoodNet was first established, the importance of food attribution in the calculation of food-specific incidence rates was recognized. Consequently, the system was designed to include ongoing case control studies to identify specific foods/food groups that might be consumed more commonly by ill persons infected with a specific

resources will be needed for further characterization of foodborne disease attribution in support of risk-based food safety management.

Simply knowing the proportion of the occurrence of a particular disease that is associated with a specified hazard is not enough. For example, contamination and agent proliferation (and inactivation) can occur at all stages throughout the food chain. There is a need for attribution estimates across the chain—for example, what proportion of salmonel-

pathogen than by well controls. Under the FoodNet program, six case control studies have been conducted. While many have yielded useful epidemiologic data (Friedman et al., 2004; Marcus et al., 2007; Varma et al., 2007), it has become apparent that this is not an effective means to determine attribution percentages: it is expensive and labor intensive, and it yields only crude estimates of the relative contribution of various food categories to disease incidence. Concern has also been raised about possible biases inherent in the selection control process (which has generally involved random digit dialing techniques).

Source Tracking: Food safety agencies in the Netherlands and Denmark have pioneered work in the source tracking of pathogens, that is, using molecular markers/typing to link human disease with animal sources. The process requires careful monitoring of isolates from food animals, with appropriate typing, and application of identical typing methods for human isolates. Data are then entered into models that permit real-time calculation of the relative public health impact of various food–pathogen combinations. These data have been used effectively, particularly in the Netherlands, to guide regulatory actions designed to deal with new and emergent problems in the national food safety system. However, this work has dealt almost exclusively with animal sources for pathogens; virtually no work has been done with pathogen contamination of produce, and produce generally has not been included in the source-tracking models. In the United States, some initial efforts were made to develop such a system, focusing primarily on salmonella. However, results have not been impressive, in part because of the incompatibility of data sets (and lack of data sharing). The U.S. Food and Drug Administration has sponsored intramural research on molecular-typing methods that might be utilized in these systems, but to date, efforts to develop appropriate risk models have not led to useful results.

losis cases attributable to the consumption of contaminated leafy greens is associated with poor personal hygiene practices of food handlers versus preharvest contamination on the farm? Likewise, because agents can be transmitted by multiple routes, more defined data on transmission are needed—for instance, what proportion of human norovirus infections is attributable to foodborne routes as compared with person-to-person transmission? These are simply examples of important questions about

TABLE 3-2 Summary of Approaches to Food Attribution

Approach	Data Needs	Advantages	Limitations	Examples
Foodborne disease surveillance Based on the use of aggregate data from epidemiologic investigation of outbreaks.	Coordinated surveillance systems with similar data collection efforts throughout a specified location, region, or country. Takes many years to accumulate sufficient data. Must include food vehicle information.	Usually applied to multiple foods and pathogens. Outbreak data are a measure of attribution at the point of consumption. Able to take into account other routes of transmission (such as travel, contact with animals). Addresses a broad range of microbes and foods. Data are collected routinely on a national basis for a large number of pathogens over many years.	Assumes equivalence of pathogen-specific contributions of each food type to disease. Adequately classifying multicomponent foods is challenging. Serious gaps in databases exist.	Batz et al., 2004; Adak et al., 2005; DeWaal et al., 2006
Case control study Analytic epidemiologic study that compares diseased (cases) with nondiseased (controls) persons with respect to previous exposures; relative role of exposure is determined by comparing frequencies in cases and controls.	Systematic review of published case control studies and case series to identify relevant risk factors for disease; calculation of population-attributable risk to estimate relative importance of different exposures.	Identification of sources of sporadic infections. Classic strengths of case control study design, including ability to explore multiple exposures (specific foods, food preparation practices, cross-contamination, travel, other risk factors).	Classic weaknesses of case control studies, including misclassification, recall bias, limited resolution for commonly consumed foods, establishment of temporality. Many cases required for adequate statistical power. Usually limited to a single microorganism rather than multiple agents. Expensive.	Multiple examples, but specific applications to food attribution are sparse (see EFSA, 2008)

Method				References
Microbial subtyping Based on a combination of strain typing collated with epidemiologic surveillance data and mathematical modeling; underlying hypothesis is that control of ultimate reservoir (usually occurring before harvest) will prevent human exposure.	Integrated, active surveillance of most major sources (food, animals); reliance on extensive collection of representative strains for comparison; information on amount of animal or food product available for consumption.	Best suited to pathogens that are clonally disseminated through the food chain. Useful in identifying original reservoir and setting priorities for interventions when contamination occurs during production.	Usually applied to a single pathogen. In current use, but not well suited to organisms that have relatively unstable DNA. Does not take into account effects of other contamination risk factors (such as human handling, cross-contamination). Assumes equivalence of relative pathogen-specific contribution of each food type to disease. Expensive. Requires extensive libraries of isolates from a range of foods or reservoirs.	van Pelt et al., 2003; Hald et al., 2004, 2007
Quantitative microbial risk assessment Yields mathematically derived estimates of risk.	Information on estimates for parameters to use in modeling and uncertainty distributions for estimates; logic model of how parameters are related to each other.	Allows a high level of detail with respect to specific food commodities. Theoretically, can integrate data obtained from national surveillance programs.	Serious data gaps. Substantial uncertainty (should be accompanied by uncertainty analysis). Resource intensive.	CFSAN/FSIS, 2003 (*Listeria monocytogenes*); Evers et al., 2008
Expert elicitation Experts combine and weigh data from different sources to estimate attribution.	More explicit, structured, quantitative methods (including well-calibrated methods and performance-based weighting) are being used and are increasing resolution and transparency.	Best suited to filling in data gaps. Able to combine information from multiple sources (different experts with different knowledge bases).	Subjective in nature. Potential for bias (based on respondent background, personal bias), although use of structured approaches decreases bias. Best methodological approaches (calibrated, highly structured) require a high degree of expertise and are resource intensive.	Hoffmann et al., 2007a,b; Havelaar et al., 2008

SOURCE: NRC, 2009b.

attribution that must be answered if food safety risks are to be understood and characterized.

Foodborne disease attribution data and models are essential to support a risk-based food safety management approach. They directly support Steps 1 (strategic planning), 2 (public health risk ranking), and 6 (monitoring and review); they also support the other steps of the process indirectly. From a planning perspective, for example, risk ranking must be based on the hazard–food combinations that generate the greatest burden of disease and/or the most significant negative impact on public health. It is difficult to perform such risk ranking without reliable foodborne disease attribution data. Similarly, it is difficult to evaluate and implement risk-based intervention approaches without knowing the most likely means by which a contaminant enters the food chain or which specific practices contribute to its proliferation and/or inactivation. Finally, in monitoring and reviewing the efficacy of risk management strategies that have already been implemented, it is necessary to determine whether public health objectives are being met. Attribution is a logical metric in this regard, perhaps the most important one, as a reduction in the burden of disease associated with a specific food–hazard combination provides the best evidence that interventions are working. The availability of comprehensive epidemiological attribution data also aids in transparency. In short, solid epidemiological attribution data form the cornerstone of risk-based prioritization, management, and evaluation.

KEY CONCLUSIONS AND RECOMMENDATIONS

The committee defined a risk-based food safety management system as "a systematic means by which to facilitate decision making to reduce public health risk in light of limited resources and additional factors that may be considered." The committee went on to define the key attributes of such a system and produced a stepwise approach to its design. The committee recognizes that some of the variables to be considered in models used to rank risks from imported foods will be different from those considered for domestic foods. Variables for models used to rank intentional contamination will be different as well. However, the committee believes the recommended risk-based approach is broad enough to apply to all hazards, whether intentionally introduced or not, and to all foods, whether domestically produced or imported. The committee recognizes that this comprehensive risk-based approach is a relatively new concept that will take time and resources to implement.

While the committee commends the FDA for recent steps taken and progress toward risk ranking and prioritization described in this chapter, the FPP falls short of providing a comprehensive vision for a risk-based food safety management system. Much of the agency's current decision-making process appears to be based on crisis management rather than a systematic preventive approach. Furthermore, although the FDA states in many of its documents that it operates under a risk-based framework, many of the attributes of a risk-based system that the committee regards as necessary (in particular, strategic planning, comprehensiveness, transparency, external review of risk assessment and intervention analysis programs, and risk communication) are not sufficient in the agency's current approach. The resources (personnel, data, models) necessary to design and support a risk-based food safety management system are extensive, and the FDA does not have the human capacity, data infrastructure, or organization to support such a function at the present time. The provision of these resources is essential to the success of the FDA's future food safety risk management activities.

The committee offers the following recommendations to enhance the management of food safety at the FDA.

Recommendation 3-1: The type of risk-based food safety approach outlined by the committee in Box 3-2 should become the operational centerpiece of the FDA's food safety program. This approach should be embraced by all levels of management and should serve as the basis for food safety decision making, including prioritization of resources dedicated to all agency functions (e.g., inspections, promulgation of regulations, research). This approach should be applied to all domestically produced and imported foods and to all food-related hazards, whether due to unintentional or intentional (i.e., with intent to harm) contamination. The FDA should work with local, state, and national regulatory partners to facilitate the incorporation of these principles into their programs.

Recommendation 3-2: The FDA should develop a comprehensive strategic plan for development and implementation of a risk-based food safety management system. The agency should also develop internal operating guidelines for the conduct of risk ranking, risk assessment, risk prioritization, intervention analysis, and the development of metrics with which to evaluate the performance of the system. The strategic plan and guidelines should include descriptions of data, methodologies, technical analyses, and stakeholder engagement. Further, the strategic plan and all guidelines for the risk-based system should be fully supported by the scientific literature and subjected to peer review. When appropriate, the FDA should adopt guidelines already established by other federal agencies or international organizations.

The following recommendations encompass essential steps that need special attention in the implementation of a risk-based approach.

Recommendation 3-3: The FDA, in collaboration with partners, should identify metrics with which to measure the effectiveness of the food safety system, as well as its interventions. The FDA should include these metrics, and plans for any related data collection, as part of strategic planning. The metrics should have a clearly defined link to public health outcomes.

Recommendation 3-4: The FDA should identify expertise needed to implement a risk-based approach. This includes training current and/or hiring new personnel in the areas of strategic planning; management of data; development of biomathematical models and other tools for risk ranking, prioritization, intervention analysis, and evaluation; and risk communication.

REFERENCES

Adak, G. K., S. M. Meakins, H. Yip, B. A. Lopman, and S. J. O'Brien. 2005. Disease risks from foods, England and Wales: 1996–2000. *Emerging Infectious Diseases* 11(3):365–372.

Batz, M. B., S. A. Hoffmann, A. J. Krupnick, J. G. Morris, D. M. Sherman, M. R. Taylor, and J. S. Tick. 2004. *Identifying the Most Significant Microbiological Foodborne Hazards to Public Health: A New Risk Ranking Model.* Food Safety Research Consortium Discussion Paper No. 1. Resources for the Future, Washington, DC. http://www.rff.org/RFF/Documents/FRSC-DP-01.pdf (accessed February 6, 2009).

Batz, M. B., M. P. Doyle, G. Morris, Jr., J. Painter, R. Singh, R. V. Tauxe, M. R. Taylor, and D. M. Lo Fo Wong. 2005. Attributing illness to food. *Emerging Infectious Diseases* 11(7):993–999.

Becker, G. S. 2008. *U.S. Food and Agricultural Imports: Safeguards and Selected Issues.* Washington, DC: Congressional Research Service.

Becker, G. S. 2009. *Food Safety on the Farm: Federal Programs and Selected Proposals.* Washington, DC: Congressional Research Service.

Behn, R. D. 2003. Why measure performance? Different purposes require different measures. *Public Administration Review* 63(5):586–606.

Bell, J. W. 2009. *The USFDA and Ensuring Food Safety Perspective of a Seafood Scientist.* Paper presented at Institute of Medicine/National Research Council Committee on Review of the FDA's Role in Ensuring Safe Food Meeting, Washington, DC, March 24, 2009.

Belton, V., and T. J. Stewart. 2002. *Multiple Criteria Decision Analysis: An Integrated Approach.* Boston, MA: Kluwer Academic Publishers.

Bevan, G., and C. Hood. 2006. Have targets improved performance in the English NHS? *British Medical Journal* 332(7538):419–422.

Bird, S., C. S. David, V. T. Farewell, H. Goldstein, T. Holt, and P. C. Smith. 2005. Performance indicators: Good, bad, and ugly. *Journal of the Royal Statistical Society Series A* 168(Part 1):1–27.

Brougher, C., and G. S. Becker. 2008. *CRS Report for Congress: The USDA's Authority to Recall Meat and Poultry Products.* Washington, DC: Congressional Research Service.

Brownson, R. C., E. A. Baker, T. L. Leet, and K. N. Gillespie. 2003. Chapter 1: The need for evidence-based public health. In *Evidence-Based Public Health*, edited by R. C. Brownson, E. A. Baker, T. L. Leet and K. N. Gillespie. Oxford, UK: Oxford University Press.

CAST (Council for Agricultural Science and Technology). 2006. *Using Risk Analysis to Inform Microbial Food Safety Decisions*. CAST Issue Paper Number 31. Ames, IA: Council for Agricultural Science and Technology.

Cavalluzzo, K. S., and C. D. Ittner. 2004. Implementing performance measurement innovations: Evidence from government. *Accounting, Organizations, and Society* 29(3–4):243–267.

CFSAN (Center for Food Safety and Applied Nutrition). 2008. *Sec. 555.320* Listeria Monocytogenes *Draft Guidance*. F. C. ORA. Rockville, MD: FDA CFSAN. http://www.fda.gov/ICECI/ComplianceManuals/CompliancePolicyGuidanceManual/ucm136694.htm (accessed March 15, 2010).

CFSAN/FSIS (Food Safety Inspection Service). 2003. *Quantitative Assessment of Relative Risk to Public Health from Foodborne* Listeria Monocytogenes *Among Selected Categories of Ready-to-Eat Foods*. Washington, DC: CFSAN/FSIS. http://www.fda.gov/ohrms/dockets/dailys/03/oct03/103003/99n-1168-ra00001-002-Assessment-vol24.doc (accessed February 9, 2009).

Charlebois, S., and C. Yost. 2008. *Food Safety Performance World Ranking 2008*. Saskatchewan, Canada: Research Network in Food Systems, University of Regina. http://www.ontraceagrifood.com/admincp/uploadedfiles/Food%20Safety%20Performance%20World%20Ranking%202008.pdf (accessed on March 13, 2010).

Consumers Union. 2008. *Increased Inspections Needed for Produce, Processing Plants to Protect Consumers from Unsafe Food*. http://www.consumersunion.org/pub/core_food_safety/005732.html (accessed January 25, 2010).

DeWaal, C. S., H. Giselle, K. Barlow, L. Alderton, and L. Vegosen. 2006. Foods associated with foodborne illness outbreaks from 1990 through 2003. *Food Protection Trends* 26(7):466–473.

EFSA (European Food Safety Authority). 2008. Overview of methods for source attribution for human illness from foodborne microbiological hazards: Scientific opinion of the Panel on Biological Hazards. *The EFSA Journal* 764:1–43. http://www.efsa.europa.eu/cs/BlobServer/Scientific_Opinion/biohaz_op_ej764_source_attribution_en.pdf?ssbinary=true (accessed February 6, 2009).

Engeljohn, D. 2009. *USDA's Approach to Ensuring Food Safety*. Paper presented at Institute of Medicine/National Research Council Committee on Review of the FDA's Role in Ensuring Safe Food Meeting, Washington, DC, May 28, 2009.

Evers, E. G., H. J. Van Der Fels-Klerx, M. J. Nauta, J. F. Schijven, and A. H. Havelaar. 2008. *Campylobacter* source attribution by exposure assessment. *International Journal of Risk Assessment and Management* 8(1/2):174–190.

FAO/WHO (Food and Agriculture Organization/World Health Organization). 2006. Food safety risk analysis. A guide for national food safety authorities. *FAO Food and Nutrition Series* 87. ftp://ftp.fao.org/docrep/fao/009/a0822e/a0822e00.pdf (accessed March 5, 2009).

Fazil, A., A. Rajic, J. Sanchez, and S. McEwen. 2008. Choices, choices: The application of multi-criteria decision analysis to a food safety decision-making problem. *Journal of Food Protection* 71(11):2323–2333.

FDA (U.S. Food and Drug Administration). 2005. *Pathogenic Vibrio Parahaemolyticus in Raw Oysters: Quantitative Risk Assessment on the Public Health Impact of Pathogenic* Vibrio Parahaemolyticus *in Raw Oysters*. http://www.fda.gov/Food/ScienceResearch/ResearchAreas/RiskAssessmentSafetyAssessment/ucm050421.htm (accessed January 26, 2010).

FDA. 2009. Office of the Commissioner reorganization; statement of organizations, functions, and delegations of authority: Action notice. *Federal Register* 74(158):41713–41734.

Friedman, C. R., R. M.Hoekstra, M. Samuel, R. Marcus, J. Bender, B. Shiferaw, S. Reddy, S. Ahuja, D. L. Helfrick, F. Hardnett, M. Carter, B. Anderson, and R. V. Tauxe. 2004. Risk factors for sporadic *Campylobacter* infection in the United States: A case-control study in FoodNet sites. *Clinical Infectious Diseases* 38(Suppl. 3):S285–S296.

GAO (U.S. Government Accountability Office). 2004a. *Federal Food Safety and Security System: Fundamental Restructuring Is Needed to Address Fragmentation and Overlap.* Washington, DC: GAO.

GAO. 2004b. *Food Safety: FDA's Imported Seafood Safety Program Shows Some Progress, but Further Improvements Are Needed.* Washington, DC: GAO.

GAO. 2004c. *Food Safety: USDA and FDA Need to Better Ensure Prompt and Complete Recalls of Potentially Unsafe Food.* Washington, DC: GAO.

GAO. 2005. *Overseeing the U.S. Food Supply: Steps Should Be Taken to Reduce Overlapping Inspections and Related Activities.* Washington, DC: GAO.

GAO. 2007. *Federal Oversight of Food Safety: High-Risk Designation Can Bring Needed Attention to Fragmented System.* Washington, DC: GAO.

GAO. 2008. *Food Safety: Improvements Needed in FDA Oversight of Fresh Produce.* Washington, DC: GAO.

GAO. 2009a. *Agencies Need to Address Gaps in Enforcement and Collaboration to Enhance Safety of Imported Food.* Washington, DC: GAO.

GAO. 2009b. *Information Technology: FDA Needs to Establish Key Plans and Processes for Guiding Systems Modernization Efforts.* Washington, DC: GAO.

Givens, J. M. 2009. *Review of FDA's Role in Ensuring Safe Food (FDA's Approach to Risk Based Inspections—A Field Perspective).* Paper presented at Institute of Medicine/National Research Council Committee on Review of the FDA's Role in Ensuring Safe Food Meeting, Washington, DC, March 24, 2009.

Gombas, D. E. 2009. *FDA's Role in Food Safety: A Produce Industry Perspective.* Paper presented at Institute of Medicine/National Research Council Committee on Review of the FDA's Role in Ensuring Safe Food Meeting, Washington, DC, March 24, 2009.

Gueorguieva, V., J. Accius, C. Apaza, L. Bennett, C. Brownley, S. Cronin, and P. Preechyanud. 2009. The Program Assessment Rating Tool and the Government Performance and Results Act: Evaluating conflicts and disconnections. *American Review of Public Administration* 39(3):225–245.

Hald, T., D. Vose, H. C. Wegener, and T. Koupeev. 2004. A Bayesian approach to quantify the contribution of animal-food sources to human salmonellosis. *Risk Analsyis* 24(1):255–269.

Hald, T., D. M. Lo Fo Wong, and F. M. Aarestrup. 2007. The attribution of human infections with antibiotic resistant *Salmonella* bacteria in Denmark to sources of animal origin. *Foodborne Pathogens and Disease* 4(3):313–326.

Hammond, J. S., R. L. Keeney, and H. Raiffa. 1999. *Smart Choices: A Practical Guide to Better Decision Making.* Boston, MA: Harvard Business Publishing.

Hartogensis, M. 2009. *Feed and Pet Food Safety at the Center for Veterinary Medicine.* Paper presented at Institute of Medicine/National Research Council Committee on Review of the FDA's Role in Ensuring Safe Food Meeting, Washington, DC, May 28, 2009.

Havelaar, A. H., J. Braunig, K. Christiansen, M. Cornu, T. Hald, M. J. Mangen, K. Molbak, A. Pielaat, E. Snary, M. Van Boven, W. Van Pelt, A. Velthuis, and H. Wahlstrom. 2006. Towards an integrated approach in supporting microbiological food safety decisions. *Zoonoses Public Health* 54(3–4):103–117.

Havelaar, A. H., A. V. Galindo, D. Kurowicka, and R. M. Cooke. 2008. Attribution of food-borne pathogens using structured expert elicitation. *Foodborne Pathogens and Disease* 5(5):649–659.

Henson, S. J., J. A. Caswell, J. A. Cranfield, A. Fazil, V. J. Davidson, S. M. Anders, and C. Schmidt. 2007. A multi-factorial risk prioritization framework for food-borne pathogens. In *Department of Resource Economics: Working Paper 2007-8.* http://people.umass.edu/resec/workingpapers/documents/ResEcWorkingPaper2007-8.pdf (accessed January 26, 2010).

Hoffmann, S., P. Fischbeck, A. Krupnick, and M. McWilliams. 2007a. Using expert elicitation to link foodborne illnesses in the United States to foods. *Journal of Food Protection* 70(5):1220–1229.

Hoffmann, S., P. Fischbeck, A. Krupnick, and M. McWilliams. 2007b. Elicitation from large, heterogeneous expert panels: Using multiple uncertainty measures to characterize information quality for decision analysis. *Decision Analysis* 4(2):91–109.

IOM/NRC (Institute of Medicine/National Research Council). 1998. *Ensuring Safe Food: From Production to Consumption.* Washington, DC: National Academy Press.

IOM/NRC. 2003. *Scientific Criteria to Ensure Safe Food.* Washington, DC: The National Academies Press.

IPCS (International Programme on Chemical Safety). 2004. *IPCS Risk Assessment Terminology.* Geneva, Switzerland: World Health Organization.

IRGC (International Risk Governance Council). 2005. *White Paper on Risk Governance: Towards an Integrative Approach.* Geneva, Switzerland: IRGC. www.irgc.org (accessed May 14, 2010).

IRGC. 2009. *Risk Governance Deficits. An Analysis and Illustration of the Most Common Deficits in Risk Governance.* Geneva, Switzerland: IRGC. www.irgc.org (accessed May 14, 2010).

Johnsen, A. 2005. What does 25 years of experience tell us about the state of performance measurement in public policy and management? *Public Money and Management* 25(1):9–17.

Lynn, L. E. 1998. *Requiring Bureaucracies to Perform: What Have We Learned from the U.S. Government Performance and Results Act (GPRA)?* Second Revised Draft. The University of Chicago Harris School Working Papers, September 1, 1998. http://harrisschool.uchicago.edu/about/publications/working-papers/ (accessed March 9, 2010).

Maczka, C. 2009. *FSIS Data-Driven Inspection.* Paper presented at Institute of Medicine/National Research Council Committee on Review of the FDA's Role in Ensuring Safe Food Meeting, Washington, DC, May 28, 2009.

Mangen, M. J., M. B. Batz, A. Kasbohrer, T. Hald, J. G. Morris Jr., M. Taylor, and A. H. Havelaar. 2009. Integrated approaches for the public health prioritization of foodborne and zoonotic pathogens. *Risk Analysis* 30:702–797.

Marcus, R., J. K. Varma, C. Medus, E. J. Boothe, B. J. Anderson, T. Crume, K. E. Fullerton, M. R. Moore, P. L. White, E. Lyszkowicz, A. C. Voetsch, and F. J. Angula. 2007. Re-assessment of risk factors for sporadic *Salmonella* serotype Enteritidis infections: A case-control study in five FoodNet Sites, 2002–2003. *Epidemiology and Infection* 135(1):84–92.

Morgan, M. G., B. Fischhoff, A. Bostrom, L. Lave, and C. J. Atman. 1992. Communicating risk to the public. *Environmental Science and Technology* 26(11):2048–2056.

NRC (National Research Council). 2009a. *Informing Decisions in a Changing Climate.* Washington, DC: The National Academies Press.

NRC. 2009b. *Letter Report on the Review of the Food Safety and Inspection Service Proposed Risk-Based Approach to and Application of Public-Health Attribution.* Washington, DC: The National Academies Press.

NRC/IOM (Institute of Medicine). 2009. *Letter Report on the Development of a Model for Ranking FDA Product Categories on the Basis of Health Risks.* Washington, DC: The National Academies Press.

Radin, B. 2006. *Challenging the Performance Movement: Accountability, Complexity and Democratic Values.* Washington, DC: Georgetown University Press.

Ruzante, J. M., V. J. Davidson, J. Caswell, A. Fazil, J. A. L. Cranfield, S. J. Henson, S. M. Anders, C. Schmidt, and J. Farber. 2009. A multi-factorial risk prioritization framework for foodborne pathogens. *Risk Analysis* 30(5):724–742.

Scallan, E. 2007. Activities, achievements, and lessons learned during the first 10 years of the Foodborne Diseases Active Surveillance Network: 1996–2005. *Clinical Infectious Diseases* 44(5):718–725.

Scott, J. 2009. *GMA Perspective on FDA's Role in Ensuring Safe Food.* Paper presented at Institute of Medicine/National Research Council Committee on Review of the FDA's Role in Ensuring Safe Food Meeting, Washington, DC, March 24, 2009.

Solomon, S. 2009. *Regulating in the Global Environment.* Paper presented at Institute of Medicine/National Research Council Committee on Review of the FDA's Role in Ensuring Safe Food Meeting, Washington, DC, March 24, 2009.

Taylor, J. 2009. Strengthening the link between performance measurement and decision making. *Public Administration* 87(4):853–871.

Taylor, M. R. 2002. *Reforming Food Safety: A Model for the Future.* Washington, DC: Resources for the Future. http://www.rff.org/rff/Documents/RFF-IB-02-02.pdf (accessed January 25, 2010).

Taylor, M. R., and S. A. Hoffman. 2001. *Redesigning Food Safety: Using Risk Analysis to Build a Better Food Safety System.* Washington, DC: Resources for the Future. http://www.rff.org/documents/RFF-DP-01-24.pdf (accessed January 26, 2010).

Treasury Board of Canada Secretariat. 2007. *Assessing, Selecting, and Implementing Instruments for Government Action.* Secretariat: Her Majesty the Queen in Right of Canada. http://www.tbs-sct.gc.ca (accessed January 26, 2010).

Tucker-Foreman, C. L. 2009. *Testimony of Carol L. Tucker-Foreman, Distinguished Fellow, The Food Policy Institute, Consumer Federation of America, before the Committee on Agriculture, U.S. House of Representatives.* Agriculture. Washington, DC.

USDA (U.S. Department of Agriculture). 2010. *FSIS National Residue Program for Cattle.* http://www.usda.gov/oig/webdocs/24601-08-KC.pdf (accessed on May 12, 2010).

van Pelt, W., M. A. de Wit, W. J. Wannet, E. J. Ligtvoet, M. A. Widdowson. and Y. T. van Duynhoven. 2003. Laboratory surveillance of bacterial gastroenteric pathogens in the Netherlands, 1991–2001. *Epidemiology and Infection* 130(3):431–441.

Varma, J. K., M. C. Samuel, R. Marcus, R. M. Hoekstra, C. Medua, S. Segler, B. J. Anderson, T. F. Jones, B. Shiferaw, N. Haubert, M. Megginson, P. V. McCarthy, L. Graves, T. Van Gilder, and F. J. Angula. 2007. *Listeria monocytogenes* infection from foods prepared in a commercial establishment: A case-control study of potential sources of sporadic illness in the United States. *Clinical Infectious Diseases* 44(15):521–528.

Wagner, R. 2009. *FDA'S Current Approach to Risk Based Domestic Inspection Planning.* Paper presented at Institute of Medicine/National Research Council Committee on Review of the FDA's Role in Ensuring Safe Food Meeting, Washington, DC, March 24, 2009.

4

Sharing the Responsibility
for a Risk-Based System:
Models of Governance and Oversight

The safety of the U.S. domestic and imported food system is a responsibility shared by suppliers, farmers, food handlers, processors, wholesalers and retailers, food service companies, consumers, third-party organizations, and government (federal and state) agencies in the United States and abroad. Given the size and scope of the system, it is unrealistic to expect the U.S. Food and Drug Administration (FDA), or any agency at the federal level, to be everywhere and to do everything necessary to ensure food safety through surveillance and inspection without the help of those who share this responsibility.

The design of approaches to governance to achieve society's goals has been the subject of much debate and experimentation in a wide range of areas, from the financial system to public safety. The published literature on the subject addresses the pros and cons of various approaches to sharing responsibility, factors to be considered, and lessons learned from the implementation of these approaches. Models of governance that deviate from the traditional enforcement of rules through the imposition of penalties include voluntary approaches whereby regulators work with industry to develop codes of practice, third-party audits, management-based systems in which firms are responsible for adhering to plans that limit harms, and performance-based approaches that emphasize results rather than the use of specific technologies or actions. These alternatives may serve to distribute accountability across all parties that might affect outcomes.

Innovative governance approaches have already been applied to the environment, building safety, consumer product safety, nuclear power plant safety, transportation safety, and health care, among many other areas, with

BOX 4-1
Examples of the Use of Alternative Governance Approaches

Nuclear Power Safety

Before the Nuclear Regulatory Commission (NRC) focused attention on issues essential to protecting public health, the Atomic Energy Commission was often criticized for its dual role in protecting public health while also avoiding imposing requirements that would inhibit the growth of the industry. With respect to nuclear reactors, the NRC took the traditional approach of creating standards and requirements to protect public health, eventually giving operators the sense that accidents would be prevented as long as compliance with these standards and requirements was verified by an inspector. This traditional prescriptive approach, however, was criticized as being unable to promote uniform levels of safety. The NRC then moved toward a risk-based system, whereby accountability is placed on the operator's side. However, the Government Accountability Office has noted major challenges to the success of this system, including the need to encourage a shift to a culture of safety, significant human capital needs and costs, and methodological challenges (GAO, 2006).

British Railway System

Potential limitations of implementing novel governance approaches in the health and safety arena may be evident in the experience of the British railway system. Hutter (2001) suggests that such a move may have led to breaches in public safety. Often, a self-regulatory regime is seen as a superior governance model in that it relies not only on government accountability, but also on the capacity of corporations to regulate themselves and develop systems tailored to their specific operations. Innovation is encouraged, and companies are more likely to follow their own rules than rules imposed on them. Hutter argues that in the case of the railway industry in Britain, enforced self-regulation was not appropriately monitored and ended up being itself the source of risk. In fact, the self-regulation was more procedural than substantive; although rules were in place, they were not well understood. Lack of communication was a major explanation for the failure of the system in a company that was fragmented functionally and geographically.

both failure and success. Examples are presented in Box 4-1. These examples illustrate that developing criteria for selecting a governance approach, making the selection, and evaluating performance outcomes are essential activities for regulatory agencies. These two examples are but a small sampling of the many models of regulation and oversight that exist, and the selection of the most appropriate model for specific circumstances is a subject of active debate. Even within the area of food safety, several different models of governance are evolving worldwide (Batz et al., 2005; Garcia-Martinez et al., 2007; Treasury Board of Canada Secretariat, 2007).

Chapter 3 describes the elements that are essential to the operation of a risk-based food safety system, as concluded by the committee. A governance model for the FDA must articulate criteria for deciding who is responsible for overseeing the various elements, for choosing and implementing policy interventions, and for evaluating the performance of the system. Defining the nature and range of shared responsibility is central to implementing several of these elements. This need for clearly reasoned models for shared responsibility and oversight is the subject of this chapter. The chapter reviews approaches to making governance decisions and developing a regulatory philosophy, as well as choosing policy interventions and assigning responsibility. The discussion includes the committee's observations on how the FDA selects models of governance.

OVERALL APPROACH TO MAKING GOVERNANCE DECISIONS AND DEVELOPING A REGULATORY PHILOSOPHY

The Food Protection Plan (FPP), written in 2007 under the leadership of the Office of Food Protection, contains the FDA's general philosophy with respect to food safety and focuses on what the agency considers to be the core elements of food safety: prevention, intervention, and response (see Box 4-2). The FPP also outlines the following four cross-cutting principles for a comprehensive food protection approach: (1) focus on risks over a product's life cycle from production to consumption, (2) target resources to achieve maximum risk reduction, (3) address both unintentional and deliberate contamination, and (4) use science and modern technology systems. To operationalize these elements and principles and to strengthen its ability to protect Americans from foodborne illnesses, the FDA proposes internal administrative changes and recognizes the need to make legislative changes (Box 4-3). The FPP is a platform for initiating a transformation at the FDA, whereby policy decisions are based on prevention and risk. However, it does not provide detail on how the principles it outlines will be achieved. The committee supports the findings of the U.S. Government Accountability Office (GAO) (GAO, 2008a,b) that the plan does not offer specific strategies for many of the actions proposed. For example, although it refers to risk-based inspections, detail on analytical risk models or even factors that will be considered in developing such models is absent. The terms "risk" and "risk-based approaches" are understood in different ways, underlining the importance of detailed articulation of such factors. Indeed, Chapter 3 explains the importance of a regulatory agency's delineating in detail a broad strategic

---

BOX 4-2
Three Core Elements of Food Safety in the
U.S. Food and Drug Administration's Food Protection Plan

Prevent foodborne contamination:
- Promote increased corporate responsibility to prevent foodborne illnesses.
- Identify food vulnerabilities and assess risks.
- Expand the understanding and use of effective mitigation measures.

Intervene at critical points in the food supply chain:
- Focus inspections and sampling based on risk.
- Enhance risk-based surveillance.
- Improve the detection of food system "signals" that indicate contamination.

Respond rapidly to minimize harm:
- Improve immediate response.
- Improve risk communications to the public, industry, and other stakeholders.

---

approach that explains its philosophy, that is, the factors it will weigh in making decisions about prioritization of efforts, allocation of resources, and selection of interventions. The committee concluded that the FPP should be supported by the kind of detailed strategic planning (both broad and specific) outlined in Chapter 3. To illustrate this shortcoming, this section describes the committee's understanding of the FPP's vision for the responsibilities of different parties involved in food safety and how it could be improved.

As part of the strategic planning process (Step 1 in the risk-based system described in Chapter 3), the responsibilities of all parties in achieving the desired level of food safety must be articulated. Because these responsibilities will vary with the situation, and new situations are always arising, there must also be a road map for assigning responsibilities based on a defined set of factors. These elements of a risk-based system constitute an agency's regulatory philosophy.

The FPP makes several statements about the responsibilities of different parties in the food safety system. A major plank of its prevention strategy is a call for promoting increased corporate responsibility to prevent foodborne illness. The plan notes that examples of enhanced corporate responsibility might include "evaluating safety and security vulnerabilities and possible impacts; when appropriate, implementing preventive measures—

BOX 4-3
Additional Protections That Involve
Legislative Changes to the U.S. Food and Drug
Administration's (FDA's) Authority

Prevent foodborne contamination:
- Allow the FDA to require preventive controls to prevent intentional adulteration by terrorists or criminals at points of high vulnerability in the food chain.
- Authorize the FDA to institute additional preventive controls for high-risk foods.
- Require food facilities to renew their FDA registrations every 2 years, and allow the FDA to modify the registration categories.

Intervene at critical points in the food supply chain:
- Authorize the FDA to accredit highly qualified third parties for voluntary food inspections.
- Require a new reinspection fee from facilities that fail to meet current Good Manufacturing Practices.
- Authorize the FDA to require electronic import certificates for shipments of designated high-risk products.
- Require a new food and animal feed export certification fee to improve the ability of U.S. firms to export their products.
- Provide parity between domestic and imported foods if FDA inspection access is delayed, limited, or denied.

Respond rapidly to minimize harm:
- Empower the FDA to issue a mandatory recall of food products when voluntary recalls are not effective.
- Give the FDA enhanced access to food records during emergencies.

---

both required and voluntary—to ensure that food is produced safely and securely; and developing a contingency plan to aid in a response in the event of contamination" (FDA, 2007a, p. 14). The plan states that an increased emphasis on prevention "will require close interaction with growers, manufacturers, distributors, retailers and food service providers, and importers. These partners have the ability to implement preventive approaches and to require them of their suppliers" (p. 11).

The FPP also states that:

[t]hose with the biggest stake in food safety, after the consumers who eat the food, are the people and companies who grow, process, and sell

food. Their livelihood depends entirely on the confidence of their customers. A poor reputation for proper food handling can drive a company to bankruptcy. Promoting increased corporate responsibility is key in shifting FDA's food protection effort to a proactive rather than a reactive one. The FDA will seek partnerships with industry to enhance consumer confidence. FDA will continue to work with industry in a) developing food protection plans that address safety and defense vulnerabilities, b) implementing prevention steps, and c) developing contingency plans to improve response to an outbreak of foodborne illness. (p. 15)

In addition, the FPP supports exploring new roles for third-party certification as part of the overall system of food safety assurance. As to working with other responsible parties, the plan states:

FDA will continue to work with industry, state, local, and foreign governments to further develop the tools and science needed to identify vulnerabilities and determine the most effective approaches. With regard to imports, FDA will also work with foreign governments, which have a greater ability to oversee manufacturers within their borders to ensure compliance with safety standards. (p. 11)

Finally, concerning consumer responsibility, the plan notes, "Consumers protect themselves and their families from foodborne illness by responding promptly to FDA alerts" (p. 23).

The above statements indicate that the FDA is focusing on the need for shared responsibility in designing its food safety program. In several exchanges with FDA staff, however, the committee did not find that the FDA has a well-thought-out approach to defining food safety responsibilities beyond these general statements. On several occasions, for example, the committee invited FDA officials to further articulate what the agency sees as the substance and consequences of the FPP's call for placing more responsibility on the corporate sector. The officials were unable to do so, nor did their answers recognize the need for a systematic approach (a road map) to making these decisions. The agency's approach appears to be ad hoc and its regulatory philosophy unclear.

Describing the role of each responsible party is an important activity for a regulatory agency and an essential element of its strategic plan. A model for choosing modes of governance is integral to the subsequent choice of interventions and their design and implementation (Steps 4 and 5 of a risk-based system). This model should account for a range of factors that will differ across risks, such as the sources and controllability of risks and the structure of the supply chain, and will affect what mix of shared responsibility will address the risks most effectively.

A generic list of governance options is a useful starting point for thinking about shared responsibility for food safety. An example of such as a list is shown in Figure 4-1 (adapted from Garcia-Martinez et al., 2007). On one end of the spectrum, food safety is entirely an individual, private responsibility, and there is no intervention by public agencies. On the other end of the spectrum is direct regulation, whereby public agencies prescribe what companies must or must not do in ensuring food safety, for example, with respect to production practices, product standards, or labeling. This end of the spectrum is frequently referred to as a "command and control" approach. Between these extremes is a range of public–private mixes. Self-regulation involves the use of industry voluntary codes of practice and farm assurance schemes with self- or third-party certification. Information and education entails the government's generating and communicating information for the use of private parties. Coregulation denotes programs in which responsibility is shared in a public–private partnership, for example, when statutes incorporate industry codes of practice. Finally, incentive-based

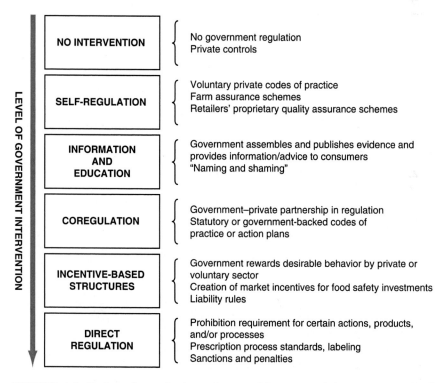

FIGURE 4-1 Options for assigning private–public responsibility to ensure food safety.
SOURCE: Adapted from Garcia-Martinez et al. (2007).

structures vary the amount and type of regulatory oversight based on how well a company performs; this is frequently referred to as a performance approach and also includes the setting of liability rules and related concepts, such as due diligence.

The nature of shared responsibility for the management of food safety risks will evolve over time as legislation is passed, new circumstances arise, knowledge grows, stakeholders express different priorities, and constraints

---

BOX 4-4
Managing the Safety of Produce:
An Example of Evolving Shared Responsibility

An example of how the U.S. Food and Drug Administration (FDA) has modified its governance philosophy over time is the case of produce safety. While the FDA has jurisdiction over produce, in the past it did not exercise this authority through direct regulation. This lack of direct oversight occurred in part because the FDA gave priority to its efforts to control contaminants in foods known to present such problems, and at the time fresh produce was not recognized as an important vehicle for pathogens. Until recently, there were no guidelines, codes of practice, or regulations directed toward ensuring the safety of fresh produce during production and processing.

The FDA started to pay more attention to produce safety when various produce items were identified as vehicles for foodborne illness outbreaks. Recent examples of FDA attempts to manage the safety of fresh produce include the Tomato Safety Initiative (FDA, 2007b), the Lettuce Initiative (FDA, 2009a), and Produce Safety from Production to Consumption (FDA, 2004). Important efforts common to all these initiatives were continuing to reach out to the produce industry, facilitating and promoting research, and working with federal, state, and local public health officials in illness detection and outbreak response. These efforts are examples of an information and education approach to intervention (see Figure 4-1).

The FDA first developed Guidelines for Agricultural Practices in 1998. They were followed by guidelines for minimizing or eliminating microbial contamination in commodities that appear to present the greatest risks: tomatoes, leafy greens, and melons. As guidelines, however, none of these documents are enforceable. To encourage the farm community to accept and adopt them, the FDA has engaged in information and education programs, for example, through dedicated efforts by cooperative extension offices.

The lack of strong regulatory action by the FDA drove some states to

shift. Based on outcomes, the mix of responsibility chosen initially may prove to be too reliant on voluntary action, at one end of the spectrum, or too focused on prescriptive government regulations, at the other end. A salient example of this evolution is the FDA's regulatory approach to the safety of produce (see Box 4-4). The committee notes that an evolving approach makes sense, but found that the FDA's approach frequently

implement stricter measures. For example, the Tomato Good Agricultural Practices (Florida Department of Agriculture and Consumer Services, 2007) are now included in a rule aimed at enhancing the safety of fresh tomatoes produced or handled in Florida; this is an example of direct regulation. Although voluntary, the California Leafy Greens Marketing Agreement (LGMA, 2010), overseen by the California Department of Food and Agriculture, is a mechanism for verifying that participating growers (99 percent of leafy green vegetable production volume) follow specific food safety practices. A similar program implemented in Arizona covers approximately 75 percent of leafy green vegetables produced in the state (AZLGMA, 2008). These efforts are a form of coregulation.

In fall 2009, the FDA announced that the agency will issue regulations setting enforceable standards for fresh produce safety at the farm and packing house, based on prevention-oriented public health principles and on current knowledge and guides (HHS/FDA, 2009). The FDA's proposed rule would establish standards for the implementation of preventive controls, emphasizing the importance of environmental assessments and recognizing the need to tailor preventive controls to particular hazards and operations. This shift in the FDA's governance approach to produce safety from an educational model to direct regulation could be due to many factors, including new research findings, an increased rate of foodborne illness that suggests higher risk attributed to produce, a low rate of implementation or effectiveness of FDA guidelines, or a change in general philosophy about the management of food safety within the agency. In fact, communications from the FDA about what is expected of industry and regulatory approaches taken over the years have not clearly articulated the rationale for changes or provided a road map that would enable stakeholders to participate in and anticipate such changes.

cannot be tied systematically to an underlying regulatory philosophy and related road map for making these decisions.

Regardless of the governance models selected or policy interventions used to achieve them, food safety will always be the responsibility of many partners. Thus cooperation and collaboration are key not only in the collection, analysis, and sharing of information and data but also in the enforcement and oversight of policies. A lack of cooperation and collaboration among the many entities with responsibility for food safety results in an inefficient food safety system. To be credible, the development of governance models must be done with transparency and stakeholder involvement.

CHOOSING POLICY INTERVENTIONS AND ASSIGNING/SHARING RESPONSIBILITY

A risk-based approach entails identifying important risks to target and stating the means that will be used to control them. Many factors enter into the selection and design of policy interventions (Steps 4 and 5 in a risk-based system). Given the complexity involved (multiple risks, multiple candidate interventions, uncertainty of information), regulatory agencies benefit from having a risk-based road map for identifying and selecting interventions. Once policy interventions have been selected, assigning responsibility to different parties in the system is an important aspect of their implementation.

The Policy Interventions Tool Kit

Governments and their regulatory agencies can chose from a broad range of possible interventions to influence the performance of markets. It is useful to think of these interventions as a tool kit offering multiple options, depending on the job at hand. In its main document on intervention choice, the Treasury Board of Canada Secretariat (2007) uses the term "policy instruments" to refer to this set of interventions, defined as follows:

> Instruments for government action are the means a government has at its disposal to achieve public policy outcomes—to govern. While several definitions of "instruments for government action" exist, this document uses a broad interpretation, defining them as the **"means by which policy objectives are pursued"** [emphasis in original]. Instruments for government action set up relationships between the state and its citizens. In some cases, such as criminal law, the relationship is of a coercive nature. In other cases, such as legal agreements, the relationship is reciprocal. (p. 3)

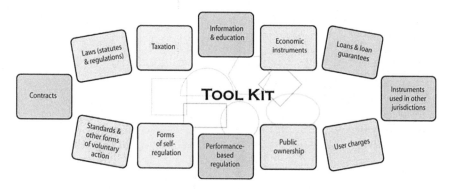

FIGURE 4-2 The interventions tool kit.
SOURCE: Treasury Board of Canada Secretariat, 2007.

Figure 4-2 shows the classes of interventions outlined in the document. These tools are frequently used in combination to achieve the desired performance outcomes.

Road Maps for Choosing Policy Interventions

Deciding what policy interventions to use in different situations and determining the associated assignment of responsibilities is facilitated by having a road map of factors to consider in the selection process. It is common for multiple interventions to be in place simultaneously. For example, processing standards may ensure food safety, while consumer labeling educates about safe use. Referring to Figure 4-1, explicitly thinking about which level of intervention or mix of levels to use and why can lead to choices that enhance the effectiveness of the food safety system.

As mentioned above, the committee asked FDA officials to explain the FDA's thought process in selecting interventions. From these discussions and a review of FDA documents, the committee concluded that the FDA does not have a systematic method for making these decisions at Step 4 of the risk-based approach. Several countries have developed road maps of the type suggested by the committee. For example, the United Kingdom's Food Standards Agency has in place a regulatory framework[1] (FSA, 2006), and a set of detailed impact assessments has been completed (FSA, 2010).[2] Box 4-5 presents an example of a road map for choosing interventions, developed by the Treasury Board of Canada Secretariat (2007).

---

[1] See http://www.food.gov.uk/foodindustry/regulation/betregs/regframe (accessed February 12, 2010).

[2] See http://www.food.gov.uk/foodindustry/regulation/betregs/ria (accessed February 12, 2010).

BOX 4-5
Example Analytical Framework for Selecting Policy Instruments

The Treasury Board of Canada Secretariat (2007) has developed a framework (see the figure below) for selecting policy instruments (its term for what this report calls interventions) for use by all departments and agencies, which may use the framework as is or as a template for developing their own framework for their respective areas of responsibility. The framework is intended to facilitate a disciplined approach to assessing, selecting, and implementing instruments. According to the Secretariat, the framework establishes a sequence of enquiry, specifies a methodological foundation, and provides guidance for each step in the instrument choice process. The benefits identified as flowing from the use of this framework are

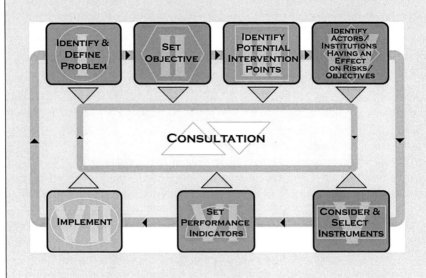

Assigning/Sharing Responsibility

The FDA or any agency charged with managing food safety must have mechanisms for overseeing food safety both domestically and internationally (for imported foods). Different intervention choices incorporate different assignments of responsibility for ensuring that the desired level of food safety assurance is achieved. The key parties to whom different levels of responsibility for food safety may be assigned include the private sec-

- greater transparency in decision making by providing an explicit rationale for instrument choices,
- greater cohesion in decision making by providing a disciplined approach for assessing and selecting instruments,
- overcoming risk aversion by using a risk-based analysis that will assist in understanding the challenges and the most appropriate means of addressing risks, and
- better outcomes by selecting an appropriate mix of instruments.

The Secretariat states that the framework is based on two overarching rationales:

(1) The process of analyzing a situation or problem and considering means by which the government could take appropriate action is iterative.
(2) The contribution of consultation (e.g., risk communication) throughout this iterative process is crucial. It enhances government transparency, promotes knowledge sharing, and supports the integrity of government action.

The framework is not intended to be a sequential road map of where and how officials should assess instruments to achieve public policy objectives. The process is inherently iterative in that the accumulation of information and knowledge concerning a problem or situation and the objectives the government is aiming to achieve will require officials to revisit each of the steps in the framework repeatedly. The framework document presents simple but complete approaches to each step of the instrument choice process.

SOURCE: Treasury Board of Canada Secretariat, 2007.

tor, third-party or other accrediting organizations, governments of other countries, and the states.

The Private Sector

A regulatory agency needs to set clear food safety standards and enforce those standards. At the same time, industry has, and must have, the primary responsibility for ensuring food safety because it is the sector that actually makes or grows the products and is in closest touch with problems as they occur. Industry has broad roles to play; for example, it conducts research on mitigation strategies to produce solutions for food safety practices. Another role of industry is to innovate and explore management approaches. For example, systems analogous to the Hazard Analysis and Critical Control Points (HACCP) system were already in existence and had been applied in some food processing operations prior to being considered by the government as a preventive approach (IOM/NRC, 2003).

In HACCP-based systems, industry formulates control plans that the regulatory agency oversees. When reviewing a HACCP plan, the agency can determine whether the technologies proposed are adequate for food safety protection and are being used appropriately.

Private-sector responsibility is carried out within the range of intervention strategies outlined above. For example, industry responsibility may vary if the government has no intervention strategy. It may take the form of complying with information interventions, for example, with the new requirement of a reportable food registry. Tort law, tax incentives, subsidies, other incentive-based interventions, and direct regulation are other strategies for producing the desired level of food safety. As noted above, the preferred choice of interventions and related assignment of responsibility evolve over time. Box 4-6 describes a current example of this evolution in the area of traceability.

Third-Party Certification

Interest has grown in the use of quality assurance by accreditation bodies (third-party certification) to ensure food safety rather than (or in addition to) relying on government agencies. These assurance/accreditation bodies may be an industry group (the self-regulation option of Figure 4-1) or a third party that is independent of individual firms or the government. They can develop and accredit standards, providing assurance to buyers in the supply chain and/or to consumers. In coregulation interventions, such bodies can partner with the government to ensure food safety. In incentive-based interventions, they can be used as a means of credibly signaling lower risk to the government and may lead to streamlined oversight (e.g., to a fast track for imports).

The use of third-party accreditation as an aspect of government interventions is controversial and, at this time, is more accepted in some countries than in others. Significant questions arise as to how and by whom the accreditation bodies themselves are audited, how transparent they are, to what extent they solicit and use stakeholder input, and whether the audits are reliable (Albersmeier et al., 2009). In the context of a risk-based food safety

BOX 4-6
Example of the Evolution of
Shared Responsibility for Traceability

The term "food traceability" can be defined generally as the ability to identify where a food comes from. In the area of food safety, traceability refers to the ability to identify a food product's history (e.g., processes, locations, manufacturers). Past experience with foodborne illness or contamination investigations has demonstrated that determining the history of a food product from production to consumption can be a daunting, time- and resource-consuming effort in the United States, but one that is absolutely necessary to making decisions during and after a crisis.

With the idea of providing food agencies with prompt, necessary information, Section 306 of the Public Health Security and Bioterrorism Preparedness and Response Act of 2002 requires the establishment and maintenance of records that allow for identification of the immediate previous sources and subsequent recipients of food.[a] This information, along with labels that identify the contents of the package and the name and address of the manufacturer, packer, or distributor must be made available to the U.S. Food and Drug Administration (FDA) within 24 hours when food contamination is suspected.

However, the lack of guidance for best practices and the fact that companies already follow their own traceability procedures for other purposes (e.g., safety, quality, marketing) have resulted in a diverse system with limited value for the FDA. Food traceability for safety purposes is an example of a situation in which simply letting individual food companies establish procedures with little guidance, coordination, or leadership has not led to a well-functioning system.

For traceability to be useful during a crisis, procedures need to be seamless and effective. Setting standards is essential. Because both industry and government play distinctive roles (i.e., the system needs to be feasible and practical for industry but also needs to be usable by government investigators), it may be necessary for them to set the standards in collaboration, with a clear definition of the roles of the partners. As this report is being written, the FDA and the U.S. Department of Agriculture have engaged in a joint dialogue with industry to address past inefficiencies by developing procedures that will be useful during investigations (*Federal Register*, 2009). Collaboration of this type can move systems forward to meet both societal and industry needs.

---

[a]*Public Health Security and Bioterrorism Preparedness and Response Act of 2002 (Bioterrorism Act)*, Public Law 107-188, 107th Cong., 2nd sess. (January 23, 2002), 306.

system, a key question is whether these systems meet standards for being risk based and, in particular, how well they address public health issues.

The rapid growth of auditing platforms (e.g., those of the Global Food Safety Initiative, the International Organization for Standardization, Safe Quality Food [SQF], the British Research Consortium [BRC], the Global Partnership for Good Agricultural Practice [GlobalGAP]) shows that supply chains see value in these systems. Interest in leveraging these systems in government regulation and oversight stems from a desire to gain possible efficiencies in the production of food safety through the elimination of duplication of effort. Increased reliance on these systems, however, requires regulatory agencies to institute a system for auditing the auditors and setting standard criteria for these operations.

The FDA has been exploring this issue. For example, as noted earlier, the FPP calls for new legislative authority to authorize the agency to accredit highly qualified third parties for voluntary food inspections. This legislation would authorize the FDA to accredit independent third parties (or to recognize accrediting bodies) to evaluate compliance with FDA requirements, allowing the agency to allocate inspection resources more effectively. According to the FPP,

> FDA would use information from these accredited third-party organizations in its decision making but not be bound by such information in determining compliance with FDA requirements. Use of accredited third parties would be voluntary and might offer more in-depth review and possibly faster review times and expedited entry for imported goods manufactured in facilities inspected by accredited third parties. Use of accredited third parties may also be taken into consideration by the FDA when setting inspection and surveillance priorities. (p. 18)

The FDA proposes to oversee these independent third parties by auditing their work to ensure that FDA requirements are consistently assessed, reviewing their inspection reports, and providing ongoing training criteria to ensure that they maintain their skills and knowledge (FDA, 2007a). It should be noted the FPP defines third parties much more broadly than is the case in this report. Included in its definition are other federal departments and agencies, state and local government agencies, foreign government agencies, and private entities without financial conflicts of interest (FDA, 2007a). The committee believes the FDA's definition is too broad (see Chapter 7).

The FDA's 2009 Guidance for Industry on Voluntary Third-Party Certification Programs for Foods and Feeds[3] describes the agency's views on the

---

[3] See http://www.fda.gov/RegulatoryInformation/Guidances/ucm125431.htm (accessed February 16, 2010).

general attributes of a third-party certification program. The FDA regards this guidance as one of the steps in its future recognition of voluntary third-party certification programs for particular product types, and it has stated that it will recognize a certification program only if it has sufficient confidence in the certification body (FDA, 2009b). The FDA also has explored the use of third-party certification for imported foods, as discussed in the following section. It should be noted that, although GAO reports on food safety programs recommend exploring the development of a third-party certification program, they also recommend taking lessons from the FDA's medical device program, in which the lack of incentives resulted in weak participation and few inspections (GAO, 2008a,b).

The potential value and legitimacy of third-party certification is a topic of debate internationally as well. For example, private standards have been on the agenda of the World Trade Organization's (WTO's) Sanitary and Phytosanitary (SPS) committee since 2005, and their role in the process of public standards setting is under discussion at the Codex Alimentarius Commission, where a position on the matter has not yet been taken. During its last meeting in 2009, Codex decided to conduct an in-depth evaluation of the role and impact of such standards, based on comments about the negative impact of private standards on economies and questions about the science and transparency of the process (Henson and Humphrey, 2009). There is published evidence of the comparatively higher costs of meeting private standards versus European Union (EU) standards (Plunkett and DeWaal, 2008). Overall, however, third-party efforts are clearly an important part of a risk-based system of shared responsibility for food safety.

Governments of Other Countries

There have been only limited, initial efforts to compare food safety performance across countries (Charlebois and Yost, 2008); therefore, no evidence exists to support the idea that vulnerability will increase with the growth of international trade in food and agricultural products and the import share of food consumption. The enforcement of food safety regulations in foreign countries is challenging.

Importing countries ensure import safety through a combination of controls in place in the exporting countries and border inspections. It is unrealistic to expect the FDA to have an effective inspectional presence in countries around the world as border inspection is a difficult, expensive, and sometimes ineffectual means of monitoring food safety. Inspectors cannot check every grape, or even every box of grapes. In this situation, a U.S. regulatory agency may leverage its efforts by verifying and then relying on the safety control systems of other countries. This approach has the added advantage of responding to the call of WTO's Agreement on the

Application of SPS Measures for recognition of equivalent systems across countries.

An additional challenge in the oversight of imported foods is the inability of a government to interfere with a foreign country's laws. Exporting countries are outside the FDA's jurisdiction, and therefore enforcing U.S. food laws with respect to their products is problematic. For example, inspecting foods and facilities in situ not only is impractical but also might not be welcomed or allowed by the exporting country. A regulatory agency needs oversight mechanisms that can overcome these barriers while remaining in line with WTO trade agreements. The current system by which the FDA manages the safety of food imports (mainly inspections at the border) is ineffective (only 1.28 percent of shipments were inspected in 2007) and could use additional tools (GAO, 2009).

As Appendix E describes, with the expansion of the global market for foods and the signing of the WTO agreements, preventive mechanisms have been instituted to ensure the safety of imported foods. Those mechanisms include monitoring and directed sampling (Canada); third-party audits, and equivalency agreements, and limited entry posts for high-risk products (EU countries); inspection based on food risk categories (Australia and New Zealand); and import certificates (New Zealand). Presentations made to the committee and its own investigation further support the existence of a broad range of approaches to allocation of responsibility and coordination with other countries to ensure food safety (Appendix E). Designing a coherent approach to working with other countries to ensure the safety of imports is clearly important.

The committee found that the FPP does not articulate a clear approach to the roles of private parties and other governments in ensuring food safety for products imported into the United States. As discussed in Appendix E, the United States maintains that its approach to imported foods stands on the same general principles as its approach to domestic foods. It is the responsibility of companies and importers to know the U.S. food laws and regulations and to comply with them. However, the U.S. government will ultimately be held accountable for a safe supply of both domestic and imported foods.

The States

Given the size, complexity, and growth of the food industry in the United States (more than 156,008 domestic food facilities [FDA, 2010], more than 1 million food establishments [including restaurants and retail stores[4]], and more than 2 million farms), it is unrealistic to expect that the

---

[4] Personal communication, Chad Nelson, FDA, October 13, 2009.

FDA could have enough resources to provide adequate surveillance and inspection of the entire U.S. food supply (Mavity, 2009). The regulations and programs of state and local (including tribal and territorial) governments have been a strong component of the U.S. food safety system for the past century. State surveys conducted in 2001 and 2009 indicate the broad scope of food safety activities conducted by the states, from collecting data on food contamination and outbreak surveillance, to performing food and feed inspections, to enforcing the laws and issuing recalls (AFDO, 2001, 2009). In fact, the FDA's food safety knowledge (and therefore management) could be enhanced by leveraging data collected by state and local authorities on food safety inspections, disease outbreak investigations, product safety, consumer perspectives, and enforcement actions. Doing so, however, would require that programs be standardized and harmonized; for example, standards for training of inspectors and data collection would need to be in place. In the absence of truly harmonized programs at the state and local levels, the FDA has instituted some mechanisms that facilitate cooperation, such as the signing of confidentiality agreements, contracts, or memorandums of understanding. Although these mechanisms facilitate shared effort, they also have limitations in that funding is not always available, and they are not always utilized.

As with the assignment of responsibility to industry, third parties, and other countries, the FDA needs an overall strategic vision for when it is desirable to rely on or partner with the states to ensure food safety as well as what allocation of appropriate areas and levels of responsibility is optimal. The committee found that the FDA lacks an overall regulatory philosophy or road map for these choices. With a clear approach, the agency might be able to expand its collaborations with state and local food safety programs so these programs would be better recognized and utilized in the national food safety system (see Chapter 7).

Examples of Mixes of Public and Private Responsibility

Clearly options for the choice and design of policy interventions (Steps 4 and 5 in a risk-based system) are broad, cutting across different mixes of public and private responsibility for ensuring food safety. Researchers have begun to analyze these diverse models for shared responsibility, particularly as several countries have expressed their interest in newer, hybrid forms of governance as a means of ensuring food safety more efficiently. As yet, there have been no comprehensive comparisons of the effectiveness of these alternative models, but several studies shed some light on the options currently in use.

The structure of private standards for food safety management has been developing particularly rapidly in the last decade (Henson, 2008). Historically, a no-intervention approach characterized by private standards set on a business-to-business basis was predominant. These approaches were either national (e.g., Nature's Choice by Tesco in the United Kingdom, Field-to-Forks by Marks and Spencer in the United Kingdom, Filière Agriculture-Raisonnée by Auchan France) or international (e.g., Wal-Mart and Nestlé). Recently, a self-regulatory approach characterized by joint standards used by a group of suppliers or retailers, frequently with third-party certification, has been gaining ground. Examples of these joint standards include, at the national level, the Dutch HACCP, the BRC Global Standard, Assured Food Standards, Qualität und Sicherheit (the "QS system"), and Integrate Keten Beheersing. At the international level, they include the International Food Standards, SQF 1000/2000/3000, and GlobalGAP (formerly EuroGAP) (Henson, 2008).

A study conducted for the Food Standards Agency in the United Kingdom documents a mix of private and public responsibility in use across the United Kingdom, the United States, Canada, and Australia (Fearne et al., 2006; Garcia-Martinez et al., 2007). The United Kingdom has been active in thinking about and experimenting with different mixes of responsibility. An example is the Zoonoses Action Plan Salmonella Programme for pigs. In this case, standards setting was private (voluntary), with funding from the government and a multistakeholder group advising on ongoing developments. Implementation was private, with funding and facilitation from the government. Enforcement and monitoring were private as well (as part of farm assurance scheme requirements), with the public sector providing on-farm support and advice to high-risk producers. A further example of exploration of alternative public–private mixes is the voluntary HACCP Advantage program in Ontario, Canada. Here, the standards setting was public–private, the system was introduced through educational programs led by the government, and enforcement and monitoring were conducted through private, third-party audits.

An example of exploration of different mixes of public and private responsibility from the United States is a series of efforts the FDA has conducted to assess the value of third-party certification systems as a tool to verify the compliance of foreign food companies with U.S. food laws. Such exploratory efforts are recommended in the *Action Plan for Import Safety: A Roadmap for Continual Improvement* (Interagency Working Group on Import Safety, 2007), as well as in the 2007 FPP. The FDA conducted a pilot study to evaluate voluntary third-party certification programs for imported aquaculture shrimp. The FDA envisioned that such a program could help the agency make decisions about the safety of imported foods, such as prioritizing inspections and sampling. The pilot program was conducted in two phases. During Phase I, participants were paper audited and selected on the basis of a set of criteria, with six certification bodies selected. Phase II, involving onsite audits and targeted sampling, was scheduled to be completed and evaluated in July 2009. The committee was not given any results of this pilot program and was unable to evaluate it as an approach to shared responsibility for food safety.

KEY CONCLUSIONS AND RECOMMENDATIONS

Food safety in the United States is the responsibility of suppliers, farmers, food handlers, processors, wholesalers and retailers, food service companies, consumers, third-party organizations, and government (federal and state) agencies in both the United States and abroad. It is, therefore, unrealistic to expect the FDA, or any government agency, to have sufficient resources to manage food safety without the help of others who share this responsibility.

A risk-based approach to the choice and design of interventions (Steps 4 and 5 in a risk-based system) requires a comprehensive understanding of the policy intervention tool kit and a road map for choosing and designing interventions. Further, developing an approach to defining the roles of other responsible parties is a component of strategic planning in a risk-based food safety system. In essence, this road map should also serve to assign shared responsibility among the federal government, the private sector, third parties, the governments of other countries, the states, and consumers. The design of novel approaches to governance to achieve food safety is currently the subject of experimentation by other governments and debate by scholars.

The committee found that the FDA has made ad hoc efforts in this direction but does not have a clear regulatory philosophy for assigning responsibility for food safety or a comprehensive strategy for choosing the level and intensity of interventions as part of strategic planning in a risk-based approach. The committee offers the following recommendations to address these shortcomings.

> Recommendation 4-1: To ensure food safety, the FDA should develop a plan for defining the extent of and form for sharing responsibilities with the states, the private sector, third parties (e.g., independent auditors), and other countries' governments.

> Recommendation 4-2: The FDA should develop a comprehensive strategy for choosing the level and intensity of policy interventions needed for different food safety risks. Criteria for choosing the level and intensity of policy interventions and a plan for evaluating the selected interventions should be developed with transparency, stakeholder participation, and clear lines of communication.

REFERENCES

AFDO (Association of Food and Drug Officials). 2001. *State Resource Survey*. York, PA: AFDO.

AFDO. 2009. *State Food Safety Resource Survey*. York, PA: AFDO.

Albersmeier, F., H. Schulze, G. Jahn, and A. Spiller. 2009. The reliability of third-party certification in the food chain: From checklists to risk-oriented auditing. *Food Control* 20:927–935.

AZLGMA (Arizona Leafy Green Products Shipper Marketing Agreement). 2008. *About AZ LGMA 2008*. http://www.azlgma.gov/about_azlgma/default.asp (accessed February 12, 2010).

Batz, M. B., M. P. Doyle, G. Morris, Jr., J. Painter, R. Singh, R. V. Tauxe, M. R. Taylor, and D. M. Lo Fo Wong. 2005. Attributing illness to food. *Emerging Infectious Diseases* 11(7):993–999.

Charlebois, S., and C. Yost. 2008. *Food Safety Performance World Ranking 2008*. Saskatchewan, Canada: Research Network in Food Systems, University of Regina. http://www.ontraceagrifood.com/admincp/uploadedfiles/Food%20Safety%20Performance%20World%20Ranking%202008.pdf (accessed March 13, 2010).

FDA (U.S. Food and Drug Administration). 2004. *Produce Safety from Production to Consumption: 2004 Action Plan to Minimize Foodborne Illness Associated with Fresh Produce Consumption*. Washington, DC: FDA. http://www.fda.gov/Food/FoodSafety/Product-SpecificInformation/FruitsVegetablesJuices/FDAProduceSafetyActivities/ProduceSafetyActionPlan/ucm129487.htm (accessed February 4, 2010).

FDA. 2007a. *Food Protection Plan: An Integrated Strategy for Protecting the Nation's Food Supply*. Rockville, MD: FDA.

FDA. 2007b. *Tomato Safety Initiative*. Washington, DC: FDA. http://www.fda.gov/Food/FoodSafety/Product-SpecificInformation/FruitsVegetablesJuices/FDAProduceSafetyActivities/ucm115334.htm (accessed February 4, 2010).

FDA. 2009a. *Lettuce Safety Initiative*. Washington, DC: FDA. http://www.fda.gov/Food/FoodSafety/Product-SpecificInformation/FruitsVegetablesJuices/FDAProduceSafetyActivities/ucm115906.htm (accessed February 4, 2010).

FDA. 2009b. *Guidance for Industry: Voluntary Third-Party Certification Programs for Foods and Feeds*. http://www.fda.gov/RegulatoryInformation/Guidances/ucm125431.htm (accessed February 16, 2010).

FDA. 2010. *Food and Drug Administration FY 2011 Congressional Budget Request: Narrative by Activity—Foods Program FY2011*. http://www.fda.gov/downloads/AboutFDA/ReportsManualsForms/Reports/BudgetReports/UCM205367.pdf (accessed June 2, 2010).

Fearne, A., M. Garcia, J. Caswell, S. Henson, and Y. Khatri. 2006. *Exploring Alternative Approaches to Traditional Modes of Food Safety*. London, UK: Imperial College/Food Standards Agency. http://www.foodbase.org.uk//admintools/reportdocuments/202-1-337_D03004.pdf (accessed February 16, 2010).

Federal Register. 2009. Product tracing systems for food. 74(211):56843–56855.

Florida Department of Agriculture and Consumer Services. 2007. *Tomato Best Practices Manual: DACS Tomato Best Practices Manual*. Tallahassee: Florida Department of Agriculture and Consumer Services. www.doacs.state.fl.us/fs/TomatoBestPractices.pdf (accessed March 30, 2010).

FSA (Food Standards Agency). 2006. *FSA Regulatory Framework*. http://www.food.gov.uk/foodindustry/regulation/betregs/regframe (accessed February 12, 2010).

FSA. 2010. *Impact Assessments 2009*. http://www.food.gov.uk/foodindustry/regulation/betregs/ria/ (accessed February 12, 2010).

Garcia-Martinez, M., A. Fearne, J. A. Caswell, and S. Henson. 2007. Co-regulation as a possible model for food safety governance: Opportunities for public–private partnerships. *Food Policy* 32(3):16.

GAO (U.S. Government Accountability Office). 2006. *Nuclear Regulatory Commission: Oversight of Nuclear Power Plant Safety Has Improved, but Refinements Are Needed.* Washington, DC: GAO.

GAO. 2008a. *Federal Oversight of Food Safety: FDA Has Provided Few Details on the Resources and Strategies Needed to Implement Its Food Protection Plan.* Washington, DC: GAO.

GAO. 2008b. *Federal Oversight of Food Safety: FDA's Food Protection Plan Proposes Positive First Steps, but Capacity to Carry Them Out Is Critical.* Washington, DC: GAO.

GAO. 2009. *Agencies Need to Address Gaps in Enforcement and Collaboration to Enhance Safety of Imported Food.* Washington, DC: GAO.

Henson, S. 2008. The role of public and private standards in regulating international food markets. *Journal of International Agricultural Trade and Development* 4(1):63–81.

Henson, S., and J. Humphrey. 2009. *The Impacts of Private Food Safety Standards on Food Chain and on Public Standard-Setting Processes.* Paper presented at Report to the Codex Alimentarius Commission, 32nd Session, Rome, Italy, June 29–July 4, 2009.

HHS/FDA (U.S. Department of Health and Human Services/U.S. Food and Drug Administration). 2009. *Produce Safety Regulation, RIN #: 0910-AG35.* http://www.reginfo.gov/public/do/eAgendaViewRule?pubId=200910&RIN=0910-AG35 (accessed May 13, 2010).

Hutter, B. M. 2001. Is enforced self-regulation a form of risk taking? The case of railway health and safety. *International Journal of the Sociology of Law* 29(4):379–400.

Interagency Working Group on Import Safety. 2007. *Action Plan for Import Safety: A Roadmap for Continual Improvement.* http://www.importsafety.gov/ (accessed April 22, 2010).

IOM/NRC (Institute of Medicine/National Research Council). 2003. *Scientific Criteria to Ensure Safe Food.* Washington, DC: The National Academies Press.

LGMA (California Leafy Green Products Handler Marketing Agreement). 2010. *About LGMA 2007.* http://www.caleafygreens.ca.gov/about/lgma.asp (accessed January 28 2010).

Mavity, S. 2009. *Safety of Imported Foods: A Perspective from a Company in the Seafood Industry.* Paper presented at Institute of Medicine/National Research Council Committee on Review of the FDA's Role in Ensuring Safe Food Meeting, Washington, DC, May 28, 2009.

Plunkett, D., and C. S. DeWaal. 2008. Who is responsible for the safety of food in a global market? Government certification v. importer accountability as models for assuring the safety of internationally traded foods. *Food and Drug Law Journal* 63(3):657–664.

Treasury Board of Canada Secretariat. 2007. *Assessing, Selecting, and Implementing Instruments for Government Action.* Ottawa: Treasury Board of Canada Secretariat.

Part III

Implementation of the
New Food Safety System

5

Creating an Integrated Information Infrastructure for a Risk-Based Food Safety System

Information science—a term that refers to the collection, organization, storage, retrieval, exchange, interpretation, and use of information— and information technology (IT) are critical to the success of a risk-based decision-making system.[1] If the U.S. Food and Drug Administration (FDA) is to implement a risk-based approach in fulfilling its regulatory mission, it must know what is happening in the arena it regulates; that is, data from the food enterprise must be appropriately collected, integrated, and analyzed. To allocate resources, understand and prevent food safety problems, and drive continual improvements in public health, a risk-based system requires accurate, reliable, secure, and timely information that is accessible, within appropriate limits, to all stakeholders in the food safety system. The importance of information to the food safety enterprise has been recognized by the White House Food Safety Working Group as one of the three principles guiding the development of a modern, coordinated food safety system: "High-quality information will help leading agencies know which foods are at risk; which solutions should be put into place; and who should be responsible" (FSWG, 2009, p. 3).

As described in this chapter, large quantities of data related to food safety are already being collected. Yet, as has been highlighted by others, the FDA is facing an information crisis and currently lacks the necessary infrastructure to efficiently process, manage, protect, integrate, analyze, and leverage the large volume of data to which it has access. This deficiency hampers the agency's ability to achieve its mission and increases both costs

---

[1] In this chapter, the terms "data" and "information" are used interchangeably.

147

and the likelihood of regulatory errors (FDA Science Board, 2007). Much of the data is "stovepiped" into stand-alone databases that are not accessible within and across government agencies, including the FDA (Taylor and Batz, 2008; FDA Science Board, 2009). A lack of resources, legal constraints, nonstandardized data collection, varied data formats, incompatible IT systems, a sense of ownership by the group that collects the data, and a culture that often uses publication rather than rapid information release as the basis for evaluating performance have been identified as contributing to the persistent problems with data sharing (Taylor and Batz, 2008; FDA Science Board, 2009). For example, the FDA apparently has the regulatory authority to require that all data be submitted electronically and to specify the format of these data submissions, but it may not have sufficient resources to implement such electronic standards (FDA Science Board, 2007). It has been noted that inspection reports are often handwritten and take a long time to enter into the electronic system, databases sometimes contain incorrect or contradictory information, and data analysis is slow (FDA Science Board, 2007; GAO, 2009). The Science Board has also stated that requirements need to be developed in conjunction with stakeholders who will be making the submissions. Finally, the FDA lacks the necessary tools to store, search, model, and analyze data (FDA Science Board, 2007).

Generating and providing timely access to the appropriate data is challenging for any food regulatory agency because of the complexity of data needs, coupled with the diverse types of information from multiple sources and scientific disciplines. Also, the committee recognizes the challenge for government officials to be expeditious about communicating with stakeholders while also ensuring accuracy. In some instances, moreover, depending on the nature of the data and the needs of the user, release to others may justifiably be delayed because of the time needed to either interpret data or mask confidential information. As explained later in the chapter, however, the committee found that some delays that occur in the current system are not justifiable.

Recognizing these challenges, moving forward with a risk-based food safety system will require the development of an integrated information infrastructure that provides a relatively uninhibited flow of high-quality, relevant information (see Chapter 3). In the context of this report, an integrated information infrastructure refers to one that is strategically designed to facilitate the systematic collection, integration, management, storage, analysis, interpretation, and communication of the information needed to support a risk-based food safety management system, and also one that has the flexibility and accessibility to meet the varied and changing information needs of a diverse set of users.

This chapter outlines the key types of data needed to support risk-based decision making. In addition, it briefly illustrates the breadth of food safety data that are being collected by government and other parties as well as gaps and challenges in the collection of these data. A particular barrier to achieving an efficient, risk-based food safety system that is discussed extensively in the chapter is the lack of data sharing. Finally, the chapter describes the elements that are critical to designing and implementing an integrated information infrastructure that can support a risk-based food safety management system. These elements include strategic planning to assess data needs and plan study designs as well as data analysis and communication, mechanisms to allow for timely sharing of quality data, a modern IT infrastructure, and the human capacity to collect, analyze, manage, and communicate the data.

THE ROLE OF DATA IN A RISK-BASED FOOD SAFETY MANAGEMENT SYSTEM

At its core, the FDA is a public health agency, and the ultimate goal of protecting the public health should be its highest priority. To support the achievement of this goal, the FDA's information infrastructure should provide a foundation for risk-based decision making in all aspects of food safety management.

Data will be needed to implement the steps in the risk-based approach delineated in Chapter 3. In strategic planning (Step 1 of the risk-based approach), the FDA will need access to high-quality and timely data to identify the key public health objectives on which its food safety program will be centered. At the highest level, these public health objectives will be consistent with national public health objectives, such as those articulated in Healthy People 2020, which include "reduc[ing] the number of outbreak-associated infections caused by food commodity group" (including dairy, fruits/nuts, and leafy vegetables)[2] (HHS, 2009). However, the FDA will also pursue specific intermediate outcomes, such as the reduction of methyl mercury in foods, that will serve as the basis for its targeted risk management programs. The establishment of these objectives should be based on data acquired in the field, such as data on contamination or foodborne illness.

The process of public health risk ranking (Step 2) will also require data. For example, as discussed in Chapter 3, foodborne illness attribution models are crucial to public health risk ranking because they provide the bridge between public health impact and risk in the food continuum. However, developing such models requires a comprehensive data collec-

---

[2] See http://www.healthypeople.gov/hp2020/Objectives/ViewObjective.aspx?Id=487& TopicArea=Food+Safety&Objective=FS+HP2020%e2%80%937&TopicAreaId=22 (accessed October 8, 2010).

tion system that integrates data from various sources and harmonizes the categorization of foods, as well as the methods used to produce, process, and distribute those foods (NRC, 2009).

Data collection and subsequent analyses are the outcomes of Step 3 of a risk-based system (targeted information gathering). In carrying out this step, risk managers must identify and consider additional criteria upon which risk-based decision making will be based and, for each high-priority and/or uncertain risk, determine the need for collecting additional information. Such additional data may encompass virtually any (and all) of the data types noted below. These data then form the basis upon which intervention analysis (Step 4) can proceed, which may also involve the collection of even more information in an effort to evaluate the efficacy and feasibility of candidate control options.

Finally, data must be collected to measure the efficacy of specific interventions, the overall food safety system, and the risk-based approach in achieving national and agency-specific public health objectives (Step 6). Crucial to this process is the collection of information that can directly relate interventions to specific public health outcomes, including epidemiological data and associated attribution models.

Ultimately, the FDA's purpose in collecting food safety data is to better understand the distribution and determinants of foodborne illness, prioritize the determinants based on their public health impact, and develop interventions for the determinants and thereby control foodborne illness. In fact, understanding the epidemiology of foodborne illness is necessary to support the ability to make informed, risk-based policy decisions and allocate food safety resources appropriately. In turn, a risk-based decision-making process will improve knowledge of the epidemiology of foodborne illness and drive continual improvements in public health. As defined by Last (1995, p. 62), epidemiology is "the study of the distribution and determinants of health-related states or events in specified populations, and the application of this study to control of health problems." As noted by Havelaar and colleagues (2006, p. 9), "epidemiology is now largely a quantitative science that extensively uses statistical (associative) models to explore the relation between risk factors and disease."

DATA NEEDS FOR A RISK-BASED SYSTEM

To meet the needs of a risk-based system, data would ideally be collected at each point along the food production continuum—on the farm, in processing, during distribution, at retail, and in the home. A variety of data sources can contribute to an understanding of the epidemiology of foodborne illness, including data collected through surveillance, behavioral studies, analytical research, and traditional epidemiological studies. The types of data collected might include foodborne pathogen levels and transmission routes in animals, plants, food products, humans, and the environment; current industry and consumer practices, including behaviors and attitudes; and the efficacy of candidate intervention approaches at all phases of the continuum. There is also a need for epidemiological data to support estimates of the overall burden of foodborne illness and the proportion of such illness associated with specific vehicles (foods) and transmission routes (i.e., foodborne illness attribution). A regulatory agency might decide to include other factors in its risk-based approach as well, such as the costs and benefits of implementing specific interventions, even though those factors are not directly related to public health. These data types can be broadly categorized as behavioral, economic, food production, and surveillance data. The importance of each type of data for a risk-based system is discussed further in the following subsections. To maximize the utility of these diverse surveillance systems, there must be an integrated information infrastructure that, through strategic planning, facilitates informed data collection and promotes standards for data exchange. Effective collection of these types of data will require active research—including basic, population, and clinical research—as outlined in Chapter 6.

Behavioral Data

Behavioral data are critical to understanding routes of transmission, implementing intervention strategies to change behavior, developing risk communications, improving public health response, and evaluating interventions. As discussed in Chapter 9, behavioral data are ultimately essential for developing strategies that will enable the FDA to communicate effectively with diverse audiences under a wide range of circumstances and through multiple communication channels. For example, the attitudes, perceptions, and behaviors of the general public and food industry personnel can impact their compliance with recommended food safety interventions, such as safe food-handling practices (Medeiros et al., 2001; Pilling et al., 2008). Likewise, understanding the attitudes, perceptions, and behaviors of public health personnel—including physicians, laboratory personnel, and government officials—can help identify ways to improve public health response.

Economic Data

In a risk-based system, data on benefits and costs are combined for use in cost-effectiveness and cost–benefit analyses of alternative policy interventions. Economic data can be used to measure and understand several important dimensions of a risk-based food safety system. These data may be thought of as measuring factors that affect the demand for safer food by individuals and by society as a whole on the one hand and factors that affect the supply of safer foods on the other. The demand for food safety arises in part from the costs of foodborne illness in terms of medical treatment, lost productivity due to mortality and morbidity, and other costs, such as loss of leisure time or burden on family members due to illness (Majowicz et al., 2004; Frenzen et al., 2005; Kemmeren et al., 2006; USDA/ERS, 2009). In addition to avoiding these costs, individuals or society may be willing to pay for (i.e., demand) improved safety based on the well-being or peace of mind associated with safer foods (Shogren et al., 1999). On the supply side, economic data can be used to measure the potential and actual costs of actions intended to supply safer foods, as well as to gain insight into incentives for countries and companies to invest in food safety. These data on incentives include domestic and international market impacts from the incidence of foodborne pathogens, from outbreak incidents in total, and as distributed across the supply chain. Examples of such impacts include the loss of market share by food producers in domestic markets due to the loss of reputation for safety and loss of export markets. Data that can help in understanding these effects include farm cash receipts, total value at retail, value of exports, value of imports, proportion of domestic consumption of food products produced domestically, and information on key export and import markets (Ruzante et al., 2009).

Food Production Data

To support risk-based decision making, the FDA needs to have information that relates to the production, processing, and storage of foods, including the size of the regulated industry and the distribution channels. For example, the FDA needs to understand current industry practices, including best practices, intervention strategies, and emerging technologies. The agency also needs to know the prevalence of foodborne pathogens throughout the food production, processing, and distribution chain. In fact, in support of the functions of the Office of Regulatory Affairs (ORA), including routine inspection activities, the FDA collects a large amount of data for both regulatory and nonregulatory purposes that may address these types of questions.

Data are also collected by the industry in support of safety control systems such as Hazard Analysis and Critical Control Points and routine microbiological monitoring. In addition, industry data collected by the academic and government research sectors are a rich source of information that can be used to estimate the prevalence and levels of pathogens and toxins in the food supply, evaluate the efficacy of intervention strategies, model risk and its mitigation, and identify consumer behaviors and market trends. All these data collected throughout the food production continuum can be used to inform attribution and risk models, aid in the allocation of agency resources, and provide evidence of data gaps to inform future data collection efforts, among many other purposes.

Surveillance Data

For purposes of this report, "surveillance" refers to the ongoing, systematic[3] collection and analysis of contaminant, public health, and molecular data throughout the farm-to-fork continuum for use in preventing and controlling foodborne illness. Surveillance is a critical component of a risk-based food safety system in that it improves overall understanding of the epidemiology of foodborne illness. Specifically, surveillance can be used to establish a baseline level of foodborne illness, identify goals for its reduction, and provide a means by which to measure the impact of interventions on its control. Given resource limitations, the risk-based approach recommended in this report is essential as a tool to prioritize surveillance efforts.

Animal, food, environmental, human, public health, molecular, and behavioral (see p. 151) surveillance are all needed to respond to food safety crises, monitor food safety outcomes, and assess the effectiveness of the food safety system. Surveillance of animal populations, the food supply, and the environment is almost always undertaken with an eye to identifying sources of contamination and their subsequent transmission from a food animal to product(s) that will ultimately be consumed by people. Surveillance of human populations is used to better characterize the burden of foodborne illness and identify the relative importance of particular exposures (e.g., foods, transmission routes). Public health surveillance provides important insights into current medical, laboratory, and general public health practices, such as reporting and outbreak investigations. Molecular surveillance systems, such as PulseNet and VetNet, combine the methods of molecular biology with those of epidemiology to establish associations between contaminated food and illness when they are separated in space or time.

GAPS AND CHALLENGES IN THE CURRENT DATA COLLECTION SYSTEMS

Implementing an effective risk-based system, and developing the foodborne illness attribution models needed to support such a system, will require a comprehensive information infrastructure that integrates data

---

[3] In this context, the term "systematic" means that the surveillance is conducted in an orderly fashion, not haphazardly. For example, under certain circumstances, passive surveillance can be considered systematic, if it is conducted under some minimum established standards.

from various sources, harmonizes the data collected through the use of data standards, and finally analyzes, interprets, and disseminates those data in such a manner that they can be used to monitor and evaluate the overall food safety system. As evidenced by the following discussion, such a comprehensive system does not currently exist in the United States, compromising the FDA's capacity to fulfill its mission of protecting public health from hazards transmitted through the food supply. Current efforts to develop a risk-based food safety system are significantly limited, despite the fact that vast amounts of food safety data are already being collected. In recent years, several studies have evaluated the state of the FDA's science and information infrastructure and identified a number of problems (see Appendix B). While these problems have been well documented, it has been suggested that they persist because of a lack of commitment and inadequate investment that stem from legislative and policy inaction (FDA Science Board, 2007; Taylor and Batz, 2008).

A detailed description of the complexity and challenges of the data collection systems currently used to ensure food safety in the United States is given in the report *Harnessing Knowledge to Ensure Safe Food: Opportunities to Improve the Nation's Food Safety Information Infrastructure* (Taylor and Batz, 2008[4]). These challenges are discussed briefly below.

Fragmented Data Collection

The data needs of the nation's food safety system are currently being met through a patchwork of diverse data collection systems and networks that generate vast amounts of food safety data (for an extensive review see Taylor and Batz, 2008). Often, the collection of data is not comprehensive or designed to support a risk-based approach. Table 5-1 illustrates the breadth of the salient data by listing examples of U.S. public health–related data collection programs and networks in which the FDA is the lead or participates. Table 5-2 shows examples of the systems currently used to collect the different types of data outlined in the previous section, including some of the systems listed in Table 5-1, as well as shortcomings of these systems identified by the committee.

As part of its food regulatory function, the FDA collects some data, including microbiological samples, for the food products it regulates. With coverage in every state and territory, the FDA's field personnel and delegates are well positioned to generate and provide data that could be used in the agency's risk-based decision making. However, because field personnel do not have a daily presence in the regulated facilities, the FDA has limited opportunities to collect data outside of its routine regulatory efforts. With

---

[4] See www.thefsrc.org.

TABLE 5-1 Examples of U.S. Public Health–Related Data Collection Programs and Networks

Aflatoxin Testing Program	Under memorandums of understanding (MOUs), the U.S. Department of Agriculture's (USDA's) Food Safety and Inspection Service (FSIS) provides appropriate U.S. Food and Drug Administration (FDA) district offices with the results of aflatoxin analysis for domestic and imported peanuts, imported in-shell pistachios, and imported in-shell brazil nuts in lots that may be subject to action under the Federal Food, Drug, and Cosmetic Act (FDCA) and with an analysis certificate on any lot upon request. The FDA will also notify the Agricultural Marketing Service (AMS) of the criteria it will use concerning total aflatoxin levels in lots to determine whether they may be subject to action under the FDCA.
CAERS (CFSAN Adverse Events Reporting System)	The Center for Food Safety and Applied Nutrition (CFSAN) Adverse Events Reporting System (CAERS) team monitors all individual postmarketing surveillance adverse event reports related to CFSAN-regulated products. Reviewers in CFSAN's program offices assess these reports and work closely with program experts and researchers throughout CFSAN and the FDA. CAERS tracks what products and ingredients may be harmful and conveys this information to industry, consumers, and other interested parties. The CAERS adverse event data permit CFSAN to do trend analysis on multiple adverse events and to track rarer product-related adverse events that may occur over several years.
CIFOR (Council to Improve Foodborne Outbreak Response)	CIFOR is a working group that seeks to improve performance and coordination among federal, state, and local agencies with respect to routine surveillance of foodborne illness, foodborne outbreak detection and response, laboratory methods for detecting and measuring foodborne pathogens, and foodborne illness prevention, communication, and education at the state and local levels. The council includes representatives of the U.S. Centers for Disease Control and Prevention (CDC), the FDA, USDA, the Association of Food and Drug Officials, the Association of Public Health Laboratories, the Association of State and Territorial Health Officials, the Council of State and Territorial Epidemiologists, the National Association of County and City Health Officials, the National Environmental Health Association (NEHA), and the National Association of State Departments of Agriculture. CIFOR also includes an industry workgroup composed of 16 leaders from food production, restaurant, and retail companies.

continued

TABLE 5-1 Continued

EHS-Net (Environmental Health Specialists Network)	EHS-Net is a CDC-coordinated collaborative forum of environmental health specialists who work with epidemiologists and laboratories to identify and mitigate environmental factors that contribute to foodborne illness and other disease outbreaks. Its goals include translating investigatory findings into improved food safety prevention efforts using a systems-based approach and strengthening relations among epidemiology, laboratory, and environmental health programs.
eLEXNET (Electronic Laboratory Exchange Network)	This web-based information network, coordinated by the FDA, allows federal, state, and local food safety officials to compare, share, and coordinate laboratory analysis findings. It is also the data capture and communication system for the Food Emergency Response Network (FERN). eLEXNET provides the necessary infrastructure for an early warning system that identifies potentially hazardous foods and enables health officials to assess risks and analyze trends.
Epi-Ready	This nationwide team-training initiative, led by CDC and NEHA, provides up-to-date foodborne illness outbreak investigation and surveillance training to public- and private-sector environmental health professionals, as well as other professionals who collaborate in conducting foodborne illness outbreak investigations.
Epi-X (Epidemic Information Exchange)	Run by CDC, Epi-X is a web-based surveillance communication tool for public health professionals. It enables public health professionals to access and share preliminary health surveillance information and notifies them rapidly of health events as they occur. Key features of Epi-X include scientific and editorial support, controlled user access, digital credentials and authentication, rapid outbreak reporting, and support for multijurisdictional peer-to-peer consultation.
FERN (Food Emergency Response Network)	FERN is a network of local, state, and federal food-testing laboratories that responds to emergencies involving biological, chemical, or radiological contamination of food. It provides a national surveillance capability designed to offer an early means of detecting threat agents in the American food supply, prepares the nation's laboratories to respond to food-related emergencies, and offers surge capacity for responding to widespread, complex food contamination emergencies. FERN is coordinated by both the FDA and USDA/FSIS.

TABLE 5-1 Continued

FoodNet (Foodborne Diseases Active Surveillance Network)	A collaboration among CDC, the FDA, USDA, and the ten states participating in CDC's Emerging Infections Program, FoodNet has the goal of providing more accurate estimates of foodborne illness associated with pathogens by conducting active, population-based surveillance for foodborne illness cases at ten sites. FoodNet has contributed to the standardization of methods among laboratories and performs targeted case control studies to identify risk factors for pathogen-specific illnesses.
FoodSHIELD	FoodSHIELD's mission is to support federal, state, and local government regulatory agencies and laboratories through web-based tools that enhance threat prevention and response, risk management, communication, asset coordination, and public education.
MDP (Microbiological Data Program)	MDP is a national foodborne pathogen database program implemented in 2001. Through cooperation with state agriculture departments and relevant federal agencies, MDP is meant to collect, analyze, and report data on foodborne pathogens for selected agricultural commodities. The FDA provides technical assistance to enhance methods used by MDP participants. Additionally, USDA/AMS informs the FDA of any positive pathogenic findings detected through MDP.
NARMS (National Antimicrobial Resistance Monitoring System)	NARMS was established in 1996 to monitor changes in the susceptibility of select bacteria to antimicrobial agents of human and veterinary importance among foodborne isolates collected from humans, animals, and retail meats. NARMS is a collaboration between three federal agencies including FDA's Center for Veterinary Medicine (CVM), CDC and USDA. NARMS also collaborates with antimicrobial resistance monitoring systems in other countries, including Canada, Denmark, France, Mexico, the Netherlands, Norway, and Sweden, so that information can be shared on the global dissemination of antimicrobial resistant foodborne pathogens. Molecular fingerprints of select foodborne bacteria (*Salmonella* and *Campylobacter*) recovered via NARMS are deposited into the CDC PulseNet databank for use in identifying sources and spread of foodborne outbreaks. The information from NARMS forms the basis for public health recommendations for the use of antimicrobial drugs in both food producing animals and humans. NARMS data also are vital in disease outbreak investigations and can be used to help create treatment guidelines for foodborne pathogens, thereby ensuring better health outcomes.

continued

TABLE 5-1 Continued

OutbreakNet/NORS (National Outbreak Reporting System)	OutbreakNet is a national CDC-coordinated network of local, state, and federal public health officials who investigate outbreaks of enteric illness, including foodborne outbreaks. State OutbreakNet members report findings of their foodborne outbreak investigations to CDC through NORS, a national web-based reporting system that tracks foodborne, person-to-person, animal contact, waterborne, and norovirus outbreaks. Prior to NORS, states reported foodborne outbreaks through the Electronic Foodborne Outbreak Reporting System. In 2008, the FDA and CDC executed an MOU under which the FDA provides two contract employees to the OutbreakNet unit at CDC for the purpose of mining and analyzing CDC data to address the FDA's policy and programmatic questions and support its regulatory mission and public health interventions. A plan of work was developed and implemented beginning in late fall 2008. Biannual reports are made to the FDA on progress in the plan's implementation. Examples of topics being addressed are attribution of outbreaks due to raw milk and raw milk cheese versus all dairy and produce attribution classified by produce type.
PDP (Pesticide Data Program) and National Residue Program	Under USDA/AMS's PDP, a collaboration with the U.S. Environmental Protection Agency (EPA), the FDA is notified of apparent food-related violations that are detected by PDP for follow-up, as warranted. Under USDA/FSIS's National Residue Program, the FDA is notified of apparent residue violations in meat, poultry, and egg products for follow-up with the responsible firms. The FDA's pesticide residue data are provided to and used by EPA to support EPA's pesticide tolerance reassessments, required under the Food Quality Protection Act of 1996. When FDA pesticide residue findings indicate pesticide misuse (a violation of the Federal Insecticide, Fungicide, and Rodenticide Act, which is enforced by EPA), the FDA notifies EPA for follow-up as warranted. Currently, as mandated by the Food and Drug Administration Amendments Act of 2007, an MOU among the FDA, USDA's AMS and FSIS, and the U.S. Department of Commerce is being developed so that AMS and FSIS pesticide residue monitoring data will be included in the FDA's pesticide residue monitoring program.

TABLE 5-1 Continued

PetNet	PetNet is a proposed network that would be developed by CVM to report disease outbreaks in companion animals or contamination incidents concerning pet food or animal feed. In March 2009, a working group—including representatives of CVM, CDC, USDA, the U.S. Department of Homeland Security, and public health and feed control officials from the states—was formed to combine expertise in epidemiology, veterinary medicine, emergency response, feed regulation, and laboratory analyses and charged with the development and implementation of PetNet. The target date for implementation is August 2010.
PulseNet (National Molecular Subtyping Network for Foodborne Disease Surveillance)	Established by CDC in collaboration with state public health laboratories, PulseNet is an early warning system for outbreaks of foodborne illness, consisting of a national network of public health laboratories that perform deoxyribonucleic acid (DNA) fingerprinting on foodborne bacteria. Comparison of DNA patterns permits analysts to connect cases to a common source.
Total Diet (TDS) Study	In this ongoing market basket survey, conducted by the FDA, samples of approximately 280 core foods in the U.S. food supply are collected and analyzed to determine levels of various contaminants (such as acrylamide and perchlorate) and nutrients in those foods. Data provided by the TDS have been used by regulatory agencies to estimate exposures to chemicals in foods, to perform risk assessments, and to establish policy.
VetNet	VetNet, a database maintained by USDA's Agricultural Research Service (ARS), was modeled after PulseNet and serves as USDA's pulsed-field gel electrophoresis (PFGE) pattern library. VetNet uses PFGE to subtype animal specimens submitted to NARMS and samples collected from federally inspected meat and poultry establishments for nontyphoidal *Salmonella* and *Campylobacter*. Combined data from VetNet and PulseNet could be used in outbreak investigations and surveillance efforts; however, data sharing issues have limited the usefulness of VetNet in this way. In 2007, an MOU among FSIS, ARS, and CDC was signed to help improve data sharing, but the effectiveness of this agreement has not been evaluated.

TABLE 5-2 Examples of Current Data Collection Systems and Associated Shortcomings

Type of Data	Examples of Current Data Collection Systems	Shortcomings
Behavioral (see Chapter 9)	Food Safety Survey	• Government funding is not adequate. • Substantial delays are incurred because of the 1990 Paper Reduction Act, which includes unnecessary barriers to approval of study designs.
Economic	Only ad hoc collection of this type of data	• Data often are not collected or are collected ad hoc to meet Office of Management and Budget requirements. • Estimates often have many uncertainties.
Food Production (nonregulatory, collected by industry)	Data on levels or presence of pathogens (or pathogen indicators) in ingredients	• Industry is reluctant to share data for fear of regulatory action if a contaminant is found. • Industry fears that competitors will derive some advantage from the information shared. • The amount and type of data collected vary among and within sectors of the food industry. • Smaller producers, processors, etc. have limited ability to collect and analyze data. • Problems with using data may occur when data standards do not exist or are not followed. • The capability for electronic reporting of data is lacking.
Food Production (regulatory or nonregulatory, but collected by government)	Data collected by industry with regard to juice Hazard Analysis and Critical Control Points or low-acid canning process Data collected on traceability to comply with Bioterrorism Act Selected pathogens in domestic and imported fresh produce	• Data collected at the state level are not utilized to drive a risk-based approach. • At the U.S. Food and Drug Administration (FDA), collection is led by the Office of Regulatory Affairs and based on an annual work plan. Participation of the FDA program centers with regard to data needs for a risk-based approach is questionable. • Data collection opportunities are minimal because of the low rate of inspection. • Problems with using data collected for regulatory purposes may occur if design or data standards are inadequate. • Adequate information technology systems with which to share and analyze data on a real-time basis are lacking.

TABLE 5-2 Continued

Type of Data	Examples of Current Data Collection Systems	Shortcomings
Surveillance	Molecular-based • VetNet • PetNet • PulseNet (National Molecultar Subtyping Network for Foodborne Disease Surveillance)	• Collection of data is especially lacking at the farm and retail levels. • VetNet consists of data on isolates obtained through the U.S. Department of Agriculture's regulatory testing program for slaughter and processing establishments. • VetNet is not integrated with PulseNet, hindering the ability to use the data to develop attribution models. • PetNet is in development, and how it will be integrated with VetNet and PulseNet is unclear. • Clinical data, which would be useful for risk ranking, are not collected. • Data cannot be used to estimate the incidence of specific pathogens.
	Contaminants • Aflatoxin testing • Pesticide Data Program • Total Diet Study • Microbiological Data Program	• Most data are not collected routinely, except for some commodities (e.g., sprouts). • Very little data are collected on farms or retail establishments.

continued

TABLE 5-2 Continued

Type of Data	Examples of Current Data Collection Systems	Shortcomings
Surveillance (continued)	Acute clinical outcomes • Center for Food Safety and Applied Nutrition Adverse Events Reporting System • Foodborne Diseases Active Surveillance Network • Epidemic Information Exchange • Norovirus Outbreak • OutbreakNet	• Resources for food safety vary by state and local jurisdiction. • There are no standard procedures, only guidelines, for investigating a local or multistate outbreak. Although guidelines often are followed as if they were legal standards, procedures and participation still vary by state and local jurisdiction. • Lack of communication between epidemiologists and laboratory analysts may delay investigations. • Communication between the FDA and relevant industries varies by state and local jurisdiction. • Etiology is not identified in more than 50% of outbreaks. • Data availability is often delayed by months or years. • The reporting rate to state or local departments varies because of various factors, including a lack of testing or reporting by physicians or others. • Although summaries are available from the U.S. Centers for Disease Control and Prevention, raw data are not easily accessible.
	Long-term clinical outcomes	• Identification of the long-term effects of foodborne illnesses is not routinely performed in the United States.

the exception of a few high-risk products, such as sprouts, the FDA generally has not required routine microbial surveillance of the foods over which it has jurisdiction.

Molecular-based surveillance of microbial pathogens in foods is sparse, particularly at the farm and retail levels. Laboratory and personnel resources have not been made available for such testing and surveillance, and the FDA has lacked the analytic capability to utilize such data optimally even if they were collected. As part of the 1997 Food Safety Initiative, the FDA did conduct companion microbiological surveys of selected imported and domestic produce to examine the prevalence of selected foodborne pathogens. While the results of these surveys were used to guide regulatory activities, they could not be used in quantitative risk assessment because of the low rate of contamination and the lack of quantitative and molecular subtyping data.

In addition to relying on its own data collection, the FDA utilizes data collected by systems (e.g., National Molecular Subtyping Network for Foodborne Disease Surveillance [PulseNet], OutbreakNet, Foodborne Diseases Active Surveillance Network [FoodNet]) managed by other groups, such as the U.S. Centers for Disease Control and Prevention (CDC). These systems, which collect data through nationwide passive or active surveillance in several sentinel sites that are representative of the whole population (IOM, 2003), are starting to address problems associated with the collection of human epidemiological surveillance data.

PulseNet is an example of a notable, albeit still imperfect, improvement in the coordination and sharing of laboratory data among states and federal agencies to conduct nationwide surveillance of foodborne pathogens. The system has been instrumental in recognizing national outbreaks by linking small numbers of cases in different states, which by themselves might not have been further investigated, to similar small clusters in other states. While other federal agencies have established companion data collection systems for animal and food isolates (e.g., VetNet), data sharing between these systems and PulseNet is inconsistent. Further, different methodologies for subtyping, naming, and classifying isolate patterns have complicated the FDA's ability to use data from these other systems even if they were to be fully accessible. As a result, it has not been possible to date to use molecular data to track specific pathogens from farm to table to patient. If PulseNet is to continue to play a significant role in the monitoring of disease occurrence, significant, ongoing funding must be committed to modernizing the system. For example, pulsed-field gel electrophoresis, the technology that serves as the basis for PulseNet, is increasingly antiquated.

OutbreakNet, another CDC system, also relies on information from state and local health departments and works in partnership with PulseNet. Foodborne outbreak reporting is useful for analyzing long-term trends for pathogens not captured in other surveillance systems and for providing summaries of outbreaks (IOM, 2003). OutbreakNet has played a pivotal role in the identification of several national, multistate outbreaks, including the 2006 *E. coli* O157:H7 outbreak associated with spinach. Recognizing the limitations of state and local data and their importance to the efficacy of nationwide foodborne illness and outbreak surveillance, the Institute of Medicine has recommended enhancements to the outbreak investigation and reporting of state and local health departments (IOM, 2003).

Unlike passive surveillance systems, CDC's FoodNet is an active population-based surveillance system that has improved foodborne illness estimates, contributed to the standardization of methods among laboratories, and identified risk factors for pathogen-specific illnesses through its targeted case control studies. In addition, FoodNet is particularly advantageous for capturing data on illnesses that are underrepresented in passive surveillance systems. For example, *Campylobacter* or *Vibrio* infections rarely appear in outbreaks and often are not reportable (IOM, 2003). Even so, FoodNet has its own limitations. For example, case ascertainment is costly and currently neither rapid nor real-time, and the sentinel site approach restricts the system's geographic scope. It is also well recognized that large numbers of cases are not identified because those affected often do not seek medical attention. If medical attention is sought, the physician frequently does not order a stool culture, or, if a stool culture is ordered, the laboratory that receives the specimen may fail to screen for the pathogen that infected the individual. FoodNet attempts to quantify underreporting of foodborne illness through regular telephone-based community surveys as well as periodic surveys of physicians and laboratories.

Regulatory agencies, such as the FDA, are highly dependent on human disease surveillance systems, which in turn depend on data provided by state and local health departments. Reporting practices, the intensity of foodborne illness investigations, and the criteria for deciding which outbreaks to investigate depend on local interests and resources, resulting in foodborne illness reporting rates that can vary more than ten-fold among states in any given year (CDC, 2009). As a result, disease surveillance data available to the FDA are often inconsistent in quality and timeliness. Reporting in general is slow, requiring weeks to months for data to be transmitted from the local to the state to the federal level. Consequently, summary data are posted and published intermittently, often many months or years after a reporting period ends. For example, CDC's 2007 Summary of Notifiable Infectious Diseases was not made available publicly until 2009. Further, because of the variability in reporting by the states, summary data cannot provide reliable estimates of disease prevalence. The lack of standardization in the collection and analysis of data and diverse state and local government capabilities have limited both the utility of these surveillance systems and the speed with which the FDA has been able to respond to recent outbreaks. Moreover, while data on public health practices among the general public, physicians, and clinical laboratories are critical to risk-based decision making, such data are collected only sporadically and usually do not include surveillance of the public health practices of federal, state, and local government agencies (e.g., reporting practices). The committee concluded that, if the FDA is to utilize state and local government data more reliably, standardization of state and local food safety programs will be necessary (see Chapter 7).

Clearly, numerous data collection systems that generate large quantities of data with direct applicability to food safety already exist. These systems were created largely in response to specific needs and often put in place with no strategic forethought as to how the data would be analyzed and/or leveraged, through integration, to achieve the goals of the broader food safety system. Once established, data collection systems frequently have become institutionalized, even if the data being collected are of questionable quality and utility. When new questions arise, there is a tendency to try to retrofit existing systems to address them. While this approach may meet short-term data needs, it often compromises the ability to evaluate trends over time and limits the generalizability and interpretability of the data overall. In some cases, data collection systems simply do not exist (e.g., surveillance for the long-term health effects of foodborne illness) or are sparse (e.g., behavioral data). Some types of data, particularly those generated by industry, have been particularly difficult to acquire and will remain so until mechanisms that can overcome these challenges are put in place.

Lack of Data Sharing Among Government Entities

A wide variety of government entities collect data on food-associated hazards to humans and animals, but significant barriers to sharing those data have been extensively documented (Taylor and Batz, 2008). One barrier is federal and state laws, regulations, and policies that sometimes restrict the sharing of data among government entities because of such concerns as the protection of patient privacy, trade secrets, and confidential business information. These laws, regulations, and policies vary markedly among—and sometimes even within—different federal agencies. Personnel from government agencies performing field investigations frequently lack a firm understanding of the laws, regulations, and policies of their own agencies (and those of their partners), and this lack of knowledge often hampers coordination of efforts and leads to excessive withholding of information.

The failure of government entities to share food safety data sufficiently within the bounds of the law appears to result not only from a misunderstanding of legal obligations but also in part from institutional culture. This observation is illustrated by the sometimes tense relationship between the FDA and CDC. The two agencies agree (in theory) that they should share all information with each other. They have entered into a memorandum of understanding (MOU) (MOU 225-03-8001) that states the following:

> Although there is no legal requirement that FDA and CDC exchange information in all cases, FDA and CDC agree that there should be a presumption in favor of full and free sharing of information between FDA and CDC. As sister public health agencies within the Department of Health and Human Services, there are no legal prohibitions that preclude FDA or CDC from sharing with each other most agency records in the possession of either agency. (FDA, 2003)

The committee learned, however, that the actual relationship between the FDA and CDC falls far short of fulfilling this presumption of full and free data sharing (Morse, 2009; Osterholm, 2009). In response to written questions about information sharing between the agencies, the Center for Food Safety and Applied Nutrition (CFSAN) provided the following statement:

> To determine what foods may be responsible for causing outbreaks, FDA relies in part on epidemiological data from the [CDC] which, in large part, relies on the states. CDC redacts confidential private patient information from these data, as required by federal privacy laws, but otherwise there are no legal constraints to the sharing of this information between CDC and FDA because there is a signed confidentiality [MOU] between the two agencies that allows for the free exchange of information. However, sometimes there are delays in FDA's receiving epidemiological data from CDC because the states need to supply CDC with the data and CDC needs time to compile the data, redact any confidential patient information, and analyze, [sic] and interpret these data before sharing.[5]

CFSAN's response illustrates the real and perceived barriers to information sharing between CDC and the FDA. CDC appears to have informed the FDA that "federal privacy laws" require CDC to redact confidential patient information before providing data to the FDA. This redaction of information delays data sharing; at worst, it prevents or delays the FDA's use of the information to protect public health. Federal law does not require such redaction. The relevant statute, the Privacy Act, 5 U.S.C. 552a,[6] prohibits federal agencies from disclosing any personal record without the consent of the person to whom the record pertains, but it contains an explicit exception for disclosures "to those officers and employees of the agency which maintains the record who have a need for the record in the performance of their duties." CDC and the FDA, as sister agencies within the U.S. Department of Health and Human Services (HHS), fall within this exception.[7] Of course, none of this is to suggest that patient-identifying information should be shared between the agencies when there is no need

---

[5] Personal communication, Chad Nelson, FDA, July 25, 2009.

[6] *The Privacy Act of 1974*, 5 U.S.C. § 552a(b)(1); The Health Privacy Rule of the Health Insurance Portability and Accountability Act would not normally limit CDC's authority to share data with anyone because CDC is not a "covered entity" subject to that rule.

[7] The Privacy Act incorporates the definition of the term "agency" from the Freedom of Information Act, which in turns defines "agency" as "any executive *department*, military department, Government corporation, Government controlled corporation, or other establishment in the executive branch of the Government (including the Executive Office of the President), or any independent regulatory agency [emphasis added]." *The Privacy Act of 1974*, 5 U.S.C. § 552a(f)(1).

to do so. But sharing of confidential information is appropriate when redaction by CDC would unduly delay the transmission of essential information to the FDA in an emergency situation or would completely deny the FDA information it needs to protect the public health. Consequently, it is important for the agencies to understand that such redaction by CDC is not legally required.

The MOU between CDC and the FDA (MOU 225-03-8001) appears to assume that such confidential information may be shared between the agencies, and it establishes a mechanism for doing so. For "routine requests for information," the agency seeking the information need only demonstrate, in writing, why it needs the requested information, and the responding agency "should only decide not to share information in response to [such] a request if it has credible information and a reasonable belief that the requesting agency may not be able to comply with applicable laws or regulations governing the protection of non-public information or with the principles or procedures set forth in this MOU." With respect to "emergency requests for confidential information," the MOU sets forth more flexible and expeditious procedures, which include oral requests. The MOU explicitly cites "a foodborne illness outbreak" as its one example of "emergency circumstances" (FDA, 2003).

CFSAN's quoted response to the committee's written questions suggests that CDC fails to live up to the MOU's presumption of "full and free sharing of information" not only because of real or perceived legal limitations but also, as suggested above, because of its institutional culture. The response states that CDC withholds food safety data from the FDA until it "analyzes" and "interprets" the data. There is no legal requirement or public health justification for such a delay. The perception among some witnesses questioned by the committee was that CDC employees are reluctant to disseminate data, even to a sister agency, if early release of those data might compromise their academic publishing opportunities.

The committee understands, but was unable to verify, that some states may have data-sharing agreements with CDC that prohibit CDC from sharing confidential data it has obtained from the states with additional parties, perhaps even sister federal agencies such as the FDA. If such provisions do in fact exist, in the new climate of a closer working relationship between federal and state food safety authorities, greater sharing of information and the development of ways to share information within the bounds of confidentiality would be beneficial. To the extent that state laws prohibit the sharing of confidential information with federal agencies altogether, even when such sharing is necessary to protect the public health, reassessing such laws to permit the creation of a truly cooperative and integrated food safety system would be warranted.

Problems also appear to exist with respect to information sharing between the FDA and the U.S. Environmental Protection Agency (EPA), which, unlike CDC, is not a sister agency within HHS. CFSAN reported to the committee that during the 2008 incident involving the melamine contamination of dairy powder imported from China, the EPA declined to share the results of a melamine exposure assessment with the FDA because that assessment "contained confidential commercial information not disclosable outside of EPA."[8]

There is also evidence of substantial constraints and delays in the flow of food safety information from the FDA to state and local governments. The FDA's responses to the committee's questions on data sharing identify several federal laws that restrict what food safety information it can share with state and local authorities. These laws include the following:

- The Trade Secrets Act, 18 U.S.C. 1905, prohibits any federal agency employee from divulging "in any manner or to any extent not authorized by law any information coming to him in the course of his employment or official duties . . . which information concerns or relates to the trade secrets, processes, operations, style of work, or apparatus, or to the identity, confidential statistical data, amount or source of any income, profits, losses, or expenditures of any person, firm, partnership, corporation, or association."[9]
- Section 301(j) of the Federal Food, Drug, and Cosmetic Act (FDCA), 21 U.S.C. 331(j), prohibits "revealing, other than to the Secretary or officers or employees of the Department, or to the courts when relevant in any judicial proceeding under this Act, any information acquired under authority of [an enumerated list of FDCA sections] concerning any method or process which as a trade secret is entitled to protection. . . ."[10]
- The Privacy Act, 5 U.S.C. 552a, prohibits federal agencies from disclosing any personal record without the consent of the person to whom the record pertains.

The restrictions on data sharing established by these laws are not necessarily as sweeping as they appear at first glance, however. For example, the Trade Secrets Act applies only to disclosures "not authorized by law," and the FDA could by regulation "authorize" its employees to share various types of information vital to food safety, provided it has been granted the requisite authority by Congress to do so. Section 301(j) of the FDCA applies, on its face, only to trade secrets and not to confidential commer-

---

[8] Personal communication, Chad Nelson, FDA, July 25, 2009.
[9] *The Trade Secrets Act*, 18 U.S.C. § 1905.
[10] *The Federal Food, Drug, and Cosmetic Act*, 21 U.S.C. 331(j).

cial information that does not qualify as a trade secret.[11] Consequently, this provision appears to bar FDA officers and employees from sharing information concerning food formulas and manufacturing processes, for example, but not from sharing distribution data needed to conduct trace-back/trace-forward activities. The Privacy Act contains a number of potentially relevant exceptions, the most important of which is the "routine use" exception. Under this provision,[12] an agency can disclose a record containing information about an individual without that individual's consent if the disclosure is for a "routine use" defined by regulation. An agency may define the disclosure of a record as a "routine use" if the disclosure is for any "purpose which is compatible with the purpose for which [the record] was collected."[13] Each agency thus has broad discretion under the Privacy Act to decide when it is appropriate to disclose personal information.

These federal laws clearly present real obstacles to information sharing between the FDA and state and local governments. One possible method for facilitating such communications in light of these legal restrictions is through the liberal use of commissioned officials in state and local governments. According to its regulations, the FDA may share "data otherwise exempt from public disclosure" with "state and local government officials commissioned pursuant to 21 U.S.C. 372(a)," which states that:

> [t]he Secretary is authorized to conduct examinations and investigations for the purposes of this Act . . . through any health, food, or drug officer or employee of any State, Territory, or political subdivision thereof, duly commissioned by the Secretary as an officer of the Department.

The FDA is understandably concerned that state and local officials

---

[11] The FDA's own regulations draw a distinction between a "trade secret" on the one hand and "commercial or financial information that is privileged or confidential" on the other. According to the regulations,

> [a] trade secret may consist of any commercially valuable plan, formula, process, or device that is used for the making, preparing, compounding, or processing of trade commodities and that can be said to be the end product of either innovation or substantial effort. There must be a direct relationship between the trade secret and the productive process). 21 CFR 20.61(a)

By contrast,

> [c]ommercial or financial information that is privileged or confidential means valuable data or information which is used in one's business and is of a type customarily held in strict confidence or regarded as privileged and not disclosed to any member of the public by the person to whom it belongs. (21 CFR 20.61(b))

[12] 21 U.S.C. 552a(b)(3) (incorporating by reference 21 U.S.C. 552a(a)(7) and 21 U.S.C. 552a(e)(4)(D)).

[13] 21 U.S.C. 552a(a)(7).

with whom it shares confidential information will disclose that information inappropriately. Under 21 CFR 20.84, commissioned officials are "subject to the same restrictions with respect to the disclosure of such data and information as any other [FDA] employee." Nevertheless, CFSAN, in its answers to the committee's questions, noted that "due to their sunshine [openness] laws, certain states are unable to keep such information confidential, which limits FDA's ability to share such information."

With regard to the provision of information by state and local governments to the FDA, CFSAN told the committee that:

> [t]here are legal restrictions on the sharing by state and local governments of epidemiological data that may contain patient information that is considered confidential. This occurs with every outbreak investigation. . . . We understand that these restrictions derive from state and federal patient privacy laws. . . .[14]

Federal law may in fact limit information sharing by state and local government entities in at least some instances. For example, the FDA public information regulations, 21 CFR 20.63(b), state that:

> [t]he names and other information which would identify patients . . . should be deleted from any record before it is submitted to the [FDA]. If the [FDA] subsequently needs the names of such individuals, a separate request will be made.[15]

The committee does not know whether this regulation has prevented or delayed the sharing of vital food safety information by state and local governments with the FDA.

One oft-cited federal statute that, regardless of perception, does not in fact appear to greatly inhibit the sharing of food safety information between state and local governments and the FDA is the Health Insurance Portability and Accountability Act (HIPAA). The HHS Privacy Rule implementing HIPAA, 45 CFR Part 160 and Part 164, Subparts A and E, applies only to "covered entities" specified in the statute, namely "health plans," "healthcare clearinghouses," and "healthcare providers."[16] Many state and local agencies possessing epidemiological data do not fall within any of these categories. To the extent that a state or local agency is a "covered entity," the Privacy Rule contains an explicit public health exception that would

[14] Personal communication, Chad Nelson, FDA, July 25, 2009.
[15] 21 CFR 20.63(b).
[16] *The Health Insurance Portability and Accountability Act of 1996*, Public Law 104-191, section 1172.

apply in the context of a food safety emergency.[17] HIPAA prevents the disclosure only of patient-identifying information, so even when the statute applies, it does not prohibit the dissemination of appropriately redacted data (although the redaction process may cause delay). However, it should be noted that state privacy laws may present a greater barrier to the sharing of food safety information by state and local governments. They may cover more types of entities and impose more stringent privacy requirements than does HIPAA.[18]

Access to Industry Data

Many food companies have carefully designed science-driven food safety systems that produce a substantial amount of data that would be of great value for risk-based decision making. Industry has, however, been reluctant to share its data with the FDA. Barriers that limit the ease with which data from industry could flow to the FDA include the proprietary nature of such data, the absence of an appropriate information infrastructure to manage the data, and potential regulatory ramifications, the latter of which is often cited as the most significant concern. In short, the FDA has generally not been successful in accessing industry data, and although the concept periodically arises as a point of discussion, the agency has made no coordinated effort to overcome the barriers involved.

MOVING FORWARD: DESIGNING AND IMPLEMENTING AN INTEGRATED INFORMATION INFRASTRUCTURE

Designing and implementing the integrated information infrastructure necessary to support a risk-based food safety system will require an investment in information science, as well as an infrastructure that improves data availability and quality and facilitates data standardization, harmonization, and analysis. In 2007, the FDA Science Board recommended that the agency collaborate with other government agencies to develop data standards and large-scale sustainable data-sharing infrastructures that would allow the timely integration and analysis of data critical to the agency's mission (FDA Science Board, 2007). Such an investment would reduce data gaps and facilitate risk-based decision making while improving communication, the integration of business processes, and interoperability. In the committee's

---

[17] 45 CFR 164.512(j). See also 45 CFR 164.512(f) (law enforcement exception).

[18] HIPAA itself does not limit how strictly states may protect patient privacy. The HIPAA Privacy Rule, by its own terms, does not preempt state law regarding the privacy of patient health information to the extent that the state law is more stringent than the federal regulations (45 CFR 160.203(b)). Moreover, some state laws may impose patient privacy limitations on state and local government entities not covered by HIPAA.

opinion, key elements necessary to initiate the transition to an integrated information infrastructure include (1) strategic data collection, (2) the accessibility of data, (3) the availability of a modern IT system, and (4) the analytic capacity to design and maintain the system as well as to analyze, interpret, and disseminate data generated by the system. These elements are discussed briefly below. Chapter 11 examines potential organizational changes to ensure that these elements are in place.

Strategic Data Collection

Accurate, reliable, secure, and timely data are the backbone of any risk-based decision-making system. The types of data collected and the methods employed in data collection should, ultimately, be driven by the specific objectives and goals of the system. The data that could be collected are virtually endless, making the strategic planning process critical. Strategic planning is readily applicable to data collection and analysis; in fact, it is necessary for the development of an integrated information infrastructure. The strategic plan must address the following:

- the goals and ultimate uses of the data (attribution, public health response, development of targeted interventions);
- the types of data needed to achieve those goals;
- an assessment of what data are currently being collected, as well as their limitations and appropriateness;
- the data issues and gaps that must be addressed to achieve the stated goals;
- the priorities for collecting additional data;
- the data collection methods and standards necessary for accessing, integrating, and analyzing the various sources of data;
- the analytic capabilities necessary for collecting, integrating, and analyzing the data; and
- the performance metrics that will be used to evaluate the data collection and analysis system, including a quality assurance system.

The first step in the strategic planning process should be a comprehensive inventory and review of existing data collection systems without regard for interinstitutional boundaries. Each data collection system should be reviewed by FDA and non-FDA scientists to evaluate its relevance, funding, productivity, and programmatic benefits as they relate to the agency's mission. Such an approach would provide valuable information for the strategic planning process and would, in essence, make data collection part of the set of risk management tools available for agency use. To be effective, the strategic planning process will require input from multiple federal, state, and local government agencies, as well industry and nongovernmental organizations (NGOs).

Data collection should not be performed simply for its own sake. Decisions on data collection systems and the exact nature of the data to be collected must be driven by the needs of the underlying risk-based decision-making process. As discussed further in Chapter 11, the development of appropriate and cost-effective data collection systems should, ideally, be done in collaboration with other agencies and departments involved in work with food safety, potentially through a single, unified center focused on data collection and analysis. Data collection systems should be developed and evaluated within the risk-based decision-making process outlined in this report. In the absence of a single food agency, it will be challenging to formulate a strategic vision for developing and implementing the integrated information infrastructure necessary to support a risk-based food safety system. The FDA can and should take an active leadership role in the development and implementation of a system that is designed to suit its needs in the years to come.

Access to Data

Many different groups collect food safety data for different purposes that could be valuable to the regulatory mission of the FDA. The system should leverage data collected for a variety of purposes by various federal, state, and local government agencies, as well as by the food industry, the academic sector, and NGOs. To this end, it is essential that data be accessible to all stakeholders in a timely manner. The FDA's ability to effectively identify, investigate, and respond to food safety issues—including outbreaks, emerging pathogens, and the choice of intervention strategies—is dependent on timely access to quality data that are often collected by others.

As described above, substantial barriers to data sharing must be addressed before a risk-based system can be implemented effectively. Relevant government agencies should examine whether they currently withhold more food safety information than is required by law, and they should correct any current misunderstandings of the law. The FDA should take a leadership role in implementing the recommendations of Taylor and Batz (2008) for improving access to currently available data necessary to fulfill its mission. Chapter 11 outlines some approaches, such as a centralized risk-based analysis and data management center, that might alleviate some of the barriers to data sharing mentioned in this section. Regardless of the establishment of these approaches, many of the actions suggested below will still be needed to overcome data-sharing barriers. To the extent that legal changes are needed to allow sufficient data sharing, especially in the case of emergencies, Congress should consider amending the law.

To facilitate the sharing of food safety data relevant to protecting the public health, the Secretary of HHS should publish guidelines, including answers to frequently asked questions, concerning data sharing between different HHS agencies. In addition, the FDA and CDC should jointly provide training to their food safety employees regarding the actual limits on such data sharing imposed by federal law. There would be some benefit in having FDA and CDC employees present at the same training sessions. This training should address in detail the data-sharing MOU entered into by the two agencies. The FDA should also assist state and local food safety agencies regarding the provision of such training to state and local employees. Further, the FDA should, as recommended elsewhere in this report, consider greatly expanding the use of its commissioning authority to create a cadre of state and local commissioned officers throughout the nation, which, in addition to increasing the size of the agency's inspectional force, would facilitate data sharing between the FDA and state and local governments. Entering into formal data-sharing agreements with other federal agencies with which the FDA has shared or might share food safety information (e.g., EPA) is also advisable. In terms of legal barriers to sharing data, the FDA should determine whether federal law preempts state openness laws with respect to information provided to FDA-commissioned state and local officers and, if necessary, ask Congress to revise the relevant statutes and regulations to ensure that the agency can share confidential data without concern that those data will later be made public under state openness laws. The FDA should also determine whether its public information regulations, such as 21 CFR 20.63(b), have prevented or delayed state and local governments' sharing of vital food safety information with the agency. If necessary, the regulations should be revised to permit state and local governments, as well as other entities, to submit records to the FDA in emergency situations or when there is a legitimate need without first redacting patient-identifying information.

In terms of accessibility of industry data, the Public Health Security and Bioterrorism Preparedness and Response Act of 2002 gives the FDA access to industry records only when they are related to food that "presents a threat of serious adverse health consequences or death to humans or animals."[19] In Chapter 10, the committee recommends that the FDCA be amended to require that every food facility prepare a food safety plan and that this plan and its implementation records be made available to FDA inspectors. The FDA should identify the kinds of industry data that are needed for risk-based decision making and develop mechanisms for collecting and ensuring the quality of those data. The FDA should also

---

[19] *Public Health Security and Bioterrorism Preparedness and Response Act of 2002 (Bioterrorism Act)*, Public Law 107-188, 107th Cong., 2nd sess. (January 23, 2002).

consider regulatory changes, to the extent necessary to ensure food safety, that would authorize it to release some trade secret and confidential commercial information under the Trade Secrets Act. To help promote the trust and cooperation of industry, advances in tracking, masking, and analyzing information should be explored to enable the FDA and its partners to protect such information while sharing information that specifically helps protect public health.

Information Technology and Personnel Needs

Information Technology

A critical component of the implementation of a risk-based decision-making system is the underlying technology necessary for the collection, processing, and delivery of information. The inability to collect, integrate, and deliver information can result in inefficient use of resources, redundancy, ineffective information sharing, and delayed or inappropriate regulatory decision making, all of which impact public health (FDA Science Board, 2007; GAO, 2009). The ability to access, integrate, and analyze numerous and varied data sources depends on the development, harmonization, evaluation, and adoption of an electronic data exchange environment that supports data standards.

Several recent reports have found critical gaps in the FDA's centralized IT infrastructure, which has been described as obsolete, redundant, and unstable (FDA Science Board, 2007; GAO, 2009). In 2007, the FDA Science Board described the agency's IT situation as "problematic at best—and at worst it is dangerous" (FDA Science Board, 2007, p. 5).The FDA's IT workforce has been deemed insufficient to meet the agency's needs (FDA Science Board, 2007). Further, the FDA's IT infrastructure lacks the necessary backup systems to provide continuity of operation in case of system failures (FDA Science Board, 2007). During the 2006 spinach-related outbreak, for example, failures in the FDA's e-mail system contributed to delays in responding to the outbreak (FDA Science Board, 2007).

Recent evidence suggests that the FDA is making progress, albeit slowly, in improving its information infrastructure (FDA Science Board, 2009). In 2008, the agency began an effort to consolidate its IT infrastructure and centralize its IT management with the creation of the Office of Information Management (GAO, 2009). As of this writing, the development of a comprehensive strategic plan for this office was under way and was expected to be completed by the end of fiscal year 2009 (GAO, 2009). Progress appears to have been made on developing an IT architecture design and on building the foundation for data standards and harmonization (FDA Science Board, 2009). Several initiatives to modernize the FDA's information infrastructure and IT systems have been undertaken, with the Predictive Risk-Based Evaluation for Dynamic Import Compliance Targeting (PREDICT) model as a relevant example (see Chapter 3 and Appendix E). Workforce assessments have also been undertaken. Further, the FDA has established a Bioinformatics Board to oversee the agency's IT investments, as well as Business Review Boards for each of the core business areas that are responsible for the day-to-day oversight of IT projects. It has also created a project management office, developed criteria for evaluating prospective projects, and documented project monitoring and control processes.

Despite this recent progress, however, substantial challenges remain, including centralizing IT, developing a scientific computing infrastructure, addressing information security issues, and conducting strategic human capital planning. Of particular concern are the lack of a detailed, comprehensive strategic IT plan and the agency's segmented approach to developing its enterprise architecture. For example, the FDA started building PREDICT, a component of its enterprise architecture, without having a detailed plan or establishing priorities for the development of the overall enterprise architecture (FDA Science Board, 2009). Such an approach is contrary to the concepts outlined in this report and may ultimately result in a fragmented enterprise architecture that is incompatible with future systems.

The committee agrees with the recommendations in the FDA Science Board report. The committee emphasizes the importance of the development of a modern IT infrastructure and investment in the FDA's IT workforce (see section below regarding Personnel Needs) to meeting the agency's public health objectives and implementing its overall strategic plan.

Personnel Needs

The problems of fragmented data collection systems and inaccessibility of data are compounded by an inadequate pool of scientific personnel that can, even in times of emergency, effectively collect, manage, analyze, interpret, and disseminate the data to which they have access. Several reports have noted the problem of insufficient staff, as well as inadequate recruitment and retention and the failure to make an investment in professional development (FDA Science Board, 2007). Recently, the U.S. Government Accountability Office (GAO) recommended that the agency manage its workforce strategically by determining the critical skills and competencies needed to fulfill its mission, analyzing the gaps between current skills and future needs, and developing strategies for filling those gaps (GAO, 2009). While the FDA has increased its training budget and is conducting workforce assessments (FDA Science Board, 2007, 2009), however, it has not yet addressed the bulk of these GAO recommendations.

The FDA is underutilizing its field personnel. For example, field assignments could be used for the collection of data (e.g., who uses a specific piece of equipment in processing frozen peas) or the analysis of samples (e.g., a statistically representative sampling of bagged salads for microbiological analysis). Prior to 1994, ORA's Minneapolis Center for Microbiological Investigation conducted analyses in the field for the FDA; however, this dedicated function no longer exists. Given the agency's limited inspection capacity, most efforts of the inspectional force are dedicated to performing legally required inspectional duties.

As mentioned in Chapter 3, one way to meet the FDA's analytical personnel needs would be to create functional teams in support of the risk-based approach. In this case, for example, a surveillance team would be responsible for interacting with other federal agencies and state and local jurisdictions and for managing centralized epidemiological databases supporting modeling efforts. Such a group would include statisticians, epidemiologists, microbiologists, behavioral scientists, economists, risk analysts, biomathematical modelers, database managers, IT personnel, risk managers, and other experts as needed. Also, the agency should start implementing the above-mentioned GAO recommendation to address its IT human resource needs (GAO, 2009). Chapter 11 describes approaches for consolidating data and risk analysis, such as a centralized risk-based analysis and data management center that would meet the needs of all agencies with responsibilities for food safety. As outlined in Chapter 11, the committee sees clear potential advantages to the creation of such a center that would have access to food safety data from multiple agencies, the analytical capacity to deal with these data, and the ability to disseminate results of its analyses to agencies for policy development. Even with such a center, however, the FDA will need to maintain a core of experts in all the disciplines noted above.

KEY CONCLUSIONS AND RECOMMENDATIONS

Decisions on data collection systems and the characteristics of the data to be collected must be driven by the needs of the underlying risk-based decision-making process. The FDA has not adequately assessed and articulated its data needs. The agency currently lacks the capability to collect and integrate the data needed for effective implementation of a risk-based approach to food safety. For example, it lacks a dedicated cadre of analytical personnel to design, implement, and manage the collection of and analyze, interpret, and disseminate the data needed to support a risk-based system. It lacks a group of epidemiologists, statisticians, and data analysts that can work with risk modelers, analysts, and managers to support risk-based decisions about food safety.

In terms of sharing data with other relevant partners (e.g., CDC, the U.S. Department of Agriculture, the food industry), it appears that the legal regime now in place would permit a substantial increase in such data sharing. However, nonlegal obstacles, both technological (e.g., inadequate IT) and cultural (e.g., unnecessary delays in sharing data or a lack of trust), continue to limit the sharing of data among partners. To protect the public health, federal, state, and local agencies and industry must share more food safety information, and share it more rapidly, than is now the case.

In support of a risk-based approach driven by data, the committee makes the following recommendations.

Recommendation 5-1: Data collection by the FDA should be driven by the recommended risk-based approach and should support risk-based decision making. It is critical that the FDA evaluate its food safety data needs and develop a strategic plan to meet those needs. The FDA should review existing data collection systems for foods to identify data gaps, eliminate systems of limited utility, and develop the necessary surveillance capabilities to support the risk-based approach. The FDA should formulate and implement a plan for developing, harmonizing, evaluating, and adopting data standards. The FDA should also establish a mechanism for coordinating, capturing, and integrating data, including modernization of its information technology systems. To coordinate, capture, and integrate data, the FDA could lead the implementation of a multiagency food safety epidemiology users group as outlined by Taylor and Batz (2008). The centralized risk-based analysis and data management center proposed in recommendation 11-3 in Chapter 11 could serve the functions of data storage and analysis in support of a risk-based approach. Mechanisms should also be instituted to build trust with industry and, in partnership, collect and analyze industry data.

Recommendation 5-2: The FDA should evaluate its personnel needs to carry out its roles in collecting, analyzing, managing, and communicating food safety data. The agency should establish an analytical unit with the resources and expertise (i.e., statisticians, epidemiologists, behavioral scientists, economists, microbiologists, risk analysts, biomathematical modelers, database managers, information technology personnel, risk managers, and others as needed) to support risk-based decision making.

Recommendation 5-3: The FDA should evaluate statutes and policies governing data sharing and develop plans to improve the collection and sharing of relevant data by all federal, state, and local food safety agencies. For example, in collaboration with other food safety agencies, the

FDA should develop and implement technologies and procedures that will ensure confidentiality and facilitate data sharing. Congress should consider amending the law, to the extent that legal changes are needed, to allow sufficient data sharing among government agencies.

REFERENCES

CDC (U.S. Centers for Disease Control and Prevention). 2009. Surveillance for foodborne disease outbreaks—United States, 2006. *Morbidity and Mortality Weekly Report* 58(22):609–615.

FDA (U.S. Food and Drug Administration). 2003. *Memorandum of Understanding Between the Food and Drug Administration and the Centers for Disease Control and Prevention.* MOU 225-03-8001. http://www.fda.gov/AboutFDA/PartnershipsCollaborations/MemorandaofUnderstandingMOUs/DomesticMOUs/ucm115068.htm (accessed May 15, 2010).

FDA Science Board. 2007. *FDA Science and Mission at Risk. Report of the Subcommittee on Science and Technology.* Rockville, MD: FDA.

FDA Science Board. 2009. *Science Board Subcommittee Review of Information Technology.* Rockville, MD: FDA. http://www.fda.gov/AdvisoryCommittees/CommitteesMeetingMaterials/ScienceBoardtotheFoodandDrugAdministration/ucm176816.htm (accessed April 14, 2010).

Frenzen, P. D., A. Drake, and F. J. Angulo. 2005. Economic cost of illness due to *Escherichia coli* O157 infections in the United States. *Journal of Food Protection* 68(12):2623–2630.

FSWG (Food Safety Working Group). 2009. *Food Safety Working Group: Key Findings.* http://www.foodsafetyworkinggroup.gov/FSWG_Key_Findings.pdf (accessed February 18, 2010).

GAO (U.S. Government Accountability Office). 2009. *Information Technology: FDA Needs to Establish Key Plans and Processes for Guiding Systems Modernization Efforts.* Washington, DC: GAO.

Havelaar, A. H., J. Braunig, K. Christiansen, M. Cornu, T. Hald, M. J. Mangen, K. Molbak, A. Pielaat, E. Snary, M. Van Boven, W. Van Pelt, A. Velthuis, and H. Wahlstrom. 2006. *Towards an Integrated Approach in Supporting Microbiological Food Safety Decisions.* Med-Vet-Net. Report No. 06-001. http://www.medvetnet.org/pdf/Reports/Report_06-001.pdf (accessed May 15, 2010).

HHS (U.S. Department of Health and Human Services). 2009. *Healthy People 2020: The Road Ahead.* http://www.healthypeople.gov/hp2020/default.asp (accessed February 18, 2010).

IOM (Institute of Medicine). 2003. *Scientific Criteria to Ensure Safe Food.* Washington, DC: The National Academies Press.

Kemmeren, J. M., M. J. Mangen, Y. T. P. H. Van Duynhoven, and A. Havelaar. 2006. *Priority Setting of Foodborne Pathogens: Disease Burden and Costs of Selected Enteric Pathogens.* Bilthoven, The Netherlands: RIVM Ministry of Public Health, Welfare and Sports. http://www.rivm.nl/bibliotheek/rapporten/330080001.pdf (accessed January 30, 2009).

Last, J. M., ed. 1995. *A Dictionary of Epidemiology*, 3rd ed. New York: Oxford University Press.

Majowicz, S. E., W. B. McNab, P. Sockett, S. Henson, K. Dore, V. L. Edge, M. C. Buffett, S. Read, S. McEwen, D. Stacey, and J. B. Wilson. 2004. The burden and cost of gastrointestinal illness in a Canadian community. *Journal of Food Protection* 69:651–659.

Medeiros, L. C., P. Kendall, V. Hillers, G. Chen, and S. DiMascola. 2001. Identification and classification of consumer food-handling behaviors for food safety education. *Journal of the American Dietetic Association* 101(11):1326–1339.

Morse, D. L. 2009. *Foodborne Disease Surveillance: Vignettes of a State Epidemiologist*. Paper presented at Institute of Medicine/National Research Council Committee on Review of the FDA's Role in Ensuring Safe Food Meeting, Washington, DC, March 24, 2009.

NRC (National Research Council). 2009. *Letter Report on the Review of the Food Safety and Inspection Service Proposed Risk-Based Approach to and Application of Public-Health Attribution*. Washington, DC: The National Academies Press.

Osterholm, M. T. 2009. *Role of Foodborne Disease Surveillance and Food Attribution in Food Safety*. Paper presented at Institute of Medicine/National Research Council Committee on Review of the FDA's Role in Ensuring Safe Food Meeting, Washington, DC, March 24, 2009.

Pilling, V. K., L. A. Brannon, C. W. Shanklin, A. D. Howells, and K. R. Roberts. 2008. Identifying specific beliefs to target to improve restaurant employees' intentions for performing three important food safety behaviors. *Journal of the American Dietetic Association* 108(6):991–997.

Ruzante, J. M., V. J. Davidson, J. Caswell, A. Fazil, J. A. L. Cranfield, S. J. Henson, S. M. Anders, C. Schmidt, and J. Farber. 2009. A multi-factorial risk prioritization framework for foodborne pathogens. *Risk Analysis*. Published online in advance of print. http://www3.interscience.wiley.com/journal/122542673/abstract (accessed May 15, 2010).

Shogren, J. F., J. A. Fox, D. J. Hayes, and J. Roosen. 1999. Observed choices for food safety in retail, survey, and auction markets. *American Journal of Agricultural Economics* 81(5):1192–1199.

Taylor, M. R., and M. B Batz. 2008. *Harnessing Knowledge to Ensure Food Safety: Opportunities to Improve the Nation's Food Safety Information Infrastructure*. Gainesville, FL: Food Safety Research Consortium.

USDA/ERS (U.S. Department of Agriculture/Economic Research Service). 2009. *Foodborne Illness Cost Calculator: Assumption Details and Citations for Salmonella*. Washington, DC: USDA. http://www.ers.usda.gov/data/FoodBorneIllness/salmAssumptionDescriptions.asp?Pathogen=Salmonella&p=1&s=4683&y=2006&n=1397187 (accessed January 30, 2009).

6

Creating a Research Infrastructure for a Risk-Based Food Safety System

The U.S. Food and Drug Administration's (FDA's) food safety research functions are performed predominantly by three intramurally funded centers—the Center for Food Safety and Applied Nutrition (CFSAN), the Center for Veterinary Medicine (CVM), and the National Center for Toxicological Research (NCTR)—with some involvement of the Office of Regulatory Affairs (ORA). The agency's food safety research mission is also supported by external research centers in formal collaboration with academic institutions as well as a few other activities. The food safety research at these intra- and extramural centers is summarized by topic in Appendix F. The research authority of the FDA's food programs encompasses two major areas (Musser, 2009): (1) support for the Code of Federal Regulations, with a focus primarily on the development of improved and/or advanced detection methods, and (2) activities in support of specific food safety initiatives, such as the Food Protection Plan, counterterrorism efforts, and appropriations conference reports (Musser, 2009).

The FDA conducts a large research program in support of its food safety mission. According to the U.S. Department of Health and Human Services' fiscal year (FY) 2010 justification of estimates (HHS, 2010), total 2009 allocated research funding for the agency as a whole was $190,070,000. This total encompasses research in support of all FDA programs, of which the foods component is only a part. For the FDA's FY 2009 food programs, the congressional budget included $30,178,000[1] (approximately

---

[1] In addition to research, these figures include funding for buildings and equipment and personnel.

181

15 percent of the agency's total research budget) in base research funding for CFSAN and ORA, reflecting an increase of $2,862,000 over the previous FY(Musser, 2009). An additional $1,683,000 was budgeted for food protection research at NCTR for 2009. For FY 2010, center-specific resource allocations for research are summarized in Table 6-1. Overall, the agency's food safety research initiatives can be categorized as follows: (1) development of rapid detection methods, (2) development of confirmatory methods, (3) biotechnology, (4) virology, (5) in vitro testing, and (6) laboratory enhancement (Musser, 2009).

This chapter provides a summary of the research currently conducted under the FDA's food programs and considers how these research efforts do or do not mesh with the risk-based approach described in Chapter 3.

TABLE 6-1 FY 2010 Resource Allocations for Research, by FDA Center

Center	Research FTEs	Total Research Funding	Increase in Funding over Last Fiscal Year
Center for Food Safety and Applied Nutrition	30 (premarket applied research)[a] 140 (postmarket applied research)[a]	$9,478,000 (premarket applied research)[a] $54,222,000 (postmarket applied research)[a]	+$374,000 (premarket applied research)[b] +$8,006,000 (postmarket applied research)[b]
Center for Veterinary Medicine	16 (premarket applied research)[a] 44 (postmarket applied research)[a]	$3,043,000 (premarket applied research)[a] $8,195,000 (postmarket applied research)[a]	+$789,000 (premarket applied research)[b] +$1,208,000 (postmarket applied research)[b]
National Center for Toxicological Research	211	$58,745,000[c] $1,625,000 specifically for Protecting America's Food Supply[c]	+$6,234,000[c] +$1,625,000 specifically for Protecting America's Food Supply[c]
Office of Regulatory Affairs	Not available	$1,100,000[d]	No increase[e]

NOTE: FDA = U.S. Food and Drug Administration; FTE = full-time equivalent; FY = fiscal year.

[a] FDA, 2010b.
[b] FDA, 2010b,c.
[c] FDA, 2010d.
[d] This number applies to food research activities only (FDA, 2010e).
[e] FDA, 2009.

Much of the information on which the discussion is based was gathered from a report provided by CFSAN, which was written in response to an FDA Science Board task to review the center's research and related support programs.[2] A review of the research and related support programs at CVM was completed by the FDA Science Board in 2009 (FDA Science Board, 2009) and was also consulted in the preparation of this chapter, as was a packet of materials from the FDA with salient information about NCTR (NCTR, 2009a,b,c). In addition, information was obtained from the FDA website and consultation with FDA staff.

INTRAMURAL RESEARCH PORTFOLIO

CFSAN[3]

The FDA's largest food safety research portfolio is housed in CFSAN. In the above-referenced report provided to the Science Board, CFSAN describes the purpose of its research program as to "conduct applied and translational research that facilitates our enforcement of the Federal Food, Drug and Cosmetic Act, the U.S. Public Health Service Act, the Infant Formula Act, and the Dietary Supplement Health and Education Act." The report further states that "CFSAN takes advantage of the research capabilities of other federal research agencies, which allows it to focus its research infrastructure on the conduct of critical problem-solving research." These statements make clear that the center's research mission is applied in nature.

As of this writing, CFSAN had 170 research full-time equivalents (FTEs). For the purposes of this report, these FTEs are classified as primary researchers, engaged in the collection of original data. Information about the proportion of FTEs dedicated to food safety as opposed to nutrition was not available, but the vast majority of the research focus is food safety, with an emphasis on chemical and microbiological public health hazards and, more recently, food defense. Individuals are rarely dedicated solely to research. CFSAN research scientists, research managers, and directors also perform regulatory functions such as reviews (petitions, compliance, guidance, and policy), risk assessments, outbreak investigations, and training. This diversity is considered advantageous to the agency as research scientists become "authoritative sources of information in areas of regulatory review and policy implementation."

Most of the scientists and staff supporting the center's research mission are located at the headquarters building in College Park, Maryland. However,

---

[2] Personal communication, Chad Nelson, FDA, October 13, 2009.

[3] The discussion in this section is based on the personal communication with Chad Nelson, FDA, October 13, 2009.

the center also operates research facilities in Laurel, Maryland; Summit-Argo, Illinois; and Dauphin Island, Alabama. About 25 agency employees are housed at the National Center for Food Safety and Technology (NCFST) near Chicago, Illinois. NCFST and the other four extramural research centers are discussed in the next section.

As with research FTEs, the committee was unable to obtain information on funding allocated for CFSAN's food safety mission alone. As noted, however, most of the research at CFSAN has been devoted to food safety.

The intramural program at CFSAN is composed of research in the disciplines of chemistry, microbiology, molecular biology, food science, toxicology, immunology, epidemiology, social sciences, education, and risk assessment. Major research thrusts include the following: (1) development and evaluation of methods to recover, detect, and identify pathogens, chemicals, and biomolecules in foods, including evaluation of emerging technologies; (2) risk assessment; and (3) economics and consumer studies (Musser, 2009). CFSAN currently has about 96 active research projects related to food protection (Musser, 2009). Virtually all of these projects are considered applied in nature; in other words, they are "investigations aimed at developing and applying standards to public health needs" (Musser, 2009). Other important components of CFSAN's research program include nonlaboratory research on risk communication, labeling, education, and the economic impact of its regulations and enforcement programs.

Each intramural research project is, at most, 3 years in duration and may be adjusted as needed during this period. CFSAN did not provide the committee with a full listing of its intramural research projects; however, a list was available online[4] (CFSAN/FDA, 2008), and a listing on the state of the science at CFSAN was also made available to the committee. Referencing the two relevant areas (food safety and food defense), the committee was able to produce the table in Appendix F. Some common themes emerge from this table. Consistent with Musser's presentation (Musser, 2009), a large proportion of the research focuses on the development of detection methods. Other important themes include (1) a greater emphasis on pathogens as compared with chemicals/allergens; (2) relatively few projects focused on risk assessment and economics/consumer studies, despite these being mentioned to the committee as priority areas (Musser, 2009); and (3) a relative absence of research on control or intervention strategies.

---

[4] See http://www.fda.gov/Food/ScienceResearch/SelectedScientificPublicationsPresentations/ucm117721.htm#fs (accessed October 8, 2010).

NCTR

NCTR is located in Jefferson, Arkansas. The committee received very little information about NCTR's food safety functions. Therefore, much of the discussion here is based on the center's webpage.[5] The center as a whole receives approximately 28 percent of the FDA's total research budget, the second largest proportion of that budget (HHS, 2010). About 35–40 of the center's approximately 200 research FTEs are dedicated to food safety (NCTR, 2009a; FDA, 2010a). NCTR states that its vision is to provide "innovative and vital scientific technology, training, and technical expertise to improve public health," with a corresponding mission statement of "conduct[ing] peer-reviewed scientific research in support of the FDA mission" (NCTR, 2009a, p. 1) (see Box 6-1). In support of the center's mission, NCTR has identified seven Centers of Excellence (see Box 6-2).

As reflected in its name, NCTR's work is dedicated largely to toxicological research. A review of the program reveals that fundamental research appears to be the driving force. For example, the center houses a wide variety of state-of-the-art equipment and is addressing most of the "omics," all considered emerging transdisciplinary approaches to biological research. Clearly, this center's mission is much broader than food safety, and many of its initiatives are designed to support the FDA's drug and devices functions (FDA, 2010a).

The committee was not provided information with which to determine the proportion of NCTR's research budget dedicated to food safety. Nonetheless, one of the center's strategic goals is to "conduct research and develop strategic technologies to protect the food supply." To that end, investigators at NCTR are conducting research in the following areas: (1) food safety, food biosecurity, and methods development; (2) antimicrobial resistance; and (3) gastrointestinal microbiology and host interactions. A list of projects in support of these research initiatives is provided in Appendix F.

The committee reviewed information received from the FDA about NCTR, including the *NCTR Strategic Plan 2009–2013, FY2009 Accepted Publications, NCTR Food Publications 2005–2009*, and a breakdown of food safety spending and food safety research FTEs for 2000–2007 (NCTR, 2009a,b,c). These materials, especially the *Strategic Plan*, are clear in delineating the center's vision and mission and its strategic goals for accomplishing this mission (Box 6-1) (NCTR, 2009a). Of the five strategic goals, Goal 3 pertains directly to food safety, while Goals 4 and 5 involve broad support for the FDA's mission, which clearly includes food safety. Goal 1, while not related to food safety, does concern nutrition, which is in the domain of CFSAN. The two lists of publications (NCTR 2009b,c) show

---

[5] See http://www.fda.gov/AboutFDA/CentersOffices/nctr/default.htm(accessed October 8, 2010).

BOX 6-1
Vision, Mission, and Strategic Goals
from the National Center for Toxicological Research (NCTR)
Strategic Plan 2009–2013

Vision

NCTR is an internationally recognized U.S. Food and Drug Administration (FDA) research center that provides innovative and vital scientific technology, training, and technical expertise to improve public health. NCTR—in partnership with researchers from government, academia, and industry—develops, refines, and applies current and emerging technologies to improve safety evaluations of FDA-regulated products. NCTR fosters national and international collaborations to improve and protect public health and enhance the quality of life for the American people.

Mission

NCTR conducts peer-reviewed scientific research in support of the FDA mission and provides expert technical advice and training that enables FDA to make sound science-based regulatory decisions and improve the health of the American people. The research at NCTR supports FDA's goals: (1) to understand critical biological events in the expression of toxicity, (2) to develop and characterize methods, and incorporate new technologies to improve the assessment of human exposure, susceptibility, and risk, and (3) to increase the understanding of the interaction between genetics, metabolism, and nutrition.

NCTR is dedicated to supporting the FDA mission to protect and promote public health by:

- providing innovative and interdisciplinary research that promotes personal and public health
- developing novel translational research approaches to provide FDA/Department of Health and Human Services (HHS) with sound scientific infrastructure and multidisciplinary scientific expertise targeted towards addressing critical Agency, Department, and public-health needs such as personalized nutrition and medicine,

that the majority of the center's work is in toxicology, but it also performs significant work in food safety. It should be noted that many of NCTR's food safety publications are on non-FDA-regulated items, such as processed eggs and poultry (e.g., Kiess et al., 2007; Khan et al., 2009).

bioimaging, systems biology, bioinformatics, nanotechnology, food protection technologies, and biomarker development
- engaging with scientists across FDA and other government agencies, industry, and academia in cooperative learning to strengthen the scientific foundations vital to developing sound regulatory policy and leveraging resources in order to promote the international standardization and global harmonization of regulatory science
- participating in or leading national and international consortia for the development of harmonized standards for technologies and methods in risk assessment and for personal and public health

Strategic Goals

To accomplish its mission, NCTR has established five strategic goals:

Goal 1: Advance scientific approaches and tools to promote personalized nutrition and medicine for the public

Goal 2: Develop science-based best-practice standards, guidance, and tools to incorporate toxicological advancements that improve the regulatory process

Goal 3: Conduct research and develop strategic technologies to protect the food supply

Goal 4: Conduct bioinformatics research and development in support of FDA's regulatory mission

Goal 5: Strengthen and improve scientific and human capital management and expand training and outreach to retain and train scientific experts critical to address FDA's scientific needs

SOURCE: NCTR, 2009a.

CVM

The mission of CVM is to protect and promote the health of animals and, in so doing, to protect the safety of meat, milk, and other animal-derived products destined for the human food supply. Research in support of CVM's mission is carried out through the Office of Research (OR) in Laurel, Maryland. The OR campus houses approximately 70 research

---

BOX 6-2
National Center for Toxicological Research's (NCTR's)
Seven Centers of Excellence

1. *Functional Genomics*—uses high-information content microarrays in the development of mechanistic and biomarker data.
2. *Hepatotoxicology*—addresses critical liver injury issues by applying a systems-toxicology approach.
3. *Innovative Technologies*—uses multi-faceted approaches to address issues such as counterterrorism, rapid detection of bacteria in food, and sensors and nanotube technology.
4. *Metabolomics*—aids in the assessment of preclinical and clinical safety issues as part of a U.S. Food and Drug Administration (FDA)-wide biomarkers-development effort.
5. *Phototoxicology*—assesses the toxic and/or carcinogenic potential of chemicals and agents when exposed to light, or when applied to photo-treated skin.
6. *Proteomics*—develops and evaluates novel proteomic technologies to facilitate the translation of basic science to medical products.
7. *Toxicoinformatics*—conducts research in bioinformatics and chemoinformatics and develops and coordinates informatics capabilities within NCTR, across FDA Centers, and in the larger toxicology community.

SOURCE: http://www.fda.gov/AboutFDA/CentersOffices/nctr/default.htm (accessed October 8, 2010).

---

scientists and support staff and is organized into 3 major sections: (1) the Division of Residue Chemistry, (2) the Division of Animal Research, and (3) the Division of Animal and Food Microbiology (FDA Science Board, 2009).

The FY 2009 CVM research budget was $9.241 million, which supported 57 research FTEs and constituted 5 percent of the agency's annual research budget (FDA Science Board, 2009). The FDA Science Board report on CVM activities states that roughly 40 percent of CVM activities are focused on food safety issues pertaining to animal feeds, pet foods, aquaculture, and antimicrobial resistance of foodborne pathogens, although research scientists are frequently diverted from this focus to address emergency issues (FDA Science Board, 2009).

As is the case for CFSAN, CVM's food safety research portfolio is diverse. Its *Three-Year Research Plan: FY2009–FY2011* (CVM/FDA, 2008) states that the center's food safety research program focuses on microbial hazards associated with the preharvest phases of the animal production environment, including animal feeds, with specific focuses on

- analysis of animal feeds for the presence of human foodborne bacterial pathogens;
- identification of factors associated with the presence and persistence of zoonotic bacterial pathogens in the animal production ecosystem;
- surveys of various food products for the presence of zoonotic foodborne bacterial pathogens;
- application of genetic typing methods to track the spread of specific zoonotic foodborne bacterial pathogens; and
- identification and comparison of antimicrobial resistance genes in foodborne pathogens isolated from different sources in an effort to characterize the spread of resistant bacteria via the food chain (CVM/FDA, 2008).

In addition, CVM supports the FDA's food safety mission by (1) developing and validating tests for drugs and drug residues, including newly prohibited drugs, and (2) conducting surveys of drug residues and pathogens in feeds and in animal-derived foods destined for human consumption. Based on the project descriptions given in the CVM *Three-Year Research Plan* (CVM/FDA, 2008), the committee itemized specific CVM projects designed to support the FDA's food safety mission (see Appendix F).

As is the case for CFSAN, many CVM projects support the applied research function of developing diagnostic methods for microbes and drug residues; a few studies address more fundamental issues, such as understanding the mechanisms by which antimicrobial resistance develops. Relatively little effort has been devoted to identifying emerging threats in the area of animal feeds and associated links to human health. While addressing analytical issues is important, some limited CVM efforts support risk-based food safety management. It could be argued that CVM's survey and microbial source tracking efforts do support the risk mission, but these efforts are minimal in comparison with its other research functions.

ORA

As explained in Chapter 2, ORA's role is to support the FDA product centers by inspecting regulated products and manufacturers, conducting sample analysis, and reviewing imported products. ORA also works with state and local (including tribal and territorial) governments, through grants and cooperative agreements, to inspect FDA-regulated food products. The resource allocation or priority for ORA research functions was not described to the committee. Although ORA's total budget for food activities conducted in laboratories is more than $90,000,000, its research budget is only $1,100,000 (with only 6 FTEs), representing just 1 percent of the FDA's total research budget.[6] ORA maintains science advisors who are special government employees serving as consultants to the specific ORA laboratories to which they are assigned. Additionally, ORA has four staff members in risk management. (The information presented here was obtained from the FDA's written statements and the ORA webpage.[7])

With a limited research budget, ORA plays only a minor role in the FDA's food safety research. Its research functions are conducted at the 13 ORA laboratories, 10 of which conduct food-related work. These 10 laboratories focus primarily on developing and validating analytical methods to meet the immediate needs of the field laboratories, work that is highly applied in nature. There are two major ORA research initiatives: the Methods Development and Validation Program (MDVP) and the Analytical Tools Initiative (Glavin, 2008; Musser, 2009).

FDA field laboratory personnel are involved in work on method development and validation through the MDVP, although that program is not identified by the agency as "research." Nevertheless, the program is intended to support regulatory testing (both screening and confirmatory) by (1) identifying needs and priorities in method development to address emerging regulatory issues and (2) improving/updating current regulatory methods. The work includes method assessment and validation aimed at rapidly moving promising methodologies into ORA field laboratories for regulatory use. ORA's Division of Field Science monitors and coordinates all MDVP activities. Current initiatives include the development of rapid detection methods for foodborne pathogens such as *Salmonella*, *Escherichia coli* O157:H7, *Shigella*, *Listeria monocytogenes*, and hepatitis A virus, as well as detection of other adulterants using chemical, radiological, and other analytical methods. To illustrate the immediacy of the MDVP work, this program was responsible for the development of a real-time polymerase chain reaction (PCR) assay for high-throughput screening of *E. coli* O157:H7 during the 2006 spinach-related outbreak. ORA mobile laboratory deployments to Salinas, California, and Nogales, Arizona, to perform rapid screening of *Salmonella* and *E. coli* O157:H7 in fresh produce provide additional examples of this program's reach.

The Analytical Tools Initiative is a program for the assessment and validation of field and laboratory analytical tools addressing such critical issues as speed of analysis, increased sample throughput, improved sampling strategies, and development of field-deployable instrumentation (Musser, 2009). The ways in which the MDVP and the Analytical Tools Initiative differ was not described to the committee.

---

[6] Personal communication, Chad Nelson, FDA, October 13, 2009.
[7] See http://www.fda.gov/AboutFDA/CentersOffices/ORA/default.htm (accessed October 8, 2010).

EXTRAMURAL RESEARCH CENTERS

The FDA has five extramural research centers devoted to specific food safety initiatives. Each of these centers is funded at the level of $1–$2.5 million per year. The centers differ by structure and function; each is described briefly below.

National Center for Food Safety and Technology (NCFST)

Supported by a memorandum of understanding between the FDA and the Illinois Institute of Technology (IIT), NCFST is the oldest extramural center.[8] It was established in 1988 and remains a partnership among IIT, CFSAN, and the food industry. NCFST also houses the FDA Division of Food Processing Science and Technology, which was established by the FDA to form a link with industry to tap its expertise in food technology. NCFST is the only center in which the FDA can work collaboratively with industry and academia on projects related to food safety and technology. A fee-based membership in NCFST allows companies to gain early insight into emerging food safety issues from the CFSAN perspective and to assess the safety of new technologies that may be important for innovation. Such early collaboration with the FDA may also facilitate regulatory approval of new food processes, thereby reducing the time required for emerging processes to reach commercialization. Funding for NCFST for FY 2009 was $2.1 million (Musser, 2009).

The research performed at NCFST is organized into four primary scientific platforms,[9] three of which are particularly applicable to food safety:

(1) The Processing and Packaging Platform focuses on investigation of the effects of processing and packaging on food safety, quality, and nutrition. Included are projects focused on validation of traditional and emerging food processing and packaging technologies and the use of food safety objectives to facilitate regulatory approval and equivalency of novel processes.

(2) The Microbiology Platform is aimed at generating knowledge of the behavior of microorganisms in food and processing environments to improve food safety and quality and public health. Included are projects on *Clostridium botulinum* and other spore formers, the use of new molecular methods for studying microbial resistance, sample preparation and detection techniques, and detection

---

[8] See http://www.iit.edu/ncfst/ (accessed October 8, 2010).

[9] See http://www.iit.edu/ncfst/world_class_food_science/(accessed October 8, 2010).

and decontamination methods for food defense–related biological threat agents.

(3) The Chemical Constituents and Allergens Platform, focused on generating knowledge of chemical constituents for use by industry and regulators in making science-based decisions that influence food safety and quality and public health. This work includes a study of the effects of processing on chemical contaminants and the development of detection and validation procedures to prevent allergen cross-contact.

The primary goal of these platforms is to develop projects based on industry's needs. Research portfolios for each platform include collaborative, leveraged, and proprietary projects that balance the short- and long-term needs of NCFST, the FDA, and industry members. NCFST is well positioned to facilitate innovation in the food industry because of its long history, its strong buy-in from the FDA (including on-site FDA scientists), and its unique state-of-the-art equipment, which includes a newly constructed biosafety level-2 pilot processing facility.[10]

Joint Institute for Food Safety and Applied Nutrition (JIFSAN)

JIFSAN was established in 1996 as a partnership among the University of Maryland, CFSAN, and CVM.[11] JIFSAN research was intended to focus primarily on risk analysis. Since 1997, CFSAN has funded three 5-year cooperative agreements, the current period expiring in July 2012. In 2008, the funding level was $1,389,140. In 2009, the funding level was $1,896,200, with an additional supplemental award of $350,000 for a CVM project. As of this writing, the funding level in 2010 will be between $1.1 and $1.4 million.

JIFSAN's program can be divided into four primary areas: (1) Research, (2) International Food Safety Training, (3) Food Safety Risk Analysis, and (4) Workshops/Symposia. The Research program includes several components: faculty research, postdoctoral research, and graduate student research in collaboration with University of Maryland faculty, as well as an undergraduate internship program. JIFSAN has also provided funding for research conducted by non–University of Maryland faculty. Since 1998 JIFSAN has funded approximately 75 research projects, 15 of which have been funded since 2008. Current research areas include fresh produce safety, consumer behavior, allergens, microbiology, and risk analysis.

---

[10] See http://www.iit.edu/ncfst/world_class_food_science/food_processing_and_packaging/people_and_facilities.shtml (accessed October 8, 2010).

[11] See http://www.jifsan.umd.edu/ (accessed October 8, 2010).

JIFSAN's International Food Safety Training includes courses on Good Agricultural Practices (GAPs), Good Aquacultural Practices (GAqPs), and Commercially Sterilized Packaged Foods. JIFSAN conducted approximately 25 GAPs training sessions through 2009. The GAqPs training program was piloted in 2006, and three additional sessions were held in 2008–2009.

A major effort at JIFSAN is devoted to supporting its Risk Analysis Training Program and maintaining the FoodRisk.org website. The aim of FoodRisk.org is to serve as an information clearinghouse for risk analysis in the area of food safety. It contains tools for risk assessment and determination of contaminant and nutrition exposure, dose–response models, and tutorials, as well as many other invaluable tools.

Agricultural Products Food Safety Laboratory (APFSL) and National Center for Natural Products Research (NCNPR)

APFSL is housed at New Mexico State University and has been funded through earmarks at annual levels ranging from $1.65 to $2.35 million since FY 2005. Its purpose is to develop and evaluate rapid-screening methods for detecting microbiological and chemical contamination in food products, including methods for regulatory and/or counterterrorism purposes (Musser, 2009). The FDA provided little information regarding its function and productivity, perhaps because it is a relatively new extramural activity, and no relevant information could be found on the Internet.

NCNPR is housed at the University of Mississippi and is also funded through earmarks. Its work focuses on the discovery, development, and commercialization of pharmaceuticals and agrochemicals derived from natural products, and therefore has only limited relevance to food safety. NCNPR funding for FY 2009 was $1.6 million.[12]

Western Institute for Food Safety and Security (WIFSS) and Western Center for Food Safety (WCFS)

WIFSS is spearheaded by the University of California, Davis, along with partners (the California Department of Food and Agriculture; the California Department of Public Health, formerly California Department of Health Services; the U.S. Department of Agriculture [USDA]; and the FDA). Its primary mission is to devise better management practices for reducing the number and virulence of pathogens in the nation's food system, to ensure a safe and secure food supply, to grow the agricultural economy, and to protect the public health.[13]

---

[12] See http://www.pharmacy.olemiss.edu/ncnpr/site/index.html (no longer accessible).

[13] See http://wifss.ucdavis.edu/ (accessed October 8, 2010).

Housed in WIFSS is WCFS, which was established in 2008 as a cooperative agreement among the FDA; WIFSS; the University of California, Davis, School of Veterinary Medicine; the College of Agricultural and Environmental Sciences; and the greater academic community. The center's efforts focus on understanding the risks associated with the interface between production practices and food safety in fresh-produce systems. Administrative oversight of the center is provided in part by WIFSS and the FDA/CFSAN. Annual funding (for a total of 5 years) is in the range of $1.0 to $2.5 million, and some of these funds have been made available to the scientific community at large by way of a targeted extramural funding program in produce safety.[14]

Extramural Funding

Although the FDA pointed out that it is not an extramural funding agency, in actuality it does fund a small number of competitive research grants as well as cooperative research and development agreements, which are almost always focused on a specific stated need of the agency. There are currently 2 projects related to food defense, 31 related to food safety, and 15 related to improving nutrition,[15] funded through contracts, cooperative agreements, interagency agreements, and grants. Some of these are awarded to the extramural research centers (e.g., NCFST, JIFSAN), while others are awarded to universities, professional associations, or private consulting firms. Examples of the latter include contracts with RTI International (to support risk analysis efforts), the Association of Analytical Communities (to support methods validation), and the Institute of Food Technologists (to support the FDA's policies through evaluation of specific topics related to food safety and processing and human health). These extramurally funded projects currently focus on support of agency risk analysis efforts, development and implementation of novel detection methods, and control of pathogens in leafy greens and seafood products. The means by which the FDA determines which research questions should be addressed and funded through its small extramural program is unclear.

CFSAN has developed an automated, web-based tracking system for its intramural and extramural research programs called the CFSAN Automated Research Tracking System. The system, designed to improve the efficiency and timeliness of the documentation of research projects, provides a means for information sharing and provides for accountability of the

---

[14] See http://wifss.ucdavis.edu/headcontent/newsletter/2008November_newsletter.php.

[15] Personal communication, Chad Nelson, FDA, October 13, 2009 (accessed October 8, 2010).

center's research efforts. The database is open to all CFSAN employees but not the general public.[16]

INTERAGENCY COLLABORATION

In addition to its intramural and extramural research programs, CFSAN maintains collaborative agreements and interactions with other federal government research organizations to facilitate the sharing of information and resources in support of its regulatory mission and its obligations regarding international trade agreements. For example, CFSAN participates in the Interagency Risk Assessment Consortium (IRAC), which comprises 19 federal agencies or offices. The mission of IRAC is to enhance communication and coordination and to promote scientific research on risk assessment. Currently, CFSAN maintains approximately 50 collaborative partnerships with other federal research organizations, including the U.S. Department of Commerce's National Marine Fisheries Service; the U.S. Centers for Disease Control and Prevention; and USDA's Food Safety and Inspection Service (FSIS), Agricultural Marketing Service, and Agricultural Research Service.[17] In its report to the Science Board, CFSAN describes the reasons for the existence of its research program separate from those of other entities with large research capabilities, such as the National Institutes of Health (NIH). In the case of NIH, the reason given is differences in the mission and scope of the research of the two organizations. Nevertheless, CFSAN and NIH collaborate on a handful of projects, such as in the area of dietary supplements and long-term exposure to bisphenol A.

WEAKNESSES IN THE FDA RESEARCH PROGRAM

The FDA food safety research portfolio is diverse and vast. Some of the research efforts are quite relevant to the agency's mission, while the relevance of others is less clear. There is no central oversight of FDA research, and currently each of the four FDA divisions (CFSAN, CVM, NCTR, and ORA) performing the bulk of the agency's food research manages its own research portfolio.[18] Although the purposes and goals of these individual research programs differ, overlap in some of the efforts is likely. The committee found no evidence of coordination to prevent duplication of effort or to leverage the efforts of one investigator with those of others having complementary skills and interests.

---

[16] Personal communication, Chad Nelson, FDA, October 13, 2009.

[17] Personal communication, Chad Nelson, FDA, October 13, 2009.

[18] Personal communication, Donald Zink, Senior Science Advisor, FDA/CFSAN, September 25, 2009.

The committee found that, in some cases, the role of the extramural research centers is poorly defined. Of these centers, NCFST has the most well-defined mission and, with its unique expertise and advanced equipment, is well positioned to continue to serve the agency into the future. It offers an invaluable service (evaluation of the efficacy of emerging processing methods with respect to foodborne pathogens), although its research portfolio appears to be somewhat haphazard. The mission of JIFSAN is admirable, and despite recent funding reductions, it continues to offer value in providing risk analysis training and serving as a data clearinghouse. However, JIFSAN's work represents a very small proportion of the risk analysis support the FDA will need to move toward a comprehensive risk-based food safety management strategy. WIFSS/WCFS is new, so predicting its performance or value is difficult; however, WCFS is addressing a high-profile food safety problem in what appears to be an aggressive manner. The remaining two extramural centers, APFSL and NCNPR, have produced little in the way of tangible results by which they can be evaluated.

Strategic planning for the FDA's food safety research needs has been limited in scope and in some instances nonexistent. The FDA Science Board reviews each center every 5 years;[19] a review was recently completed for CVM (FDA Science Board, 2009), and the review of CFSAN is currently under way.[20] CVM produced an extensive strategic plan for this review, a document that was made available to the committee (FDA Science Board, 2009). CFSAN did the same—its first strategic planning effort in more than a decade. NCTR also has a strategic plan (NCTR, 2009a). The status of strategic planning for ORA and the extramural research centers is unknown. Apparently the strategic planning process includes both "formal" and "informal" scientific planning, both within the agency and with other agencies having a food safety mission, but the means by which this is accomplished is unclear. In any case, it is apparent that no coordinated strategic planning initiative exists in which all FDA food safety research programs are addressed in a unified way.

In the absence of a coordinated agencywide strategic planning effort for food safety research, key questions have not been addressed, including the following:

- What is the tangible value of the FDA's food safety research program with respect to supporting the agency's mission?
- What is the appropriate balance between basic and applied research? Should the agency even be conducting basic research?

---

[19] Personal communication, Donald Zink, Senior Science Advisor, FDA/CFSAN, September 25, 2009.

[20] Personal communication, Chad Nelson, FDA, October 13, 2009.

- What are the agency's research needs, and do they address critical data gaps?
- Is the current organizational structure for management of the FDA's research functions appropriate? If not, what structure would be more so?
- How is research prioritized, and how are research resources allocated?
- Is the current approach to managing researchers effective? For example, does it make sense to divert researchers to other functions when a crisis arises? Or would it be better to have some individuals devoted solely to research and some devoted to other agency functions?

The committee believes that, until these basic questions are answered, a unified vision for the FDA's food safety research will not be achievable. The lack of such a vision results in a poorly coordinated research mission that does not support the development and implementation of a risk-based food safety management system.

USING RESEARCH TO SUPPORT A RISK-BASED FOOD SAFETY MANAGEMENT APPROACH

The committee recommends a risk-based approach to managing the agency's food safety research portfolio, as it does for virtually all FDA functions. Not only would this approach fulfill the mission of characterizing and acting on risks from food contaminants, but it would also target research to answering the most pressing (highest-risk) food safety questions and problems. Thus, management of the agency's research portfolio would benefit from application of the principles outlined in Chapter 3 and from implementation of the recommendations regarding information infrastructure in Chapter 5.

From a strategic planning standpoint (Step 1 in a risk-based food safety management system; see Chapter 3), it is important to address the role of the research mission as a whole, which entails identifying agencywide public health objectives and determining how research can contribute to achieving these objectives, as well as what proportion of total resources should go to research relative to other agency functions. Central to these deliberations should be a consideration of the importance of research in supporting risk-based food safety management and what specific role(s) research should play. It could be argued that the development of analytical capabilities (e.g., data analysis, risk and decision modeling) is a research function, and over the next 5 years, extensive resources will be required to develop these tools. Once such tools have been developed, public health risk ranking (Step 2 of the risk-based approach in Chapter 3), which identifies and prioritizes the most pressing risk management issues, can be used to support the allocation of research resources. Although unlikely, it may be that the management of high-priority risks is best approached without the need for additional research, in which case the FDA's research portfolio could be substantially reduced. It is more likely, however, that research will be needed to address some high-priority issues that the FDA now does not study, and efforts carried out under Step 2 will direct resources to the areas of greatest need and relevance.

Research can also be used as a tool in support of targeted information gathering and analysis of interventions (Steps 3 and 4 of the risk-based approach, respectively). For example, information necessary to fill data gaps in risk-ranking or risk-assessment efforts is frequently collected as a research activity. Research can also be conducted to evaluate the efficacy of potential interventions or to aid in determining the feasibility of their implementation. Research can even be applied in monitoring and review (Step 6 of the risk-based approach) as the FDA seeks to evaluate the efficacy of interventions after their implementation. Finally, the identification and design of new and innovative ways to apply risk analysis methods to food safety management is a research function that underpins the entire risk-based structure.

On a more focused level, research can be used to address unanswered questions for any specific risk. An example is the almost decade-long problem of *Salmonella* in tomatoes. This would likely be a relatively high-priority issue in a public health risk-ranking exercise. However, there are key research questions, such as the reservoir(s) for the organism, contamination routes, and the persistence of *Salmonella* in the contaminated fruit, that will take substantial resources to tackle. Yet a decision to devote research resources to the problem of *Salmonella* contamination in tomatoes as opposed to another problem (e.g., hepatitis A in green onions) is inherently risk based. To take the argument a step further, if research is directed to the *Salmonella*/tomato problem, will the FDA get the most value for its investment if it focuses on identifying the reservoir(s) for the organism or on evaluating potential interventions during the postharvest phase? And how does the FDA identify the various ongoing research projects in the academic community that address its priority research areas? If answering such questions is supported by a risk-based approach, the decisions made become more transparent and justifiable even as the use of limited agency resources is optimized.

MOVING FORWARD

The first step in applying a risk-based approach within the context of the FDA's current food safety research portfolio should be to undertake a comprehensive inventory and review of the agency's existing research program without respect for interinstitutional boundaries (e.g., CFSAN, CVM, NCFST, ORA). Thereafter, each research area should undergo a comprehensive peer review, conducted by FDA and non-FDA scientists, whose purpose should be to evaluate such issues as relevance, funding, productivity, and programmatic benefits in direct support of the agency's mission. This review might be performed with tools similar to those used in cost–benefit analysis of interventions (Chapter 3) and would provide much-needed information before the strategic planning phase was initiated. Research would then become part of the set of risk management tools available for agency use. Although the documents provided to the committee included a list of priority areas of food safety research, the process used to arrive at this list was not clear.

The committee believes that reorganization of the FDA's research function is warranted and that such reorganization should be risk based. This reorganization may necessitate a creative approach to the management of research resources. A critical initial consideration is preventing duplication of effort. One area of concern for the committee that has also been highlighted by others (GUIRR/NAS, 2009) is the lack of coordination of the food safety and defense research portfolios in the nation. Better coordination will entail communication with other federal regulatory and research agencies (e.g., USDA's FSIS, the Department of Defense, the National Science Foundation, NIH) that conduct salient activities or projects. Coordination of research efforts between the FDA and other entities could be expanded to the international sphere as well. Within the agency, the research function should not be organized around specific areas of expertise—such as microbiologists who specialize in particular organisms (e.g., *Salmonella*, viruses) or scientists who specialize in certain techniques (e.g., molecular biology, biosensors)—or pet projects, but should be focused on key unanswered questions and problems whose resolution will have the greatest impact on improving the safety of the food supply by reducing the most significant public health risks. This means that well-trained researchers with specific disciplinary expertise will need to work interdependently in multidisciplinary teams that are designed to deal with particularly complex food safety issues. Individual research professionals will likely serve as members of more than one team. As is the case in academia, the FDA's research program should evolve to become multidisciplinary, interinstitutional, collaborative, translational, and flexible.

At the same time, it is essential that certain key research thrusts be continued, with an eye to their use in support of risk-based decision making. An example is the development and application of advanced mathematical modeling techniques. Likewise, qualified research staff will be needed to interpret data for appropriate use in support of risk-based food safety management. Other research areas may support the risk-based system tangentially and might better be outsourced. For example, improved analytical methods are critical to the generation of quantitative data that can be used in risk modeling and to the monitoring of production and processing control points. In fact, a large proportion of the research done by CFSAN and NCFST is in the area of methods development. However, these centers may not be the best places for such work. It could be argued that FDA scientists have worked on methods development for decades with only limited success. Perhaps the methods development function would best be outsourced to the academic and private sectors, where cross-cutting innovative approaches ultimately lead to scientific and commercial success.

It is also important to recognize that certain research efforts will be beyond the scope of current agency resources. For example, the collection of information on the prevalence or concentrations of microbes or chemical contaminants across the farm-to-fork continuum and research on the efficacy of candidate interventions may require collaboration with industry. Likewise, the agency cannot be expected to have all the necessary in-house expertise to develop novel risk-modeling techniques, support advanced information technology capabilities, or keep pace with the rapidly developing fields of proteomics and bioinformatics. Under these circumstances, the FDA should consider alternative means by which to foster research, such as interagency personnel agreements (for short-term expertise), public–private centers, and formalized extramural funding alternatives (e.g., cooperative agreements, grants and contracts, research institutes). Although the agency occasionally uses these mechanisms, the committee believes that additional efforts to reach out to the scientific community at large would provide much-needed expertise to solve complex food safety problems using innovative, multidisciplinary approaches. Further, engagement of entities outside of the FDA would go a long way toward promoting transparency of the agency's research agenda.

In conclusion, maintaining the appropriate balance between fundamental and applied research is critical. The FDA should be true to its research mission, which focuses on applied and translational research in support of science-based decision making. The entire research program should be viewed as supporting the risk-based function; in other words, research should not exist just for its own sake. This means any fundamental research that is undertaken should be aimed at answering questions relevant to controlling the highest-priority risks, and the outcomes anticipated from such research must have relevance to risk management decision making. FDA scientists with interests in fundamental research should be encouraged to collaborate with academia, but the FDA's research resources should be used mainly to support risk-based food safety priorities.

KEY CONCLUSIONS AND RECOMMENDATIONS

Results from research allow the FDA to fill data gaps and address uncertainties and thereby help refine its risk-based decision making. The committee applauds the recent consultation of the Science Board with regard to reviewing the research portfolios of CFSAN and CVM. Based on the information provided by the FDA, however, the committee concluded that the FDA's current food safety research program is unfocused and fragmented. For almost a decade there has been no coordinated strategic planning initiative addressing all FDA food safety research programs as a whole. Coordination and leveraging of research at CFSAN, CVM, NCTR, ORA, and the five extramural research centers appear to be insufficient, and some overlap in their efforts is likely as a result. Many basic questions, such as the size of the overall research program or the balance of basic and applied research, need to be addressed if the FDA is to have a unified vision that reflects the recommended risk-based approach. The committee concludes that, in addition to enhancements to the FDA's research portfolio, better coordination of the food safety and defense research conducted in the nation by government agencies, industry, and academia is needed.

The committee offers the following recommendations to enhance the FDA's research portfolio.

> **Recommendation 6-1: The FDA should have a food safety research portfolio that supports the recommended risk-based approach. To this end, the agency's current food safety research portfolio should undergo a comprehensive review. Following this review and with consideration of the agency's broad strategic plan, the FDA should examine the relevance and allocation of its research resources by using public health risk ranking and prioritization. Future research should address the most pressing public health issues and directly support further characterization of risk and selection, implementation, and evaluation of interventions. In addition, research should be coordinated to prevent duplication of effort, especially for cases in which research efforts are better suited to the academic or medical sector.**

Once the review and planning of the agency's research program have been completed, the committee recommends the following key implementation actions.

Recommendation 6-2: Implementation of recommendation 6-1 requires reorganization of the FDA's research portfolio, including reallocation of resources from irrelevant or poorly performing initiatives; hiring of new staff in critical areas and, where appropriate, retraining of existing staff; and identification of future resource needs to support risk-based food safety management. Although the committee recognizes the difficulty of transferring scientists from one research focus to another, the FDA should foster an environment of fluidity in which teams of scientists can be formed with ease to address different research initiatives as necessary.

Recommendation 6-3: Keeping in mind that the FDA will not be able to address all important research needs, the agency should continue to utilize alternative funding mechanisms (e.g., cooperative agreements, university-based centers, contracts) based on a competitive, peer-review process. These efforts could be expanded by establishing a competitive extramural research funding program.

REFERENCES

CFSAN/FDA (Center for Food Safety and Applied Nutrition/U.S. Food and Drug Administration). 2008. *Food 2008 Intramural Research Portfolio.* Rockville, MD: FDA.

CVM/FDA (Center for Veterinary Medicine/U.S. Food and Drug Administration). 2008. *Three-Year Research Plan: FY 2009–2011.* Washington, DC: FDA.

FDA (U.S. Food and Drug Administration). 2009. *FY 2009 Congressional Justification: FDA Research Activities.* http://www.fda.gov/downloads/AboutFDA/ReportsManualsForms/Reports/BudgetReports/2009FDABudgetSummary/ucm116249.pdf (accessed January 22, 2010).

FDA. 2010a. *About the National Center for Toxicological Research.* http://www.fda.gov/AboutFDA/CentersOffices/nctr/default.htm (accessed March 2, 2010).

FDA. 2010b. *FDA Functional Activity Tables: FY 2010 Estimated.* http://www.fda.gov/downloads/AboutFDA/ReportsManualsForms/Reports/BudgetReports/UCM153841.pdf (accessed January 22, 2010).

FDA. 2010c. *FDA Functional Activity Tables: FY 2009 Omnibus.* http://www.fda.gov/downloads/AboutFDA/ReportsManualsForms/Reports/BudgetReports/UCM153840.pdf (accessed January 22, 2010).

FDA. 2010d. *FY 2010 Congressional Justification: National Center for Toxicological Research.* http://www.fda.gov/AboutFDA/ReportsManualsForms/Reports/BudgetReports/ucm153374.htm (accessed January 21, 2010).

FDA. 2010e. *FY 2010 Congressional Justification: FDA Research Activities.* http://www.fda.gov/downloads/AboutFDA/ReportsManualsForms/Reports/BudgetReports/UCM153845.pdf (accessed January 22, 2010).

FDA Science Board. 2009. *Research Planning, Program and Facilities of the Center for Veterinary Medicine.* http://www.fda.gov/AdvisoryCommittees/CommitteesMeetingMaterials/ScienceBoardtotheFoodandDrugAdministration/ucm176816.htm (accessed March 22, 2010).

Glavin, M. 2008. *Revitalizing ORA: Protecting the Public Health Together in a Changing World: A Report to the Commissioner.* Washington, DC: FDA.

GUIRR/NAS (Government-University-Industry Research Roundtable of the National Academy of Sciences). 2009. *Technology Workshop on Food Safety and National Defense.* http://sites.nationalacademies.org/PGA/guirr/PGA_053569 (accessed April 7, 2010).

HHS (U.S. Department of Health and Human Services). 2010. *FY 2010 President's Budget for HHS.* http://www.hhs.gov/asrt/ob/docbudget/index.html (accessed January 29, 2010).

Khan, S. A., K. Sung, M. S. Nawaz, C. E. Cerniglia, M. L. Tamplin, R. W. Phillips, and L. C. Kelley. 2009. The survivability of *Bacillus anthracis* (Sterne strain) in processed liquid eggs. *Food Microbiology* 26:123–127.

Kiess, A. S., P. B. Kenney, and R. R. Nayak. 2007. *Campylobacter* detection in commercial turkeys. *British Poultry Science* 48:567–572.

Musser, S. 2009. *Food Safety Research at FDA.* Paper presented at IOM Committee on Review of the Food and Drug Administration's Role in Ensuring Safe Food Meeting, Washington, DC, March 24, 2009.

NCTR (National Center for Toxicological Research). 2009a. *NCTR Strategic Plan: 2009–2013.* Jefferson, AK: NCTR.

NCTR. 2009b. *FY 2009 Accepted Publications.* Jefferson, AK: NCTR.

NCTR. 2009c. *NCTR Food Publications 2005–2009.* Jefferson, AK: NCTR.

7

Integrating Federal, State, and Local Government Food Safety Programs

The regulations and programs of state and local (including tribal and territorial) governments have been a strong component of the U.S. food safety system for the past century. Their key regulatory programs in food safety address food and public health surveillance as well as food inspection and analysis.

The U.S. Food and Drug Administration (FDA) is responsible for more than 156,008 domestic food facilities (FDA, 2010), more than 1 million food establishments[1] (including restaurants and retail establishments), and more than 2 million farms (Mavity, 2009). Given the size, complexity, and growth of the food industry in the United States, both domestic and imported, it would be unrealistic to expect the FDA to have enough resources to provide adequate surveillance and inspection of the entire U.S. food supply and to encompass all areas of policy currently overseen by state and local agencies. In fact, the FDA has repeatedly been criticized by organizations and individuals both inside and outside government, including the U.S. Government Accountability Office (GAO) and the Congressional Research Service, for the lack of adequate surveillance and inspection of the U.S. food supply (GAO, 2004a,b,c; 2005a,b, 2008a,b,c,d, 2009a,b; CRS, 2007; Hutt, 2007, 2008; Becker, 2008, 2009).

In this context, it is clear that the FDA could better leverage its food safety knowledge through improved access to, and utilization of, data from state and local authorities (e.g., data from food safety inspections, disease outbreak and product safety investigations, enforcement actions).

---

[1] Personal communication, Chad Nelson, FDA, October 13, 2009.

The idea of integrating federal, state, and local agencies into a national food safety system has been espoused in reports of the Association of Food and Drug Officials (AFDO) (Hile, 1984; AFDO, 2001, 2009a,b), in the Institute of Medicine (IOM)/National Research Council (NRC) report *Ensuring Safe Food: From Production to Consumption* (IOM/NRC, 1998), by consumer representatives (DeWaal, 2003), and more recently in the report *Stronger Partnerships for Safer Food: An Agenda for Strengthening State and Local Roles in the Nation's Food Safety System* (Taylor and David, 2009).

The committee understands an integrated system to be one that (1) minimizes duplication of food safety activities (e.g., inspection, education, data collection) by leveraging efforts at the state and local levels; (2) follows a common risk-based approach to prioritize activities at all levels of government; (3) meets a minimum set of standards at all levels of government in various areas (e.g., collection, utilization, and reporting of data; equivalency of laws and regulations and their implementation; inspection procedures and training; foodborne illness investigations); and (4) accesses and utilizes data and information collected at the state and local levels. For the purposes of this report, the terms "collaboration" and "cooperation" are used interchangeably to mean "interaction between [entities] that is largely beneficial to all those participating."[2]

This chapter presents the committee's rationale for supporting an integrated food safety system and describes the steps necessary to facilitate such integration. It also delineates the role and responsibilities of the FDA and the actions necessary to achieve integration and cooperation with state and local food safety programs. Other chapters offer recommendations whose implementation would facilitate the integration proposed in this chapter. For example, the chapters on internal organizational changes (Chapter 11), increased the efficiency of inspections (Chapter 8), and the adoption of a risk-based approach to food safety (Chapter 3) provide the basis for the harmonization and integration recommended herein. For the majority of the committee's recommendations on this subject, the literature base is sparse. Most of the evidence supporting these recommendations was derived from information received from the FDA at the request of the committee, conversations with federal government employees, individual committee members' regulatory and other experiences, and past reports addressing this topic.

---

[2] Definition found at http://www.merriam-webster.com/.

PREVIOUS RECOMMENDATIONS FOR THE INTEGRATION OF FOOD SAFETY PROGRAMS

Many individuals and organizations are calling, once again, for reform of the nation's food safety system across all levels of government (local, state, and federal) and all phases of the food production continuum, including both domestic and international products. Multiple congressional and regulatory initiatives are aimed at making proposed reforms a reality (Hogan & Hartson, LLP, 2009). This section reviews the recommendations for integration offered by the IOM/NRC (1998) and Taylor and David (2009), who expanded upon previous recommendations by providing a road map for an integrated food safety system. The committee supports these recommendations, which are presented in greater detail in Appendix B.

Recommendations of the IOM/NRC

The IOM/NRC (1998) report *Ensuring Safe Food: From Production to Consumption* calls for an integrated, risk-based food safety system and modernization of federal food safety laws (IOM/NRC, 1998). The report further recommends that Congress provide the agencies responsible for food safety with the tools necessary to integrate and unify the efforts of authorities at the state and local levels to enhance food safety. While the report addresses the federal role in the food safety system, it states that "the roles of state and local government entities are equally critical" (pp. 14, 97, 99) and cites the need to ensure nationwide adherence to minimum standards.

In addressing the need for improved integration of federal, state, and local food safety programs, the report notes the lack of adequate integration among the activities of the main federal agencies involved in implementing the 35 primary statutes that regulate food safety and the activities of state and local agencies, as well as the need for reorganization (IOM/NRC, 1998). These findings remain true today, and the recommendations offered in that report, which were directed to Congress, have not been implemented.

After the 1998 IOM/NRC report was issued, and in response to the Clinton Administration's Food Safety Initiative, the FDA cooperated with other federal, state, and local agencies to improve partnerships by hosting a 50-state meeting in 1998, whose purpose was to examine the long-held vision of an integrated national food safety system (HHS, 1998). That meeting included a series of workshops that continued into 2001 with the purpose of identifying key areas in need of integration. These areas included laboratory operations, information sharing, outbreak investigation, the establishment of national uniform criteria for food safety programs, and the clarification of roles and responsibilities (NFSSP, 2001). One positive outcome was the implementation of the FDA's Electronic Laboratory Exchange Network (eLEXNET), discussed later in the chapter.

In 2008, the FDA convened a similar 50-state meeting titled the Gateway to Food Protection. Its purpose was to reflect on progress and accomplishments made since the initial 1998 meeting (FDA, 2008) and to identify ways of strengthening the food safety system in a manner consistent with the FDA's 2007 Food Protection Plan (FPP) (FDA, 2007a). Both the 1998 and 2008 meetings were chaired by then Deputy Director of the Center for Food Safety and Applied Nutrition Janice Oliver, who stated: "We recognized that the states, the local governments, we all needed each other. Then, as now, we weren't trying to re-invent the system but to improve the system we had, and to work better together doing it" (FDA, 2008, p. 6).

The 1998 meeting led to a more cooperative relationship between state and federal agencies, which contributed significantly to the implementation of the Bioterrorism Act of 2002, in which the states had a key partnership role (see also Appendix D). On the negative side, the security threats of that decade caused agencies to rethink openness and sharing of sensitive information related to food safety (Strickland, 2005).

Recommendations of Taylor and David (2009)

The Taylor and David (2009) report *Stronger Partnerships for Safer Food* reiterates the vision of an integrated food safety system. The report was funded by the Robert Wood Johnson Foundation and spearheaded by the School of Public Health and Health Services at the George Washington University in collaboration with AFDO, the Association of State and Territorial Health Officials (ASTHO), and the National Association of County and City Health Officials (Taylor and David, 2009). During workshops leading up to the report, Michael Taylor, one of its authors, was quoted as saying, "State and local agencies occupy the critical frontline in the nation's food safety system. Food safety reform at the federal level will be incomplete and insufficient unless it strengthens state and local roles and builds true partnership across all levels of government." Dr. Paul Jarris, executive director of ASTHO, continued, "Protecting Americans and assuring them that the food they eat is safe is a fundamental responsibility of state and local health departments." Joseph Corby, executive director of AFDO and former state food regulatory official, further supported integration by saying, "Integrating the food safety efforts of federal, state, and local agencies is key to dramatically improve this country's food safety system. This report provides a clear plan for accomplishing this integration."[3]

The report begins by recognizing progress in integration: "Since the

---

[3] Personal communication, Joseph Corby, executive director of AFDO, August 25, 2009.

1990s federal, state, and local agencies have expanded their collaboration in some areas—such as illness surveillance and inspection—and there exists today among food safety officials at all levels a widely shared vision of an integrated national food safety system that operates as a full partnership among federal, state, and local agencies" (Taylor and David, 2009, p. 1). The report then presents 19 strategic recommendations for strengthening the system, which are detailed in Appendix B. A common theme is the dispersal of functions across many federal, state, and local agencies and recognition that while the states' systems are a valuable asset, challenges are associated with such a decentralized system. The need for strengthened collaboration, partnerships, standardization, and oversight is clearly articulated. The committee fully supports those 19 recommendations.

While the FDA has recently made progress toward implementing the recommendations in the Taylor and David report, the majority of the issues raised remain unresolved. Those recommendations on which significant progress has been made include the following:

- "Recommendation for Congress to establish and fund an intergovernmental Food Safety Leadership Council (FSLC) through which the federal government would collaborate with state and local governments to design and implement an integrated national food safety system including the development of a five-year integration and capacity-building plan to meet high priority state and local capacity needs" (Taylor and David, 2009, p. 2). The FDA is already moving to implement a new plan, the Integrated Food Safety System (IFSS), that focuses on instituting standards and mechanisms for data sharing, with oversight by a new FDA organizational structure (Steering Committee) (Solomon, 2009a). The White House Food Safety Working Group (FSWG) not only should be informed about progress on this plan but, with the enhancements outlined in Chapter 11, also could function as the proposed FSLC and provide leadership to the FDA Steering Committee to ensure integration of state programs in the next 5 years.

- "State and local governments should collaborate on the development and widespread adoption of a model state and local food safety law to parallel pending reforms at the federal level, clarify the role of state and local agencies in a more integrated system, and legally empower state and local agencies to work more collaboratively among themselves and with the federal government" (Taylor and David, 2009, pp. 17, 59). In 1984, the states, working through AFDO, crafted a Model Food, Drug, and Cosmetic Act for adoption by state legislatures, which continues to be updated for state adoption (Burditt, 1995). At the request of the Tomato Forum in

2006, AFDO began working with federal agencies and industry to draft the recently completed Model Code for Produce Safety for adoption by the states. States cooperate to provide positions and recommendations to the FDA on regulatory changes in food safety through their official representation in the Conference for Food Protection. The shellfish industry (through the Interstate Shellfish Sanitation Conference) and dairy producers (through the National Conference on Interstate Milk Shipments) have also embraced the conference mechanism as a means to foster collaborative partnerships between state and federal agencies and provide model food safety programs for widespread adoption. Although the level of success of these conferences varies, these conferences have provided a mechanism of past cooperation with the FDA.

- The U.S. Department of Health and Human Services (HHS), "in collaboration with the [FSLC], should establish a Food Safety Leadership and Training Institute focused on building among food safety professionals at all levels a common vision for the nation's food safety system and the leadership skills, network of relationships, and trust needed for an integrated system to succeed" (Taylor and David, 2009, p. 45). Although this recommendation was not meant to duplicate existing efforts in technical training, it called for greater coordination and support in developing training curricula, including those for inspectors. In 2009 AFDO received a $2 million grant from the Kellogg Foundation to create a food protection training institute. Established in collaboration with the International Food Protection Training Institute (IFPTI) in Michigan, it began offering a course in managing retail food safety in 2009. Congress provided a $1 million appropriation to establish a permanent home for this new institute in 2009 "to ensure that food safety inspectors would have the training and skills necessary to do their jobs and to keep consumers safe" (Upton, 2009). Many other organizations and governments offer food safety training. For example, the states help ensure that personnel are trained to implement seafood Hazard Analysis and Critical Control Points (HACCP) through the Seafood HACCP Alliance. See Chapter 9 for further discussion of training.

- "Congress should establish traceability requirements that permit federal, state, and local officials to rapidly obtain from food companies reliable information on the source of commodities, ingredients, and finished products" (Taylor and David, 2009, p. 17). Although some traceability systems are in place and others are in development for specific commodities, such as produce, concerns remain regarding many aspects of traceability. Most notable among these concerns are the ability to link internal (within a company) and external traceability and the identification of key elements needed for an effective traceability system (IFT, 2009). Collaborative efforts between the FDA and the U.S. Department of Agriculture (USDA) have recently been initiated to advance widespread implementation of traceability, but many barriers remain. For example, in 2009 the FDA and USDA hosted a public meeting (HHS/FDA, 2009) to gather information on and engage stakeholders in the development of efficient and feasible food and feed tracing systems. The FDA acknowledged that with the current system, tracing the source of foodborne illness outbreaks at each step of the chain can be time-consuming and inefficient; hence a mandate to maintain records is critical (HHS/FDA, 2009). Many efforts are currently being devoted to developing traceability systems through collaboration among the FDA, academic institutions, and industry. An example of industry efforts is the Produce Traceability Initiative, sponsored by the United Fresh Produce Association, the Produce Marketing Association, and the Canadian Produce Marketing Association, which is working to develop a standardized electronic traceability system for all fresh produce (PTI, 2008).

STATES CALL FOR INTEGRATION

The states have historically called for greater partnership and integration with the federal food safety program and have sought to counter a lack of trust and acceptance. Many factors have contributed to this situation, such as the fact that state and local food regulatory programs are highly variable in quality, expertise, and resources. In addition, there is a pervasive federal view that only federal data or inspections will suffice for regulatory purposes. Further, there is a lack of willingness on the part of the states to surrender certain controls to meet what they believe to be bureaucratic and inflexible federal requirements.

The states have formed informal yet strong relationships through such joint associations as AFDO (established in 1896) and ASTHO (established in 1879), in which food regulatory officials from all states are represented. AFDO intensified its pressure for federal recognition of state programs in 1984 during an annual conference with the FDA, with a focus on creative partnerships between state and federal officials. Then associate commissioner for regulatory affairs Paul Hile spoke of the need to gain the FDA's acceptance of state inspectional and analytical findings beyond the limited case of contamination by the pesticide ethylene dibromide (Hile, 1984). At the time, the FDA had a limited pilot program with the Association of American Feed Control Officials that involved 10 to 12 states participating in a cooperative agreement on data sharing. Hile viewed the necessary components of federal–state cooperation to be based on the willingness of the parties to share knowledge, avoid unnecessary confrontations, fine-tune respective roles, foster understanding, build credibility, and establish an atmosphere of mutual trust. In the October 1984 *AFDO Quarterly Bulletin*, Hile went on to state: "These are the building stones on which effective partnerships of any kind are built. They are the attitudes that must prevail in our organizations if we are to achieve the efficiencies these times of fiscal restraint demand of us" (Hile, 1984).

ADEQUACY OF STATE AND LOCAL GOVERNMENT FOOD SAFETY REGULATORY PROGRAMS

Trust in the adequacy of state and local programs remains an issue. In a statement to the committee, Dr. Steven Solomon, Deputy Associate Commissioner for Compliance Policy, Office of Regulatory Affairs (ORA), FDA, said: "As we move with further integrating with the states [on the recommendations included in the Taylor report] we really need to build up an enhanced FDA infrastructure to meet the demands and maintain adequate oversight to make sure there is credibility in these programs" (Solomon, 2009a). Solomon further identified two major barriers to integration: (1) sustainability of resources and information and (2) difficulties with data sharing (see Chapter 5 for recommendations to minimize barriers to data sharing). When the committee asked Solomon how he envisioned being able to move from utilizing the limited data from state contract inspections to utilizing the vast amount of data and resources from all state inspections and data analyses, he responded: "The basis for that is standardization . . . there needs to be an accreditation program that oversees that and says, yes, everyone that's doing this work is up to these standards whether this is a laboratory, whether this is an inspector, whether this is a system. We need to have a robust auditing system to make sure there is credibility in such a program." Lack of trust in the ability of state and local programs also exists among groups representing consumers, supported by published reports indicating that, taken as a whole, food safety activities such as outbreak investigations and restaurant inspections have not been adequate (Kelly et al., 2007; Klein and DeWaal, 2008; CSPI, 2009; DeWaal et al., 2009; Moran, 2009).

Regulatory Structures and Laws for State and Local Food Safety Programs

The FDA's origins can be traced back to the analysis of agricultural products in the U.S. Patent Office around 1848, a function that was transferred to USDA upon its creation in 1862. The FDA became known by that name in 1930 and was transferred to the Federal Security Agency in 1940, which became the Department of Health, Education and Welfare in 1953. Although the FDA is the oldest and most comprehensive food safety agency in the federal government, food safety programs in the states are also of long standing. For example, Florida enacted a food law in 1905, a year prior to passage of the 1906 Pure Food and Drugs Act. Even before that, Massachusetts passed the first general food law in 1784, and in 1850 California enacted "a pure food and drink law" (Darby, 1993).

The FDA is responsible for the safety of all foods in the United States, whether produced domestically or internationally, with the exception of meat, poultry, and unshelled egg products, which are under the legal authority of USDA. Likewise, each state food regulatory program is responsible for the safety of foods in its jurisdiction, whether produced domestically or internationally. However, state regulatory authority exists only within the borders of the state. Regulatory actions outside the state for products that enter interstate commerce are referred to the FDA for enforcement follow-up in other locations.

Table 7-1 lists the various sources of information on state agencies involved in food safety regulation. Currently, the food safety regulatory programs in most of the 50 states are either the responsibility of state departments of health or departments of agriculture (Table 7-2) (FDA, 1993; NASDA, 1999; AFDO, 2001, 2009b). State food regulatory programs, which have varying resources, conduct public health and food surveillance, inspections, and sample analyses on food products grown, processed, packed, held, or sold within the state. Where the food safety program is located in the state department of health, the epidemiological and outbreak investigation function also resides in that state agency as well as with the local county health departments (AFDO, 2009a,b).

Likewise, the FDA has the responsibility to conduct inspections in each state for any product (food, drug, cosmetic, or device) under its jurisdiction that will be, is, or has been in interstate commerce. The FDA's inspections and regulatory actions on foods can be duplicative of those of the states, and there is insufficient planning or coordination between federal and state agencies to prevent multiple agency inspections of food plants. The result may be, for example, the use of limited state or federal resources to inspect one facility multiple times; more important, other facilities remain with no regulatory oversight. Generally, the FDA has delegated enforcement activities at food retail and service establishments to state and local jurisdictions utilizing the Food Code (FDA, 2009a,b), which is published and updated periodically by the FDA. The Food Code provides a framework that local, state, and federal regulators can (but are not required to) apply to be consistent with national food regulatory policy. The FDA and AFDO now report

TABLE 7-1 Sources of Information on State Agencies Involved in Food Safety Regulation

Source	Year	Content
FDA, Office of Federal–State Relations	1993[a]	Details on state food safety laws; 45 states have laws based on the 1938 Federal Food, Drug, and Cosmetic Act; food safety law in Alabama, Iowa, Mississippi, Pennsylvania, and West Virginia was patterned after the 1906 Pure Food and Drugs Act.
FoodSafety.gov (interagency federal government website about food safety information)	2010	No clear delineation of state agencies' responsibilities on current site; links to state departments of health and agriculture.
National Association of State Departments of Agriculture Research Foundation Project (http://www.nasda.org/nasda/nasda/Foundation/foodsafety/index.html)[b]	1999	Detailed description of how foods are regulated in each state by agency.
FDA, State Retail and Food Service Code Regulations	Ongoing updates at www.fda.gov/Food/FoodSafety/RetailFoodProtection/FederalStateCooperativePrograms	Specific information on state agencies that enforce the Food Code at food retail establishments.
Individual State Agencies	Ongoing updates	Individual agency websites outline responsibilities.

[a] Until 1995, the FDA produced annual reports on state food safety laws. These surveys were discontinued because of a lack of resources. The last survey for which a record exists was conducted in 1993.

[b] Records for each state are located at the following address (with pertinent state inserted): http://www.nasda.org/nasda/nasda/Foundation/foodsafety/WestVirginia.pdf (accessed October 8, 2010).

TABLE 7-2 State Food Regulatory Programs: Leading Agencies Involved

Department of Agriculture[a]	Department of Health[a]	Other Agencies
Alabama	Arizona	Department of Environmental
Florida	Arkansas	Conservation (Alaska)
Georgia	California	Departments of Consumer
Maine	Colorado	Protection (Connecticut)
Michigan	Delaware	Split between Departments of
Minnesota	Hawaii	Health and Agriculture (Idaho)
Nebraska	Illinois	Department of Inspections and
New York	Indiana	Appeals (Iowa)
North Carolina	Kansas	Split between Departments of
Ohio	Kentucky	Commerce and Agriculture
Oregon	Louisiana	(South Dakota)
Pennsylvania	Maryland	
South Carolina	Massachusetts	
Tennessee	Mississippi	
Utah	Missouri	
Virginia	Montana	
Washington	Nevada	
Wisconsin	New Hampshire	
Wyoming	New Jersey	
	New Mexico	
	North Dakota	
	Oklahoma	
	Rhode Island	
	Texas	
	Vermont	
	West Virginia	
Total: 19 states	Total: 26 states	Total: 5 states

[a] Agency housing the predominant portion of food safety regulatory programs. Most states have some divided authorities between agencies.
SOURCES: FDA, 1993; NASDA, 1999; AFDO, 2001, 2009b.

that all 50 states have adopted all or portions of the Food Code (AFDO, 2009b; FDA, 2009c).

There appear to be no major fundamental differences between state and federal food safety laws, although some state laws are based on the 1906 Pure Food and Drugs Act and others on the 1938 Federal Food, Drug, and Cosmetic Act (FDA, 1993). The states, however, possess some authorities that are absent from the 1938 act. By 1993, for example, 48 states had the statutory authority to embargo or stop the sale of food products, but the FDA does not have that authority under federal statutes. In addition, many states have the authority to revoke licenses or permits for food companies that violate food safety requirements or to require destruction of contaminated products. The FDA's Office of Federal–State Relations confirms that all states now have some form of legislative authority for food and drugs; however, there are wide variations among states, such as in the number of personnel. Because of a lack of resources, no annual surveys of state regulatory authorities have been conducted since 1995; the last survey of state food laws for which there is a record was conducted by the National Association of State Departments of Agriculture in 1999.[4]

State feed programs are an integral part of the food safety system since feed contamination, either chemical or microbiological, becomes a food safety issue for humans through the consumption of food animals or exposure to the contaminated feed. Likewise, humans are exposed to certain zoonotic diseases (those transmitted from animals to humans) through the food and feed chain. Surveillance for zoonotic diseases is a responsibility of state veterinarians. Coordination of state efforts to monitor food animals' feed supply and conduct surveillance for human exposure to zoonotic diseases is part of an integrated food safety system. The FDA has reported that it is currently developing process control regulations for animal feeds similar to the voluntary national Retail Food Regulatory Program Standards and Manufactured Food Regulatory Program Standards (FDA, 2007b, 2009d).

Nearly all feed mills manufacture medicated feeds; however, only those that produce medicated feeds with specific drugs and drug concentrations are inspected routinely by the FDA or contract state inspectors. Feed mills making nonmedicated feeds are generally regulated only by states; the exception is federal regulations concerning bovine spongiform encephalopathy (BSE). Most of these mills either produce organic feed or are species specific (e.g., horse feeds). The FDA stated during testimony to the committee that regulations addressing medicated animal feed are not uniform at the state level, and therefore medicated feed inspections under FDA contracts are conducted under federal law.

Level of Regulatory Activity in the States

Several publications have reported on the number of activities (e.g., inspections, enforcements) conducted at the local, state, and federal levels (AFDO, 2001; HHS/FDA, 2009), including food- and feed-related activities. AFDO is currently finalizing an additional survey of state and local food safety regulatory programs to update previous statistics (AFDO, 2009a,b). The preliminary results (corresponding to 64 of the total 75 state agencies in 47 states at the time of this writing) show that, as in

---

[4] Personal communication, Richard Barnes, Director, Division of Federal–State Relations, FDA, June 2009.

TABLE 7-3 State and Local Food Safety Activities

Food Safety Activity	2001
Inspections	
Food processing/repackaging facilities (including dairy)	68,162
Farms	159,794
Food service establishments (institutional and retail)	1,229,638
Retail food stores	516,033
Animal feed (feed manufacturers and distributors, bovine spongiform encephalopathy inspections, rendering plants)	23,984
Other (food warehouses, food transportation vehicles, food salvage operations, etc.)	47,697
Investigations	
Foodborne illness outbreaks	3,075
Other (trace-backs, complaints, chemical residues, etc.)	86,840
Enforcement (embargo, warning letters, food recalls, etc.)	128,430
Samples analyzed (food chemistry, microbiology, pesticide residue)	328,065

SOURCE: AFDO, 2001.

2001, the states conduct a substantial number of activities.[5] For example, 2.5 million state and local food safety inspections were reported for foods regulated by the FDA, with the majority being conducted in food service and retail stores, categories the FDA has delegated to the states. In all states, food processing and repackaging establishments are far fewer in number than these categories (Table 7-3).

Florida and Texas are two examples of states that devote substantial resources to food safety. In 2008, the state food regulatory program of the Florida Department of Agriculture and Consumer Services conducted 55,364 food safety inspections in various categories (Aller, 2009).[6] The department supports 184.5 full-time equivalents (FTEs) dedicated to food safety inspection and investigation and 62 FTEs providing administrative support. In 2008, the Texas Department of Health Services conducted 24,829 food sample analyses and took 1,918 enforcement actions (Sowards, 2009).[7] Both state food laboratories are International Organization for Standardization (ISO) 17025 certified.

As noted, state food safety programs are diverse. Data from the 2001

---

[5] Personal communication, Joseph Corby, Executive Director of AFDO, August 25, 2009.

[6] Personal communication, Marion Aller, Director of the Division of Food Safety, Florida Department of Agriculture and Consumer Services, April 20, 2009.

[7] Personal communication, Dan Sowards, Food and Drug Safety Officer, Division for Regulatory Services, Texas Department of State Health Services, May 19, 2009.

AFDO State Food Safety Resource Survey (AFDO, 2001) show that the numbers of inspections, enforcement activities, and foodborne illness outbreaks differ greatly among the states. Although these disparities could be due to the numbers of facilities/establishments in each state, they also suggest that the emphasis on food safety varies by state. AFDO collected data on inspections of all types of establishments and activities: food processing/repackaging facilities, dairy plants, milk plants, dairy farms, retail food service establishments, retail food stores, wholesale meat processors, meat plants, slaughterhouses, feed manufacturers and distributors, BSE inspections, rendering plants, food transportation vehicles, food salvage operations, farm production, and food warehouses. Based on this survey, the total number of inspections conducted in 2001 ranged from 80 in one state to more than 100,000 in others; the average number of inspections was approximately 50,000 per state.

Information on statutory and enforcement activities (embargo/seizure, stop sale, health advisories, monetary penalties, license/permit revocations, injunctions, criminal prosecutions, warning letters, and informal hearings) was also collected in the AFDO survey. Some states reported fewer than 20 activities, while others reported thousands. Likewise, 13 states reported 10 or fewer outbreaks of foodborne illness, while others reported hundreds (AFDO, 2001).

In contrast with the number of state and local inspections in processing and repackaging facilities (more than 50,000 reported in 2001), the FDA reported only about 16,000 food establishment inspections and 8,000 inspections of animal drug and feed programs for 2008 (HHS/FDA, 2009). The states performed about 60 percent of the food establishment inspections for the FDA and 73 percent of the animal drug and feed program inspections.

Public Health Surveillance and Outbreak Investigations

As stated in Chapter 3, rapid detection and investigation of foodborne illnesses, whether sporadic or outbreak associated, are critical to public health management and risk-based decision making. Development of the epidemiological surveillance system necessary to support this function requires effective and efficient communication and cooperation among a large number of partners, including scientists and laboratories at the local, state, and federal levels (see also Chapter 5). A further complicating factor is the high degree of variability in funding and data collection at the state level. This variability was illustrated in a recent survey conducted by Safe Tables Our Priority, which demonstrated wide variation in response to foodborne illness outbreaks. Nearly 60 percent (23 of 39) of the responding states reported that they did not have electronic capabilities to link investigative data (Produce Safety Project, 2009). This finding is similar to that cited in the December 2009 report of the Council of State and Territorial Epidemiologists: while 90 percent of the 46 states reporting had databases compliant with the National Electronic Disease Surveillance System, only 53 percent had automated electronic laboratory reporting and 41 percent web-based provider reporting. The report also documents a reduction in the workforce, with 10 percent fewer epidemiologists working in state health departments in 2009 than in 2006 (CSTE, 2009). Since the first-line response to foodborne illness outbreaks is investigations conducted primarily by county and state health departments, with pertinent information eventually flowing to federal agencies such as the FDA or the U.S. Centers for Disease Control and Prevention (CDC), this decrease in regional professional personnel is disturbing.

Food Analysis Data

Some states routinely analyze food samples for contaminants. These data can be invaluable in measuring the effectiveness of industry preventive programs and in providing much-needed information to support risk-based food safety efforts. If these data are to be used in a national food safety system, their quality must meet defined standards of sampling and analysis. To this end, AFDO recently completed a Food Laboratory Accreditation Survey designed to gather information on what is needed for acceptance of analytical results between allied state and federal food safety regulatory agencies (AFDO, 2009a,b). Many state laboratories are equivalent to federal laboratories with regard to staffing numbers and qualifications of both inspectional and analytical personnel and analytical capabilities (e.g., facilities, instrumentation). Some states' food analytical laboratories have achieved ISO/International Electrotechnical Commission (IEC) 17025[8] accreditation, while others are progressing rapidly through this demanding process (AFDO, 2009a,b). Solomon reported in November 2009 that all FDA laboratories were ISO 17025 accredited, as were nine states' food safety laboratories.[9]

Sharing food safety data remains a challenge for various reasons, both technical and cultural (see also Chapter 5), although some valuable initiatives to this end have been undertaken. The eLEXNET system, for example, is a web-based information network that allows the FDA to compare laboratory analyses of contaminants in food or food-producing animals from

---

[8] ISO/IEC 17025 is the main standard used by testing and calibration laboratories, originally issued by ISO in 1999 and revised thereafter. Laboratories use ISO/IEC 17025 to implement a quality system aimed at improving their ability to produce valid results consistently.

[9] Personal communication, Steven Solomon, ORA, FDA, November 17, 2009.

different laboratories. It is also used as a repository for method validation and serves other roles in support of the Food Emergency Response Network (FERN) (FERN, 2009).[10] This initiative, coordinated by the FDA, began as a pilot with 8 participating laboratories and has grown to include 135 laboratories representing federal, state, and local government agencies in all 50 states. A needed enhancement and a specified goal of the FDA's ORA (FDA, 2009c,e) is for eLEXNET to have the capability to alert other users of the system about any significant findings (e.g., a contaminant in a food or a finding outside the normal parameters indicating a potential event) that might necessitate a rapid response.

Another initiative of note is an innovative database developed by the National Center for Food Protection and Defense in collaboration with AFDO, with the purpose of facilitating data sharing in the area of food defense (AFDO, 2009a,b). FoodSHIELD is designed as a web-based platform with a communication portal, a training center, and two databases that capture the capabilities, capacity, technology, and expertise of agriculture, health, environment, and emergency response agencies and their supporting laboratories. Users of FoodSHIELD are varied but are mainly government public health officials (FoodSHIELD, 2009).

FDA INTERACTIONS AND COLLABORATIONS WITH THE STATES

The FDA maintains various interactions and joint programs with state and local regulatory agencies involved in food safety. These include such activities as annual scope-of-work planning sessions, training courses, contracts for food and feed inspections, grants, cooperative agreements, confidentiality agreements, commissioning, inspector and program audits, and joint inspections. In addition, the FDA has memorandums of understanding (MOUs) with the states for various functions, which are issued chiefly to facilitate cooperation and planning.

Training of Inspection Personnel

The adequacy of state and local food safety inspectional programs and the associated training is poorly documented. Solomon (2009a,b) stated that the Office of Regulatory Affairs University (ORAU) offers 130 training courses to state food safety programs, but they are not mandatory. Since 1993, the ORAU program was initiated, 10,700 professionals have participated, and more than 83,000 courses have been completed. In 2009, for example, 37 courses were offered in food protection, including at the retail level and for milk and shellfish, 34 on manufactured foods, 6 on feed

---

[10] See www.fernlab.org (accessed December 30, 2009).

and veterinary medicine, and 23 on investigative responses, including incident command, rapid response, and farm investigations. However, access to this training is far from ideal, since an individual state has only one or two training slots available in locations far from home districts. In addition to the efforts of ORA, AFDO is now providing education and training to food protection professionals through the IFPTI, established by a $2 million grant from the Kellogg Foundation.[11] The establishment of minimal training requirements and the provision of appropriate training opportunities to meet those requirements are essential if state personnel are to be integrated successfully into the federal food safety program (see Chapter 8). The FDA Manufactured Food Regulatory Program Standards (discussed below) could serve as a basis for providing such minimal requirements as standards for state employees.

Grants, Cooperative Agreements, and Contracts

The FDA has awarded grants, cooperative agreements, and contracts to the states for more than three decades. A grant provides financial assistance to an eligible individual or group to carry out an approved project or activity in which the agency will have no substantial programmatic involvement with the recipient. In 2009, FDA grants provided $17.5 million in state funding to design and implement response, intervention, innovation, and prevention food safety programs—the four key tenets of the FPP. Cooperative agreements are similar to grants in that they give state and local governments the opportunity to enhance existing programs or develop new programs to improve public health. Currently, cooperative agreements are used in cases of substantial federal programmatic involvement.

According to Solomon (2009a,b), the FDA currently has about 43 contracts in 41 states covering a total of about 10,500 inspections. Of these inspections, 9,000 are related to Good Manufacturing Practices (GMPs), 1,100 to seafood HACCP, 47 to juice HACCP, and 53 to low-acid canned foods (see also Chapter 8). However, the total number of FDA-sponsored state contract inspections represents only 0.4 percent of the more than 2.5 million state and local food safety inspections conducted each year (AFDO, 2009a,b). In addition, 37 states currently have contracts or cooperative agreements to conduct feed inspections for the FDA. In fiscal year 2008, those states performed more than 6,000 contracted feed inspections (including GMP and BSE inspections), or approximately 76 percent of all FDA feed inspections. The FDA also has 18 contracts with states to perform tissue residue testing; the states have reported conducting 635 such

---

[11] Personal communication, Joseph Corby, Executive Director of AFDO, August 25, 2009.

inspections (Solomon, 2009a,b). The number of federal-led inspections is low compared with the number of state-led inspections.

States provide information on contract inspections through electronic access to the Field Accomplishments and Compliance Tracking System. For example, the FDA has a goal to audit 7 percent of contract inspections to determine their equivalency to FDA food inspections and ensure the proper performance of state partners. The FDA has been criticized in the media, most recently in 2009 (Burke, 2007; Schmidt, 2009; Scott-Thomas, 2009), for not meeting this oversight goal. If state and local programs were fully integrated, with adequate standardization and oversight, the FDA could raise its rate of inspection from once every 3–10 years to annually. Once state and local programs have been integrated, the committee suggests that the FDA meet this goal to ensure appropriate inspection and enforcement procedures. If this goal is met, and if the FDA increases its reliance on state and local inspections, the goal can be increased to a higher auditing rate.

State-led food inspections under FDA contracts are performed under state law since states have greater authority than the FDA to embargo shipments, remove licenses, or destroy products (Barnes, 2009). On the other hand, many states lack sufficient regulatory authority in the feed area, so they perform feed inspections under the FDA's commissioning (see below).

Cooperative agreements with the states fund rapid response teams and FERN. The rapid response teams are funded for a specified amount of time with the purpose of enhancing regulatory and surveillance programs for food protection at the state level. The agreements typically provide funds for program assessment, additional equipment, supplies, personnel, and training. The success of the teams depends on their ability to support the infrastructure needed to sustain extensive cooperation and coordination with FDA district offices, especially during emergencies. The first team was the California Food Emergency Response Team, established in 2003; since then, eight additional states (Florida, Massachusetts, Michigan, Minnesota, North Carolina, Texas, Virginia, and Washington) have been granted funds to establish such teams.

FERN encompasses state agricultural, environmental, public health, and veterinary diagnostic laboratories in partnership with federal agencies, including the FDA; CDC; USDA's Food Safety and Inspection Services, Animal and Plant Health Inspection Service, and Agricultural Marketing Service; the U.S. Department of Defense; the Federal Bureau of Investigation; the U.S. Environmental Protection Agency); and the U.S. Department of Homeland Security (FERN, 2009). FERN is organized into a national program office with regional coordination centers that, together with the laboratories, coordinate responses and ensure integration within the network. The FERN laboratories have assisted with method development and technical expertise on limited occasions. The FERN system has been activated only on a limited basis, including the 2006 outbreak of *E. coli* O157:H7 in spinach, the 2007 outbreaks associated with melamine in infant formula and pet food, the 2008 outbreak of *Salmonella* Saintpaul in Mexican peppers, and the 2008 outbreak of *Salmonella* in peanut butter.

Confidentiality Agreements and Commissioning

Forty-four states are covered by annual confidentiality agreements. The individuals signing the agreements are bound to keep confidential any information designated as such by the FDA.

Commissioning of state officials is the process by which the FDA allows the sharing of confidential information between parties, such as between the agency and a state department of health or agriculture. Commissioning has historically been reserved for high-ranking officials, and only about 1,200 state officials and 9,500 Customs and Border Protection officials are commissioned (Solomon, 2009a,b). The program was designed to better utilize state and local officials in the performance of specific functions subject to federal jurisdiction and confidentiality requirements (e.g., the conduct of examinations or inspections). Commissioning is usually limited to a specified period of time.

In its deliberations, the committee discussed the limited benefits of the current commissioning mechanism. In particular, restricting the number of high-ranking officials commissioned by the FDA in each state leads to barriers in information sharing at the state level. The committee suggests expanding the use of the commissioning process as a mechanism in order to better leverage and integrate the resources of state inspectional personnel (see Chapter 8). The committee believes that expanding use of the FDA's authority to commission both food and feed inspectors would provide an excellent mechanism for delegating agency functions and, when combined with funding mechanisms to promote sustainability of state food safety programs, would facilitate the overall integration of state and federal food safety efforts.

Memorandums of Understanding

The FDA has MOUs with the states for various functions, chiefly to facilitate cooperation and planning. However, MOUs are not binding; are written in general language expressing broad goals, such as a commitment to joint planning and coordinated inspections; and often are not utilized. Previously enacted MOUs between the FDA and the states have basically been general statements of intent; GAO has previously reported on the underutilization of the FDA's interagency agreements (GAO 2004a,b,

2005b). The committee suggests that the FDA develop and utilize more detailed formal agreements, outlining specific expectations, with all states on all food and feed safety matters.

INTEGRATION THROUGH STANDARDIZATION AND OVERSIGHT OF FOOD SAFETY PROGRAMS

The integration and analysis of food safety information and data derived from the inspections and analyses of all partners and stakeholders are of the utmost importance for (1) understanding the food safety system in its totality, (2) ensuring the trust of the consuming public, (3) providing the public with the appropriate level of regulatory scrutiny of the U.S. food supply, (4) allowing the goals of the FDA's FPP to be accomplished, and (5) implementing nationwide the risk-based approach recommended by the committee in Chapter 3. Further, collaboration, partnerships, and data sharing with the states are essential when resources need to be prioritized, but these cannot occur without an adequate foundation in legal authority, standardization, and harmonization of FDA, state, and local programs. The recommendations offered in this report, as well as those of Taylor and David (2009), outline the steps necessary for such collaboration and partnership to occur and encourage the FDA to implement an integrated national food safety system. The FDA cannot be expected to fully achieve the goals of its FPP, in which the states are partners, without fundamental intra-agency changes in culture, structure, and function, as well as interagency integration with state and local partners.

Strategic Planning, Leadership, and Cooperation

Increasing FDA funding or personnel without incorporating the fundamental changes recommended by the committee will not be sufficient to enhance food safety as outlined in this report or to allow the goals of the FPP to be accomplished. Careful strategic planning is necessary before an integrated approach can be implemented. The FDA has produced a report of recent activities toward establishing an integrated national food safety system (FDA, 2009c,e). This document recognizes that "to be successful, an integrated national food safety system must build upon the work currently being done by FDA and our regulatory and public health partners" (FDA 2009c, p. 4).

Constructive changes in federal food safety programs are under way, such as the formation of the FSWG, new leadership in the FDA, creation of the agency's Office of Foods under the Office of the Commissioner, regulatory changes proposed by the FDA, and proposed congressional actions. Efforts are under way to establish task groups internal to the FDA in the areas of national work planning, policy and procedures, national standards, training and certification, oversight, emergency response, performance outcomes and measures, and laboratories, with implementation expected over the next 5 years (FDA, 2009c,e). According to the FDA, a steering committee was established to maintain necessary communication with the FSWG via the deputy commissioner for foods (see Chapter 11). The committee supports this initiative and concludes that the FSWG, with the enhancements outlined in Chapter 11, needs to maintain a leadership role to ensure that these changes are accomplished. The committee also recognizes that integration will likely not be completed for some years, and it looks forward to seeing progress toward the system's ultimate implementation. The success of this initiative will depend on sustainable support and cooperation among the various organizational structures created (e.g., steering committees, coordinating committees, task groups, partnership for food protection work groups).

The process of integration will require a sustained spirit of collaboration. In the past, successful cooperation has depended mainly on personal relationships and trust among individuals and agencies. The committee recognizes the various ways in which cooperation is being attempted and the recent improvements in sharing of regulatory responsibilities among various jurisdictions (federal, state, and local). The committee recognizes the barriers to collaboration (including the fact that it cannot be mandated), and it emphasizes the importance of strong leadership in achieving and sustaining this important goal.

Standardization of State Programs

State and local governments have jurisdiction over the safety of food products that do not cross state or local boundaries. As noted above, despite similarities in the legal foundation for food safety, state and local programs vary. To integrate food safety as defined by the committee, these programs and their implementation must be evaluated against a minimum standard and ultimately standardized and harmonized. Two programs currently exist within the FDA for assistance that, if enforced, could be used in state standardization.

First, the Voluntary National Retail Food Regulatory Program Standards were introduced as a guide to designing and managing retail food regulatory programs. In 1998, as a pilot test, the states used these standards to assess their retail programs. However, many states failed to adopt the standards because, if the assessment indicated that a program was inadequate, there were implications for state appropriations (FDA, 2007c). Nonetheless, states have expressed the desire for a review and modification of this program.[12]

Second, in 2000, the HHS Office of the Inspector General reported on the FDA's oversight of state contracts and recommended that the agency take steps to promote equivalency between federal and state food safety standards, inspection programs, and enforcement practices (Brown, 2000). Subsequently, the FDA worked with the states to formulate the Manufactured Food Regulatory Program Standards, which were intended to establish a uniform foundation for the design and management of state programs that are responsible for the regulation of food processing plants. The standards cover ten areas: regulatory foundation, staff training, inspection, inspection audit, food-related illness and outbreaks and food defense preparedness and response, compliance and enforcement, industry and community relations, resources, program assessment, and laboratory support (FDA, 2007b). In 2008, 5 states evaluated their programs against these standards, followed by an additional 25 states in 2009. The principles of this program have also been applied to evaluate foreign food safety programs, such as those in China (Solomon, 2009a,b). Solomon (2009b) reported that the FDA had used these standards in establishing agreements with China's Administration of Quality Supervision, Inspection, and Quarantine to enhance the regulatory structure in that country. The increased participation of states is promising, and the FDA should be encouraged to review the scope of the program to ensure that it covers all phases of the food chain from production to consumption.

The committee agrees with previous recommendations for standardization of all state programs (FDA, 2007b) that are established by the FDA to foster nationwide equivalence with respect to food safety management. As of this writing, 25 states are implementing the Manufactured Food Regulatory Program Standards, which leads the committee to conclude that the integration process is feasible (Solomon, 2009a). For other states, an infusion of resources, as well as increased training, will be necessary to meet those minimal federal standards.

Oversight of State Programs by the FDA

Once standards have been established, methods for standardization are in place, and integration has been achieved, the FDA's major role should be to maintain and revise the standards as necessary; to provide professional expertise, training, and oversight; and to audit the inspections and

---

[12] Personal communication, Marion Aller, Director of the Division of Food Safety, Florida Department of Agriculture and Consumer Services, April 20, 2009.

programs of its food safety partners. The FDA already performs limited oversight of state programs through either inspector or program audits. In an inspector audit, an FDA inspector observes a state inspector at work; a program audit consists of the FDA's evaluation of a state program. As noted earlier, the FDA has established a goal of auditing 7 percent of state contract inspections and has been criticized for not meeting this goal (FDA, 2006). To the committee's knowledge, there are no FDA audits of local food inspections.

The FDA's FPP (FDA, 2007a) proposes third-party auditing as a means by which oversight of food safety programs and of adherence to regulations and standards can be conducted (see Chapter 4). Large food retailers now require third-party auditing to confirm that food safety practices are being followed by their suppliers. This type of oversight is being conducted by industry in part because the FDA currently is unable to provide such auditing (GAO, 2008b).

In the FPP, the FDA recognizes the significant role third-party auditors now play and hence seeks to provide some level of standardization for these audits. Of interest, other federal, state, and local agencies are also proposed to have a role as third-party auditors (FDA, 2007a). In practice, the committee recommends that the FDA serve as auditor of all state inspections and food safety programs. However, the committee also concludes that there is a fundamental difference between the auditing role of other government agencies and commercial third parties in that other government agencies should be considered equal partners in governing food safety. Thus, the committee objects to the reference to other government agencies, including state and local agencies, as "third parties" in the FPP because the term implies that the FDA will not consider those agencies equal partners in ensuring food safety.

Equivalency of State and Federal Inspections

Regulatory officials are frequently asked to delineate the differences between state and federal food inspections in an effort to establish the meaning of equivalency. Although the legal requirements are roughly the same for state and federal food safety inspections, program implementation, resources, and capabilities vary substantially among the states, as suggested by the AFDO surveys. For example, both state and FDA inspections are based on the applicable Code of Federal Regulations (CFR), Title 21, requirements as they have been adopted by the states. Although states have adopted the CFR, they may have their own regulations as well. Examples are a standard of identity for honey, syrup, or some other food not present in the federal regulations (FDACS, 2009) or the requirement of HACCP plans for sprout production in the state of Florida.

In terms of program implementation, there are differences not only among states but also between the states and the federal government. As a relevant example, most states are unlike the FDA in that inspectors are dedicated solely to food safety, with no responsibility to perform drug or device inspections. An additional difference between federal and state inspections is that the latter focus primarily on reviewing operations in progress rather than on reviewing records, which is more often the focus of FDA inspections. As a result, federal inspections usually take longer than state inspections.[13] One similarity is that both federal and state inspections require internal auditing of inspectors by supervisors to ensure that appropriate inspectional methods are being used. Also, like federal inspectors, state inspectors are often trained through FDA courses; an important difference in this area in that the courses currently are not mandatory for states.

Given these differences, and in the absence of criteria for standardization, there appears to be a legitimate concern within the FDA about the quality of state relative to federal inspections as well as the qualifications and training of state inspectors. As detailed in Chapter 8, the committee recommends a review and update of the inspectional procedures and training curricula for both federal and state inspections and the standardization of all state food safety inspectional programs, including inspector training. The FDA should review and update curricula specific to general food inspections as well as to particular types of inspections (e.g., seafood HACCP) for state and federal inspectors and provide sufficient resources to deliver this training. As mentioned in Chapter 8, the committee supports the partnership of the FDA with others, such as the IFPTI, for the delivery of training for inspectors and auditors.

Risk-Based Approaches at the State and Local Levels

The states apply some of the concepts embraced by a risk-based approach to making regulatory decisions. For example, some use qualitative and quantitative risk assessments and prioritization models produced by the FDA and the academic sector, such as published risk assessments on *Listeria monocytogenes* and methyl mercury. Most state programs prioritize inspections and regulatory scrutiny based on the perishability or known contamination of a food, previous inspectional and analytical history for a firm, published problems with a particular food product, publication of federal recall records, and other knowledge. However, the implementation of a common risk-based approach to food safety management is

---

[13] Personal communication, John T. Fruin, Florida Department of Agriculture and Consumer Services, 2009.

unlikely until such an approach is instituted at the federal level. Once a risk-based approach is in place at the FDA, the agency should work with state and local governments to facilitate a uniform implementation of that approach.

KEY CONCLUSIONS AND RECOMMENDATIONS

State and local government food safety regulations and programs— including food and public health surveillance and data analysis, inspection, and outbreak investigation—remain a mainstay in protecting the U.S. food supply from unintentional and intentional contamination. An integrated food safety system would have many advantages, such as leveraging efforts, minimizing unnecessary duplication, improving responsiveness when crises occur, and ensuring a reasonable frequency of regulatory scrutiny.

Despite past calls for integration of local, state, and federal food safety programs, only limited progress has been made in this regard. Most of this progress has been accomplished just recently, as evidenced by the IFSS announced by the FDA in fall 2009. This delay has been largely a function of barriers including funding limitations; state-to-state variability in food safety programs, goals, and support; past legal interpretations that integration was not possible; and institutional resistance to change and cultural barriers. Also hampering full integration is the lack of a formal federal process to support, evaluate, or guide state and local food safety programs. Nonetheless, the FDA does have standards in place that, if broadened and properly implemented, could serve as a basis for the harmonization of state and local food and feed safety programs as well as their integration with federal programs. Based on the number of states that are implementing the Manufactured Food Regulatory Program Standards, it appears that the integration process is feasible. The FDA, working with the states, is moving forward to establish core competencies and the credentialing process necessary to ensure adequate performance by inspectors (Brown, 2000; Solomon, 2009a).

The committee recognizes that there will be initial and ongoing costs associated with the integration proposed in this chapter. Certain states will have difficulty achieving the recommended levels of funding and resources. However, mechanisms within the FDA (e.g., contracts, grants, incentives) can be used to enable state programs to meet federal standards in a relatively short period of time. The committee recognizes that questions of legal authority regarding the roles of the states, CDC, and the FDA in the investigation of foodborne illness could impede the flawless, full integration of all local, state, and federal food safety activities. The committee recommends that an appropriate panel perform an overarching analysis of the relevant authorities and that, if necessary, Congress provide clear authorities to the

FDA to achieve the goal of a full integration of local, state, and federal food safety activities to the benefit of the nation's public health.

> **Recommendation 7-1: The FDA should utilize the surveillance, inspection, and analytic systems and resources of state and local governments in a fully integrated food safety program.** As a prerequisite to such integration, the FDA should work with the states and localities to harmonize their programs by providing adequate standards and overseeing their implementation, beginning with those states that meet such standards. Standardization and integration of state and local food safety programs should be conducted in an evolutionary fashion, with intermediate goals and associated performance measures. The White House FSWG should make integration of federal and state food regulatory programs a priority and provide leadership to the already established IFSS Steering Committee. The agency should provide training, auditing, and oversight of state and local programs and should facilitate nationwide implementation of the recommended risk-based approach.

Joint responsibilities of the FDA and the states should include the following:

- Both the states and the FDA should review the state statutory authorities in food and feed safety to ensure adequate protection. If deficiencies are found, the FDA should provide specific recommendations for any additional authorities needed by the states.
- The FDA should work with state and local governments to ensure that the risk-based approach is embraced at all levels.
- The FDA and the states should ensure integration of the feed regulatory program and, through the state veterinarians' offices, actively integrate surveillance of zoonotic diseases into the overall food safety program of each state.
- The FDA and each state and local government should enact formal agreements to delineate the responsibilities of each party and develop a timetable for integration. The FDA should also provide a mechanism (e.g., contracts, grants, incentives) whereby the funds necessary to support full integration are provided to each state government on the basis of its needs to achieve national standards. State programs will not be equal in size or inspection activity, as the location of food establishments is concentrated in certain geographic areas, and the supportive mechanism may be needed for multiple years based on the state's available resources and the number and nature of food firms within its boundaries.

The responsibilities of the states should include the following:

- The states should cooperate with the FDA in standardization processes and commit to obtaining sufficient resources and expertise to achieve standardization.
- The states should work with the FDA to ensure compatibility of communication systems and information technology to allow timely sharing of inspection findings and analytical data.
- The states should work to achieve certification of analytical and inspection programs and, when necessary, seek additional funding through the FDA to assist in this process.

The FDA's responsibilities should include the following:

- The FDA's role in food safety should focus on standards setting, nationwide implementation of the recommended risk-based approach, and training and oversight of state and local food safety regulatory programs, not on increasing internal resources to conduct all regulatory activities at the federal level.
- Accordingly, the FDA should provide appropriate training to state and local surveillance and inspection personnel, with a focus on supporting the risk-based food safety management approach.
- The FDA should provide the necessary standards. As a first step, a review of the Voluntary National Retail Food Regulatory Program Standards and Manufactured Food Regulatory Program Standards should be undertaken to ensure that they are adequate for all areas of food and feed regulatory programs, not just the retail and processing areas.
- As recommended in Chapter 8, after review by an independent body, the FDA's inspection procedures should be revised to promote greater efficiency and should be adopted as standards for all food and feed inspections.
- The FDA should oversee state and local food safety programs by performing regular audits of their inspections and other activities as appropriate at a prescribed annual rate. The agency should also work with the states to ensure coordination with regard to inspection of food facilities to avoid unnecessary duplication of effort.
- The FDA should immediately utilize analytical data from appropriately ISO 17025–certified state food laboratories. For those states not yet ISO-certified, the FDA should work, and assist with funding if necessary, to facilitate ISO 17025 certification over the next 10 years.

- State and local food safety programs should be fully recognized as partners in the nation's food safety program and not as third parties. The FDA's FPP needs to be revised to reflect this philosophical change.
- The FDA should identify intermediate goals with associated performance measures for the process of standardization and integration of state and local food safety programs as part of the plans for implementation. In addition, the FDA should certify and integrate state and local government programs as they meet the standards.

REFERENCES

AFDO (Association of Food and Drug Officials). 2001. *State Resource Survey.* York, PA: AFDO.

AFDO. 2009a. *State Food Safety Resource Survey.* York, PA: AFDO.

AFDO. 2009b. *AFDO Food Laboratory Standard Methods Accreditation Survey.* York, PA: AFDO. http://www.afdo.org/Resources/Surveys/Lab2009.cfm (accessed February 26, 2010).

Aller, M. 2009. *Florida Submission to AFDO State Food Safety Resource Assessment.* York, PA: AFDO.

Barnes, R. 2009. *Discussion Panel: FDA and State Inspections of Food.* Institute of Medicine/National Research Council Committee on Review of the FDA's Role in Ensuring Safe Food Meeting, Washington, DC, March 24, 2009.

Becker, G. S. 2008. *U.S. Food and Agricultural Imports: Safeguards and Selected Issues.* Washington, DC: Congressional Research Service.

Becker, G. S. 2009. *Food Safety on the Farm: Federal Programs and Selected Proposals.* Washington, DC: Congressional Research Service.

Brown, J. G. 2000. *FDA Oversight of State Food Firm Inspections: A Call for Greater Accountability.* Boston, MA: U.S. Food and Drug Administration.

Burditt, G. M. 1995. The history of food law. *Food & Drug Law Journal* 50:197–201.

Burke, G. 2007. Spinach recall sparks oversight calls. *USA Today,* August 31, 2007.

CRS (Congressional Research Service). 2007. *Federal Food Safety Systems: A Primer.* Report number RS22600. www.nationalaglawcenter.org/assets/crs/RS22600.pdf (accessed March 18, 2010).

CSPI (Center for Science in the Public Interest). 2009. *CSPI Finds a Troubling Decline in Foodborne Outbreak Investigations by State Health Officials.* Washington, DC: CSPI. http://www.cspinet.org/new/200912231.html (accessed March 31, 2010).

CSTE (Council of State and Territorial Epidemiologists). 2009. *2009 National Assessment of Epidemiology Capacity: Findings and Recommendations.* Atlanta, GA: CSTE.

Darby, W. 1993. Symposium: Historical overview of the safety of the food supply: Introduction. *The Journal of Nutrition* 123:277–278.

DeWaal, C. S. 2003. Safe food from a consumer perspective. *Food Control* 14(2):75–79.

DeWaal, C. S., X. A. Tian, and D. Plunkett. 2009. *Outbreak Alert! Analyzing Foodborne Outbreaks 1998–2007.* Washington, DC: Center for Science in the Public Interest. http://cspinet.org/new/pdf/outbreakalertreport09.pdf (accessed March 31, 2010).

FDA (U.S. Food and Drug Administration). 1993. *State Law Data.* Rockville, MD: FDA.

FDA. 2006. *State Contracts-Evaluation of Inspectional Performance: Appendix H Model Standard Agreement ORA Field Management Directive No. 76.* Washington, DC: FDA.

FDA. 2007a. *Food Protection Plan. An Integrated Strategy for Protecting the Nation's Food Supply*. Rockville, MD: FDA.

FDA. 2007b. *Manufactured Food Regulatory Program Standards*. http://www.fda.gov/downloads/RegulatoryInformation/Guidances/UCM125448.pdf (accessed February 26, 2010).

FDA. 2007c. *Voluntary National Retail Food Regulatory Program Standards*. http://www.fda.gov/Food/FoodSafety/RetailFoodProtection/ProgramStandards/ucm124968.htm (accessed March 18, 2010).

FDA. 2008. *Gateway to Food Protection. Federal, State, and Local Partners National Meeting, St. Louis, MO*. Rockville, MD: FDA.

FDA. 2009a. *FDA Releases the 2009 Edition of the Food Code*. http://www.fda.gov/Food/NewsEvents/ConstituentUpdates/ucm189688.htm (accessed December 30, 2009).

FDA. 2009b. *Food Code 2009*. College Park, MD: FDA.

FDA. 2009c. *Establishing a Fully Integrated National Food Safety System with Strengthened Inspection, Laboratory and Response Capacity*. http://www.fda.gov/downloads/ForFederalStateandLocalOfficials/UCM183650.pdf (accessed March 2, 2010).

FDA. 2009d. *Retail Food Protection: A Cooperative Program*. http://www.fda.gov/Food/FoodSafety/RetailFoodProtection/default.htm (accessed December 30, 2009).

FDA. 2009e. *Combined ORA Performance Goals*. http://www.fda.gov/AboutFDA/ReportsManualsForms/Reports/BudgetReports/2007FDABudgetSummary/ucm112775.htm (accessed January 25, 2010).

FDA. 2010. *Food and Drug Administration FY 2011 Congressional Budget Request: Narrative by Activity—Foods Program FY2011*. http://www.fda.gov/downloads/AboutFDA/ReportsManualsForms/Reports/BudgetReports/UCM205367.pdf (accessed June 2, 2010).

FDACS (Florida Department of Agriculture and Consumer Services). 2009. *Bronson Announces First Regulation in the Nation Banning Additives in Honey*. http://www.doacs.state.fl.us/press/2009/07132009.html (accessed December 30, 2009).

FERN (Food Emergency Response Network). 2009. *Uniting Federal, State, and Local Laboratories for Food Emergency Response*. http://www.fernlab.org/ (accessed December 30, 2009).

FoodSHIELD. 2009. *FoodSHIELD: United in Protecting & Defending the Food Supply*. http://www.foodshield.org/ (accessed February 26, 2010).

GAO (U.S. Government Accountability Office). 2004a. *Federal Food Safety and Security System: Fundamental Restructuring Is Needed to Address Fragmentation and Overlap*. Washington, DC: GAO.

GAO. 2004b. *Food Safety: FDA's Imported Seafood Safety Program Shows Some Progress, but Further Improvements Are Needed*. Washington, DC: GAO.

GAO. 2004c. *Food Safety: USDA and FDA Need to Better Ensure Prompt and Complete Recalls of Potentially Unsafe Food*. Washington, DC: GAO.

GAO. 2005a. *Overseeing the U.S. Food Supply: Steps Should be Taken to Reduce Overlapping Inspections and Related Activities*. Washington, DC: GAO.

GAO. 2005b. *Oversight of Food Safety Activities: Federal Agencies Should Pursue Opportunities to Reduce Overlap and Better Leverage Resources*. Washington, DC: GAO.

GAO. 2008a. *Federal Oversight of Food Safety: FDA Has Provided Few Details on the Resources and Strategies Needed to Implement Its Food Protection Plan*. Washington, DC: GAO.

GAO. 2008b. *Federal Oversight of Food Safety: FDA's Food Protection Plan Proposes Positive First Steps, but Capacity to Carry Them Out Is Critical*. Washington, DC: GAO.

GAO. 2008c. *Food Labeling: FDA Needs to Better Leverage Resources, Improve Oversight, and Effectively Use Available Data to Help Consumers Select Healthy Foods*. Washington, DC: GAO.

GAO. 2008d. *Food Safety: Improvements Needed in FDA Oversight of Fresh Produce.* Washington, DC: GAO.

GAO. 2009a. *Agencies Need to Address Gaps in Enforcement and Collaboration to Enhance Safety of Imported Food.* Washington, DC: GAO.

GAO. 2009b. *Information Technology: FDA Needs to Establish Key Plans and Processes for Guiding Systems Modernization Efforts.* Washington, DC: GAO.

HHS (U.S. Department of Health and Human Services). 1998. *White House Fact Sheet: President Clinton Signs Executive Order Creating Council on Food Safety.* Washington, DC: HHS. http://www.hhs.gov/news/press/1998pres/980824.html (accessed February 26, 2010).

HHS/FDA (U.S. Food and Drug Administration). 2009. Product tracing systems for food. *Federal Register* 74:56843–56855.

Hile, P. 1984. The annual FDA report to the association. *Association of Food and Drug Officials Quarterly Bulletin* 48:210–215.

Hogan & Hartson, LLP. 2009. *Key Provisions in Select Food Safety Legislation (The Durbin, Dingell, and Costa Bills; and Current Law), March 10, 2009.* Washington, DC: Hogan & Hartson, LLP.

Hutt, P. B. 2007. *The State of Science at the Food and Drug Administration. FDA Science and Mission at Risk.* Appendix B1–B40 in Report of the Subcommittee on Science and Technology. Rockville, MD: FDA.

Hutt, P. B. 2008. *Science and Mission at Risk: FDA's Self-Assessment.* Testimony before the Subcommittee on Oversight and Investigations of the Committee on Energy and Commerce, House of Representatives. http://energycommerce.house.gov/images/stories/Documents/Hearings/PDF/110-oi-hrg.012908.Hutt-Testimony.pdf (accessed May 13, 2010).

IFT (Institute of Food Technologists). 2009. Making decisions about the risks of chemicals in foods with limited scientific information. *Comprehensive Reviews in Foods Science and Food Safety* 8:269–303.

IOM/NRC (Institute of Medicine/National Research Council). 1998. *Ensuring Safe Food: From Production to Consumption.* Washington, DC: National Academy Press.

Kelly, K., C. S. DeWaal, E. Newman, F. Bhuiya, and C. Everett. 2007. *Making the Grade: An Analysis of Food Safety in School Cafeterias.* Washington, DC: Center for Science in the Public Interest. http://www.cspinet.org/new/pdf/makingthegrade.pdf (accessed March 31, 2010).

Klein, S., and C. S. DeWaal. 2008. *Dirty Dining: Have Reservations? You Will Now.* Washington, DC: Center for Science in the Public Interest. http://cspinet.org/new/pdf/ddreport.pdf (accessed March 31, 2010).

Mavity, S. 2009. *Safety of Imported Foods: A Perspective from a Company in the Seafood Industry.* Paper presented at Institute of Medicine/National Research Council Committee on Review of the FDA's Role in Ensuring Safe Food Meeting, Washington, DC, May 28, 2009.

Moran, A. 2009. *Survey of State Health Departments Underscores Gaps in Foodborne Illness Response.* Washington, DC: Produce Safety Project. http://www.producesafetyproject.org/admin/media/files/PSP-STOP-Survey-Release-Final-102909R.pdf (accessed March 31, 2010).

NASDA (National Association of State Departments of Agriculture). 1999. *Food Safety: State and Federal Standards and Regulations.* Washington, DC: NASDA Research Foundation. http://www.nasda.org/nasda/nasda/Foundation/foodsafety/index.html (accessed April 6, 2010).

NFSSP (National Food Safety System Project). 2001. *Multistate Foodborne Outbreak Investigations. Guidelines for Improving Coordination and Communication.* Rockville, MD: FDA.

Produce Safety Project. 2009. *State Surveillance of Foodborne Illness.* Washington, DC: The Pew Charitable Trusts at Georgetown University.

PTI (The Produce Traceability Initiative). 2008. *The Produce Traceability Initiative. Produce Marketing Association 2009.* http://www.producetraceability.org/ (accessed February 26, 2010).

Schmidt, J. 2009. Broken links in food-safety chain hid peanut plants' risks. *USA Today,* April 28, 2009.

Scott-Thomas, C. 2009. *FDA Fails to Reach State Food Safety Audit Targets.* http://www.nutraingredients-usa.com/Regulation/FDA-fails-to-reach-state-food-safety-audit-targets (accessed January 20, 2010).

Solomon, S. 2009a. *FDA and State Inspections of Foods.* Paper presented at Institute of Medicine/National Research Council Committee on Review of the FDA's Role in Ensuring Safe Food Meeting, Washington, DC, May 28, 2009.

Solomon, S. 2009b. *Regulating in the Global Environment.* Paper presented at Institute of Medicine/National Research Council Committee on Review of the FDA's Role in Ensuring Safe Food Meeting, Washington, DC, March 24, 2009.

Sowards, D. 2009. *Texas Submission to AFDO State Food Safety Resource Assessment.* York, PA: AFDO.

Strickland, L. S. 2005. The information gulag: Rethinking openness in times of national danger. *Government Information Quarterly* 22(4):546–572.

Taylor, M. R., and S. D. David. 2009. *Stronger Partnerships for Safer Food an Agenda for Strengthening State and Local Roles in the Nation's Food Safety System: Final Report.* San Francisco, CA: School of Public Health and Health Services, The George Washington University.

Upton, F. 2009. *Schauer, Upton, Stabenow & Levin Introduce Bills to Improve Food Safety, Protect Consumers.* http://www.house.gov/upton/press/press-05-21-09.html (accessed December 30, 2009).

8

Enhancing the Efficiency of Inspections

The word "inspection" is used by Congress, the U.S. Government Accountability Office (GAO), industry groups, individual scientists, and consumers as though it is a standard term. According to the *Business Dictionary*, the term denotes "critical appraisal involving examination, measurement, testing, gauging, and comparison of materials or items. An inspection determines if the material or item is in proper quantity and condition, and if it conforms to the applicable or specified requirements" (*Business Dictionary*, 2010). In reality, however, notions of just what the term means vary widely, and few understand what a U.S. Food and Drug Administration (FDA) inspection entails or what procedures are followed. As elaborated below, the FDA states that inspections are conducted with the purpose of enforcing regulations or collecting information in a processing or production setting. Instructions to investigators for how to conduct establishment inspections are contained in the *Investigations Operations Manual*[1] (FDA, 2009a). According to the FDA website, "The Investigations Manual is the primary guidance document on FDA inspection policy and procedures for field investigators and inspectors," last updated in June 2009 (FDA, 2009a), with numerous specific issuances from the Office of Regulatory Affairs (ORA).

As described in Chapter 2, ORA is the broad compliance and enforcement arm for all FDA-regulated products. It is the lead office for all FDA field activities, including inspections, sample analysis, enforcement, and development of policy on compliance and enforcement. In addition to

---

[1] See http://www.fda.gov/ICECI/Inspections/IOM/default.htm (accessed March 2, 2010).

staff located at headquarters, more than 85 percent of ORA staff work in 5 regional offices, 20 district offices, 13 laboratories, and more than 150 resident posts and border stations. In a presentation to the committee, the FDA clarified that ORA's work to foster compliance is often done in partnership not only with the FDA centers but also with industry. During an outbreak, for example, ORA field investigators work closely with the affected center, conduct investigations, and decide on courses of action (Kraemer, 2009; Wagner, 2009). In addition to its inspectional and enforcement activities, ORA hosts an online university that offers required basic courses and specialized training, such as seafood certification for federal investigators. Numerous courses, both web- and classroom-based, are also available to state investigators; however, the FDA has no requirement for state investigators to take them. The training covers such areas as retail establishments, food protection, milk, shellfish, manufactured foods, feed and veterinary medicine, investigation response, incident command systems, rapid response teams, and on-farm investigations (Solomon, 2009).

Prior reports have evaluated the adequacy and efficiency of U.S. food inspections and determined that inspections are insufficient, the basis for determining which facilities to inspect is poor (GAO, 2004; HHS, 2010), and there is a critical need to leverage resources to provide for a more efficient system (GAO, 2005a,b). Testimony offered to the U.S. Congress on numerous occasions has also spoken to this concern. An inefficient inspection process results in public health risks that could be avoided with appropriate inspection (for example, inspection of peanut facilities should have prevented the recent outbreak associated with contaminated peanuts). This chapter presents an analysis of the inspection process and explains the committee's conclusion that the process is inefficient for reasons that range from the cultural to the organizational. It should be noted that a full evaluation of the efficiency of the food safety inspection process cannot be conducted in isolation from similar processes performed by other government agencies, such as the U.S. Department of Agriculture and the National Oceanic and Atmospheric Administration (see Table 2-1 in Chapter 2). In accordance with its statement of task, however (see Chapter 1), the committee evaluated only the FDA's inspectional activities and refers to the inspectional activities of others only to the extent that they could contribute to improving the efficiency of inspections performed by the FDA. In this chapter, then, the committee offers recommendations for enhancing oversight of the food production system by improving the efficiency of the FDA's inspections and leveraging its inspectional resources. The committee comments as well on the FDA's potential use of third-party inspections (also discussed in Chapter 4).

BACKGROUND

As noted above, the FDA uses establishment inspections for either enforcement or information-gathering (surveillance) purposes. Inspections may be used "to obtain evidence to support legal action when violations [of the law] are found," or "they may be directed to obtaining specific information on new technologies, good commercial practices, or data for establishing food standards or other regulations" (FDA, 2009a, Subchapter 5.1, p. 213). Although this chapter focuses on the use of inspections as an enforcement tool, the collection of food safety data is essential to the implementation of the risk-based approach to food safety management recommended in Chapter 3.

The typical inspection begins when an inspector issues a Notice of Inspection (FDA form 482) to the management of a company to be inspected and presents his/her credentials. Inspections may be carried out by a single inspector or, if specialized techniques (e.g., microscopy, x-ray) are required, by a team. Inspectors begin by becoming familiar with the establishment's operations and products, its compliance history, pertinent safety factors, and the reporting requirements for the type of inspection to be undertaken. Other preinspectional activities are described in the *Investigations Operations Manual* (FDA, 2009a, Subchapters 5.4–5.9). General inspectional activities include observation, discussion with establishment management, label review, note taking, audio/video recording, sample collection (when appropriate), and reporting. Management of the establishment being inspected may invite outside observers as long as they do not impede the investigation. The sources of general inspectional procedures and techniques are given in the following quotation from the *Investigations Operations Manual*:

> The procedures and techniques applicable to specific inspections and investigations for foods, drugs, devices, cosmetics, radiological health, or other FDA operations are found in part in the Investigations Operations Manual (inspectional and investigational policy/procedure), various Guides to Inspections of . . . (a "how to" guidance series), and the Compliance Program Guidance Manual (program specific instructions). (FDA, 2009a, Subchapter 5.1, p. 216)

The *Investigations Operations Manual* describes the inspectional approach in general terms as follows:

> An establishment inspection is a careful, critical, official examination of a facility to determine its compliance with laws administered by FDA. Inspections may be used to obtain evidence to support legal action when violations are found, or they may be directed to obtaining specific informa-

tion on new technologies, good commercial practices, or data for establishing food standards or other regulations. In order to facilitate on-the-job training, multiple points of view, and perspectives of firms being inspected whenever practical, those with assignment authority should consider assigning different Investigator/s or different Lead Investigators at different times. This is recommended particularly when there have been multiple sequential NAI (no action indicated) inspections or when the firm's management has been uncooperative. (FDA, 2009a, Subchapter 5.1, p. 213)

The investigation of an establishment ends with the issuance of FDA form 483, Inspectional Observations. That form is

... intended for use in notifying the inspected establishment's top management in writing of significant objectionable conditions, relating to products and/or processes, or other violations of the Federal Food, Drug, and Cosmetic Act and related Acts . . . which were observed during the inspection. These observations are made when, in the Investigator's "judgment," conditions or practices observed, indicate that any food, drug, device, or cosmetic have [sic] been adulterated or are [sic] being prepared, packed, or held under conditions whereby they [sic] may become adulterated or rendered injurious to health. The issuance of written inspectional observations is mandated by law and ORA policy. (FDA, 2009a, Subchapter 5.2, p. 224)

The FDA defines two types of inspections—a comprehensive inspection and a directed inspection. Comprehensive inspections "direct coverage to everything in the firm subject to FDA jurisdiction to determine the firm's compliance status." Directed inspections "direct coverage to specific areas to the depth described in the program (compliance program), assignment (field assignment), or as instructed by [the] supervisor" (FDA, 2009a, Subchapter 5.2, p. 213). It is unclear what proportion of inspections is typically comprehensive and what proportion is directed. There are also two types of functionally distinct inspections: those based on Good Manufacturing Practices (GMPs) regulations and those based on Hazard Analysis and Critical Control Points (HACCP) regulations.

EFFICIENCY OF INSPECTIONS

Based on past authoritative reports alluding to this problem, the committee questioned the efficiency of the FDA's food safety oversight system. Further analysis of FDA-led inspectional activities revealed various reasons for this deficiency. Some of these reasons relate to the division of responsibilities between the FDA centers and ORA, which results in the centers' lack of authority over inspectors and inspectional priorities and procedures.

Also, inspectors are trained as generalists and do not specialize in, for example, food facilities. As a result, they cannot keep up with technological changes in all areas of FDA jurisdiction. Others reasons are related to the inspection procedures, which have not changed over time other than to become more burdensome with regard to paperwork and have not been adapted to the complexities of modern manufacturing establishments. The *Investigations Operations Manual* has not been reviewed externally to determine, for example, whether it is up to date, overly prescriptive, or otherwise less than ideal. Likewise, the time required for an establishment inspection either has not changed or has increased over time; thus, the number of inspections conducted annually has declined even though more inspectional full-time equivalents (FTEs) have been hired. Finally, the FDA's organizational structure, whereby ORA and the centers have various responsibilities from enforcing the law to writing risk-based regulations, is not conducive to the efficient implementation of regulations. This issue is of particular concern when roles and processes for collaborating are not completely clear and depend on maintaining good relationships between individuals.

The Role of the Inspector as an Investigator

One could argue that the inspector is the key to any required preventive food safety procedure (Gombas, 2009). As described by Givens (2009), the inspection process is part of a larger system that promotes compliance within the industry and sensitizes the industry to its responsibilities for ensuring that its products are safe. Inspectors are told which facility to inspect and are instructed that, in addition to following regulations and a compliance program, they are investigators. Thus, they must be observant, noting anything that appears irregular and following up on it while they are in the facility (Givens, 2009). Clearly, then, the instincts, judgment, and training of an inspector are valuable components of the inspection process. The committee concluded, therefore, that the FDA's food inspectors need the best available, up-to-date training in food safety. For example, although the agency has not proceeded rapidly with modernizing the GMPs, inspectors should receive training that is up to date with regard to the latest epidemiological intelligence, the latest information on pathogens, and any new technologies or techniques salient to the inspection process. Likewise, the FDA should have procedures in place to ensure that its auditors have the necessary experience, competencies, education, and continued training to perform their tasks.

In addition, inspectors have an educational function that is linked to the FDA's role in training the food industry in food safety and the interpretation of rules (see Chapter 9). This function includes directing food industry managers to relevant FDA sources (websites or other information repositories). As recommended in Chapter 9, the FDA should develop a centralized repository for food safety educational materials for industry personnel, promote the accessibility of these materials, and provide technical support for the interpretation of rules and regulations. Inspectors should be trained in improving their communication skills so the transfer of their knowledge and communication with food managers will be effective. Inspectors should also be trained in communicating effectively with industry managers when they are requesting nonregulatory data. The purpose and terms for collecting the data, as well as whether regulatory action will be taken if a contaminant is found, need to be clearly stated (see Chapter 5).

Currently, inspectors are trained to inspect establishments that represent the breadth of FDA-regulated products (i.e., drugs, devices, foods, and sometimes animal feed), and specialization is lacking. For example, an inspector who is trained and certified to inspect food processing and storage facilities may be cross-trained to inspect feed facilities. In the past, regulations and manufacturing processes were simpler, and this approach may have had benefits (i.e., a flexible inspectional force capable of being deployed to address any emergency related to any FDA-regulated products). In today's more complex world, however, those benefits pale in comparison with the benefits of a more specialized inspectional force. Manufacturing operations have become more complex, automated, and computerized over time, and new hazards have been identified. To continue training inspectors in all FDA-regulated products results in inspectors who are generalists and lack the specialized training and knowledge to deal with this context. FDA inspectors are not unlike criminal investigators in this regard. Police departments are divided into specialty areas, allowing investigators to focus their talents and knowledge in one area (e.g., homicide, auto theft). FDA inspectors, like criminal investigators, must be trained to look for clues to violations, some of which may not be readily apparent given the technical complexities of manufacturing. The committee believes that, to have adequately trained inspectors now and in the future, the FDA must begin training inspectors within a single major commodity area (i.e., food or feed) of FDA responsibility.

The FDA should review and update curricula specific to general food inspections as well as to particular types of inspections (e.g., seafood HACCP). This specific training is essential so that inspectors will be readily available and prepared to conduct an inspection in any food facility. The committee supports the partnership of the FDA with others, such as the International Food Protection Training Institute, established in 2009, to deliver career-spanning food protection training for state and local food protection professionals. Federal employees with auditing responsibilities should also be provided with specific training.

Risk-Based Inspections

Since its inception, the FDA has lacked the manpower to place an inspector in every food manufacturing facility under its jurisdiction, let alone all facilities that pack, store, and sell such products. Therefore, the agency has used its inspection authority as a deterrent (Kusserow, 1991; Busta, 2009) since an inspection could occur unannounced at any time. The FDA has suggested prioritizing inspections based on such criteria as history of compliance (Chapter 3). At a more basic level, however, the attributes of a risk-based approach as outlined in Chapter 3 are not clearly incorporated in FDA's approach to inspection of food facilities.

The *Investigations Operations Manual* defines the "depth of inspection" (FDA, 2009a, Subchapter 5.1, p. 213), noting that the attention given to various operations in a firm depends on information desired or on violations suspected or likely to be encountered. The FDA suggests that inspectors consider the following: (1) current company compliance with regulations, (2) nature of the specific assignment (inspection or investigation), (3) general knowledge of the industry and its problems, (4) firm history, and (5) conditions found as inspection progresses. A walk through is suggested early in the process so the inspector can "become familiar with the operation and plan the investigation strategy" and determine the depth of inspection necessary (FDA, 2009a, Subchapter 5.1, p. 213). Thus in theory, an inspection could be limited to a walk through and expanded as needed for further investigation depending on findings. Giving inspectors flexibility with respect to the length and depth of inspections would make it possible to conduct shorter inspections of compliant establishments while maintaining an adequate presence in all firms, thus preserving the deterrent function of the inspection process. While it appears that the FDA has the statutory authority to allow shorter inspections, there are other barriers to doing so, related to resistance to changing conventional procedures.

In a way, risk-based inspections have always existed. However, such approaches need to be adapted to new knowledge in food safety. Before microbiological, chemical, and physical analyses became more or less routine, FDA inspectors used personal observations to detect possible problems with the basic hygienic conditions in an establishment and relied primarily on two of the adulteration provisions of the Federal Food, Drug, and Cosmetic Act for authority to take action on any findings of unhygienic conditions.[2] The GMPs for foods,[3] which include special provisions for infant formulas, were finalized in the 1980s. GMPs form the basis for many international standard procedures and principles (for example, the Gen-

---

[2] *Federal Food, Drug, and Cosmetic Act of 1938*, 342(a)(3) and 342(a)(4).

[3] *Current Good Manufacturing Practice in Manufacturing, Packing, or Holding Human Food*, 21 CFR Part § 110.

eral Principles of Food Hygiene of the Codex Alimentarius Commission) and provide the foundation for establishment inspection based on sound hygienic principles, facility design, and product handling and processing. GMP inspections may generate adverse findings that are documented by the inspector and presented to a responsible individual in the establishment. Such adverse findings are expected to be corrected, and a follow-up inspection may be conducted to determine what actions were taken to that end. A criticism of GMP-based inspections, however, is that they constitute a "snapshot in time," and do not necessarily reflect the day-to-day operations of a facility (Givens, 2009).

In 2002, the FDA formed the Current Good Manufacturing Practices Working Group to determine whether the GMPs needed updating. The FDA solicited public comment, and the working group issued a report detailing areas in which modernization might be needed, such as training for supervisors and workers, food allergen control, environmental pathogen control, and written sanitation procedures. A major question was whether the food GMP regulations should be extended to facilities (such as farms) involved solely in harvesting, storing, or distributing raw agricultural commodities. To date, no apparent progress has been made on modernizing the GMPs (CFSAN/FDA, 2005), despite the fact that industry has asked the FDA to "revise its GMPs to include requirements for written sanitation plans, allergen controls, environmental monitoring programs for certain production facilities, and supervisor, manager, and employee training in hygiene and food safety measures" (Scott, 2009). The FDA itself has acknowledged the need to revise the GMPs for feed. *Fourth Draft: Framework of the FDA Animal Feed Safety System* (FDA, 2010) describes the need to update the GMPs for medicated feed. The committee recognizes that there is currently not enough information to justify separate GMPs for nonmedicated feed. As part of a risk-based system, if data indicate that the safety of nonmedicated feed is a concern, GMPs for this category of feed should be considered.

Since the promulgation of HACCP rules in the 1990s, in addition to a GMP inspection, a HACCP inspection is required for establishments that make HACCP-regulated products (seafood and juice). GMPs are one prerequisite for HACCP, since basic hygiene underlies specific preventive procedures (Scott, 2009). Because an establishment's HACCP plan, along with mandatory record keeping, is intended to reflect its daily preventive activities, inspection is viewed as more than the GMP-based inspection's snapshot in time. However, HACCP inspections are based on "snapshots" provided by the establishment's management; an inspector sees what management claims to be standard procedure within the facility.

For establishments that make HACCP-regulated products, a HACCP inspection is required in addition to a GMP inspection. HACCP inspections are lengthier than GMP inspections because of the required analysis of the establishment's HACCP plan and its implementation and review of records for each day of operation (Kraemer, 2009). Some in industry believe that "while conducting a hazard analysis and implementing preventive controls should be required of industry, these activities may or may not be in the form of a HACCP plan" (Mavity, 2009). Others believe that for those processes without a kill step (critical control point), such as for preparing fresh-cut produce, a HACCP plan may be unnecessary. While it is true that not all industry processes will have critical control points, control points and limits in the form of performance standards might be possible, thus preserving the essence of HACCP. In Chapter 10, the committee recommends that the FDA be granted the authority to request preventive controls for all food facilities, mindful of the many forms such controls can take and the fact that their adequacy depends on the type of product and process.

As noted in Chapter 3, the FDA presented the committee with information on its efforts to develop models for a risk-based inspection system. The committee did not evaluate these models, but it noted the lack of stakeholder involvement in the process.

The Inspection Process

The committee deliberated about the criticism the FDA has received for the paucity of inspections it conducts on food establishments annually (GAO, 2004, 2005a,b; Halloran, 2009; HHS, 2010). This number appears to be decreasing even as both the number of establishments in the agency's inventory and the number of food program FTEs steadily increase (GAO, 2008). This paucity of inspections is also seen with animal feed. As noted in Chapter 7, feed mills making nonmedicated feeds are generally regulated only by the states, except in the case of the FDA's bovine spongiform encephalopathy regulations. These mills are relatively small in number and produce organic feed or are species specific (e.g., horse feeds). Currently, only feed mills that produce feed with specific concentrations of medication in the premix need a license and are inspected routinely by the FDA or contract state inspectors. The committee believes any feed mill that manufactures medicated feed should be subject to the same inspectional processes regardless of the concentration of medication in the premix.

One way to increase the number of inspections without new resources is to improve the efficiency of inspections. As stated in testimony to the committee, "inspection time can certainly vary on a number of factors—the type of operation, the complexity of the process and the product, the risk of the product, and the controls that the firm may have in place." Furthermore, with regard to a firm with a poor history of compliance, an inspector "might want to spend some time, because that firm is not getting it—that may require some more time and attention to that facility" (Givens, 2009). Thus, as suggested earlier, the individual inspector's training, judgment, and intuition may also play a role in the length of an inspection. An applicable analogy might be a police officer making a traffic stop for a missing tail light. The officer sees the driver is nervous and asks more questions. During that extra time, the officer sees something in the car that prods him or her to ask the driver for access to the trunk, where drugs are found, making the stop a regulatory/legal activity that will take more time than usual.

The *Investigations Operations Manual*, developed mainly by ORA, is the primary guidance document on FDA inspection policy and procedures for field inspectors. There is no specific mechanism for obtaining input on inspection procedures from the centers, states, or other agencies. The committee is not aware of reviews of (or congressional requests to review) the *Investigations Operations Manual* and the efficiency of inspections, even in the face of the above-noted decrease in annual inspections despite increasing numbers of personnel (Plunkett, 2009). It is possible that, as new requirements have been added to the manual to prevent a specific new problem from recurring, the manual has become unnecessarily lengthy and the inspections costly. A single establishment inspection can take one or more inspectors many days to complete, even if the establishment has a history of compliance or appears to be in compliance when the inspector enters the facility. Likewise, an inspection of a facility that may be in violation because of the presence of insect fragments in food, for example, could be far more abbreviated than one for an establishment in which salmonella is thought to reside.

Inspections have become more complex and more onerous over time (Givens, 2009; Kraemer, 2009). Guidelines for inspectors have accumulated to reflect legal amendments, making the paperwork burden on the investigator increasingly time-consuming (Halloran, 2009). There has been no external study of inspection procedures in the United States, and there is no evidence of any innovative thinking applied to those procedures (Plunkett, 2009). By contrast, in 2005 the UK Treasury published a report reviewing the financial burden of government inspections and enforcement on businesses and offering recommendations for improving the efficiency of the country's inspection system (Hampton, 2005). These recommendations include devoting more resources to riskier businesses, streamlining data-sharing methods, and communicating clearly with businesses about how to comply with regulations. In the absence of such a study in the United States, questions arise as to whether it would be reasonable and more efficient to categorize inspections based on criteria that would take into consideration an inspector's experience and intuition. ORA appears to have thought about the latitude an inspector may have with regard to its high-risk product–hazard combination list (which was developed to prioritize inspectional resources), asking what the inspector should do with this information—perform an inspection, collect samples, or conduct a field exam.

ORA also appears to have thought about "regulatory testing" versus "screening" with regard to sample testing. Solomon (2009) stated to the committee that "FDA is a regulatory agency and needs to have regulatory tests—but that's not a reason that we don't have rapid screening tests that we can use to quickly . . . focus on issues and then follow up with more regulatory tests." For example, the burden of some inspections could be alleviated by making a distinction between inspections conducted to oversee a facility's compliance with all food-related regulations and those conducted to screen a facility's food safety status more rapidly by determining adherence to GMPs.

Although the committee did not conduct a review of inspectional procedures, it concluded that such a review is warranted to identify approaches, including risk-based approaches, that could increase the efficiency of the inspection process. Such a review should include examining procedures and techniques employed by other federal, state, and local government agencies, both regulatory and law enforcement, as well as those used in other countries, to determine whether they might be of value to FDA inspectors.

Organizational and Cultural Barriers to Efficient Inspections

As mentioned in Chapter 2, policy setting for FDA food regulation resides in the Center for Food Safety and Applied Nutrition (CFSAN) and the Center for Veterinary Medicine (CVM), which are both headed by directors, while enforcement of policies and regulations is carried out by ORA, which is headed by an associate commissioner. The district offices and resident posts are staffed primarily by inspectors charged with conducting inspections of establishments' producing, packing, or holding products regulated by the FDA, including foods, cosmetics, medical devices, and drugs. ORA works with CFSAN and CVM to develop an annual work plan that provides overall guidance to the field on the types and levels of inspections and surveillance activities to be conducted. There are also five field committees, one for each product category regulated by the FDA, composed of field managers and field program experts. The Food Field Committee and the Veterinary Field Committee are expected to work with CFSAN and CVM, respectively, in preparing the annual work plan, and they continue to collaborate during the year as issues arise. In practice, however, the committee questions whether this arrangement results in decisions that meet the regulatory responsibilities of CFSAN and CVM. The committee reviewed testimony and reports suggesting that this organizational structure creates barriers to improving inspection procedures.

In a report on revitalizing ORA, Glavin (2008, p. 23) states that "ORA is perceived as being too rigid, resistant to change, . . . unresponsive to new or different ideas, and too concerned with losing its span of control or turf." If this observation is true, it does not bode well for effecting meaningful efficiencies in inspection procedures or establishing a system of science-based, policy-driven enforcement.

One expert, familiar with the FDA's component organizations through extensive dealings with both CFSAN and ORA, expressed the opinion that it is extremely difficult to work with those organizations during emergency situations, such as outbreaks, as communication and coordination between the two appear obscure (Osterholm, 2009). Industry-associated groups in particular have alluded to perceived friction between CFSAN and ORA. Interorganizational problems occurring during emergency situations such as disease outbreaks may be somewhat understandable; however, CFSAN and ORA have had decades to develop procedures to prevent or mitigate misunderstandings. The lack of clarity and procedures for their roles constitutes a barrier to efficient management, especially during times of crisis. It is quite likely that the split in administration of the FDA's food programs between CFSAN and ORA, or between enforcement and policy, fuels such internal miscommunication and misunderstanding (Osterholm, 2009).

In conversations with former FDA employees, including counsels, it became clear to the committee that the relationship between ORA and the centers depends largely on the personalities of the individuals who occupy leadership positions in those organizations as well as interpersonal relationships among many individuals at lower echelons of each organization. Natural competitive relationships have evolved as a result of perceptions of the value of field versus scientific experience; in addition, different missions, such as enforcement versus policy development and management, limit the sustainability of good relationships (Osterholm, 2009). Misunderstandings and inconsistencies with regard to an enforcement matter are known to occur not only between district offices within ORA itself but also between district offices and CFSAN. These occurrences are of concern, especially in cases when delaying a decision could jeopardize public health.

CAPITALIZING ON FOOD INSPECTIONS:
USE OF STATE INSPECTORS AS PRIMARY FOOD INSPECTORS

In addition to the use of a risk-based approach, gains in inspection efficiency would be realized if food safety inspection activities at the federal, state, and local levels were coordinated (see Chapter 7). With regard to coordination at the federal level, the committee supports the GAO recommendations (GAO, 2004, 2005a,b) calling for concerted efforts in coordination of the inspectional activities of the various responsible federal agencies (see Appendix B). This section is focused on the utilization of inspectional resources at the state and local government levels.

The role of the states in the inspection of food establishments is discussed in detail in Chapter 7. Considered here is whether a system could or should be envisaged in which federally trained state inspectors would assume the role of primary food inspectors, with the FDA serving as auditor of state-conducted inspections. If such a governance model is explored, some functions in addition to auditing should remain in the FDA, such as maintaining experience in inspection methods, providing instructional materials and specialty expertise to state inspectors, developing and evaluating new inspection techniques and training, and serving as a backup corps in times of special need.

Preliminary data for 2008 indicate that states performed approximately 2,520,000 inspections (AFDO, 2009), including more than 50,000 in processing/repackaging facilities; the FDA performed only about 16,000, about 60 percent of which were conducted under contract with the states (FDA, 2009b). The committee concluded that recognition of the states as full partners in food safety assurance would be an effective way of greatly increasing the frequency of establishment inspections. Under current law, state inspectors can be commissioned as federal agents, a step that is usually taken for special assignments and is limited in time and scope. With appropriate training and oversight, state inspectors could assume a full-time role as federal deputies. The number of FDA inspectors would be limited to those required for training and auditing, and perhaps for playing an expanded role in import and export (foreign) food establishment inspections or certifying the equivalency of systems between the United States and exporting countries. The FDA would provide training to state inspectors, review inspectional procedures, and ensure that state inspections were equivalent to FDA inspections. The FDA could also defer to the states for inspection of animal feed mills. In most cases, feed mill inspectors are already from the states' departments of agriculture and are specifically trained and contracted to perform federally required GMP inspections. They also conduct state feed mill audits for label compliance, weights and measures, and sanitation.

FDA regional and district offices are spread across the U.S. mainland, but as the food industry shifts over time, they are not necessarily located in the same places as the industry (Fraser, 2009; Givens, 2009). Thus, the number of inspectors in each district office may not align with the number of establishments that need to be inspected. An individual state is in a better position to know what food establishments are within its borders (Osterholm, 2009). Therefore, a system whereby each state receives a pro rata share of inspectional resources based on the number of establishments requiring inspection might ensure more homogeneity with regard to numbers and quality of inspections. The FDA currently funds state inspections by contract; this pool of funds could be adjusted based on the inspection burden within the states and in lieu of changing the number of federal inspector positions. The agency should include in its budget a line item to fund these state contracts and partnerships to ensure their sustainability.

USE OF THIRD-PARTY AUDITS AS A SUBSTITUTE FOR INSPECTIONS

There has been a proliferation of both auditing and certifying bodies in the United States and elsewhere, and the data gathered by these third parties could be useful for enhancing the science behind the FDA's risk-based approach to food safety management. Third-party auditing evolved in the European Union when large retailers demanded certain character-istics from their suppliers, such as quality, safety, limited environmental impact, and animal welfare (see Chapter 4). In Europe, an association of retail chains, EuroGAP, was formed in 1999, changing its name in 2007 to GlobalGAP (GAP = Good Agricultural Practice) (Yudin and Schneider, 2008). Many European buyers will buy only from suppliers that can provide a certificate demonstrating compliance with rules such as those of GlobalGAP. Inspection of the suppliers is carried out by a certification body, a group of third-party auditors who are accredited by an accredita-tion body. Usually the accreditation body is a technical committee com-prised of experts from the retail and supplier sectors (Albersmeier et al., 2009). Further discussion of the potential value of third-party auditing as a governing model for managing food safety can be found in Chapter 4.

Third-party auditing was not developed originally to supersede gov-ernment oversight of food production and manufacture. In Europe, the producer of food must conform to both legal and third-party audit require-ments. Private certification is characteristic of the European food industry, whereas public certification schemes still predominate in the United States, Canada, and Japan (Albersmeier et al., 2009). However, private certifica-tion is catching up in the United States. For example, the Global Food Safety Initiative (GFSI) was created in 2000 to set common benchmarks for different national and industry food safety programs, and GFSI standards are now used widely around the world, including in the United States. Likewise, the California Leafy Greens Marketing Agreement, operating with oversight from the California Department of Food and Agriculture, provides a mechanism for verifying that the U.S. produce industry (farmers, shippers, and processors) follows appropriate food safety practices in pro-ducing leafy greens.

In response to a new challenge, private standards can be implemented more quickly than public standards, which are enacted by a government or an organization such as Codex (DeWaal and Plunkett, 2007; Henson and Humphrey, 2009). However, private standards may result in unnecessarily higher food prices. DeWaal and Plunkett (2007) conclude that a government accreditation requirement might be a better solution.

The FDA is taking some steps to assess the value of third-party auditing. In 2009, for example, the FDA released its *Guidance for Industry on Voluntary Third-Party Certification Programs for Foods and Feeds*,[4] describing the general attributes the agency believes third-party certification programs should possess whether they are administered by private entities or by federal, state, local, or foreign regulatory bodies (FDA, 2009c). However, the FDA goes further to state that it will recognize a certification program only if it has sufficient confidence in the certification body. Although this stance appears to be directed toward ensuring the safety of imported foods, it could also apply to domestic certification bodies in the future.

The committee deliberated about the legitimate role of information from third-party audits as a tool for the FDA to use in overseeing food safety. This question is also being examined at an international level, and an easy answer is unlikely (Henson and Humphrey, 2009). Although third-party certification may drive the industry to a higher standard that benefits everyone, the public acceptance of third-party auditors that are paid for by the industry needs to be evaluated. With appropriate standards in place, these audits could be of value for a risk-based approach. Therefore, before accepting third-party food safety audits, the FDA should develop standards and oversight procedures as necessary to ensure the credibility of the audit results. In particular, the FDA should set minimum standards for auditors and audits with a view to eventually having oversight by an accreditation and standards body. Further, if the type of information gathered during these audits could be of value for a risk-based approach, the FDA should seek ways to determine whether it can legally be mined from third-party audits/auditors.

KEY CONCLUSIONS AND RECOMMENDATIONS

Irrespective of the potential gains from allocating more funds to the FDA's inspection capacity, the committee concluded that a more basic and valuable exercise would be for the agency's inspection procedures to be reviewed for efficiency. The committee believes that, especially in light of resource limitations, the efficiency of the FDA's inspectional activities could be improved. The committee deliberated on ways to improve inspections with this perspective in mind.

---

[4] See http://www.fda.gov/RegulatoryInformation/Guidances/ucm125431.htm (accessed March 2, 2010).

The committee identified the following barriers to improved efficiency of FDA inspections: (1) the FDA's food programs do not have direct authority over the work of inspectors and inspectional procedures, resulting in substantial delays in policy implementation in the field; (2) inspectional procedures themselves may be inefficient; and (3) the FDA underutilizes other sources of information, such as state inspections. These barriers may result in the duplication of inspections, unnecessary targeting of resources, gaps in model coverage, and misunderstandings about priorities and highest risks, all with the potential to affect public health. (Recommendations for overcoming cultural and organizational barriers to the increased efficiency of inspections are presented in Chapter 11 in the context of other organizational changes.) Gains in efficiency would be realized if food safety inspection activities at the federal level were coordinated, and the committee supports the GAO recommendations to this end (GAO, 2004, 2005a,b; see Appendix B). In keeping with its statement of task, however, the committee did not analyze the inspectional activities of other federal agencies; it focused on formulating recommendations for overcoming the above barriers.

In addition to the need for a risk-based approach, the recommendations in this chapter reflect the conclusions presented in Chapter 7 with regard to the need to integrate all food safety activities at the federal, state, and local levels: (1) all food safety programs need to be standardized and harmonized; (2) state and local agencies are conducting many inspections, some of them under contract with the FDA, that need to be standardized and follow a risk-based approach; (3) once inspections (and other aspects of food safety programs) become standardized, the FDA will be able to capitalize on the work the states are already doing in many food safety areas, including inspection, to drive their risk-based models and make policy decisions; and (4) once food safety programs in states meet standards for food safety governance, the role of the FDA in standards setting, education, evaluation, oversight, and audit can be augmented.

Finally, the recommendations below apply to feed inspections with a caveat. Although GMPs should be extended for all medicated feed, there is currently insufficient information to justify separate GMPs for non-medicated feed.

Recommendation 8-1: The FDA should work toward an inspection system in which the frequency and intensity of inspection of each facility are based on risk, with minimum standards for the frequency and intensity of inspection of all facilities. To support the establishment of such a system, an outside panel should review the potential legal and cultural roadblocks to streamlining inspections and revise the *Investigations Operations Manual* so as to enhance efficiency and protection of the public health. As a prerequisite for a risk-based inspection system, the FDA should update its GMPs, including those for medicated animal feed, now and hereafter as necessary.

Based on the number of food safety inspections already conducted at the state and local levels and on the need for national integration of food safety activities, the committee makes the following recommendation.

Recommendation 8-2: As alternative regulatory models emerge, the FDA should evolve toward conducting fewer inspections, instead delegating inspections to the states and localities (including territories and tribes). The FDA should maintain a cadre of inspectors for several critical tasks, such as auditing inspections, providing specialty expertise, developing training and instructional materials for inspectors, identifying and evaluating new inspection techniques, and serving as a backup corps in situations of special need. In preparation for this move, the FDA should review and update curricula specific to general food inspections as well as to particular types of inspections (e.g., seafood HACCP). Agency employees with responsibility for auditing inspections by others should also be provided with specific training. An FDA-sponsored food safety certification program should be established whereby inspectors become certified as they meet agency standards. The agency should include in its budget a line item to fund state contracts and partnerships to help the states move toward and maintain full certification. Plans for implementation of the suggested changes should proceed in an evolutionary fashion, with intermediate goals and associated performance measures.

The committee also recommends that the FDA continue to consider the use of third-party certifications.

Recommendation 8-3: The FDA should fully consider the implications of accepting inspection data from an auditing program in which third-party auditors would inspect facilities for compliance with food safety regulatory requirements. If this approach is utilized, the FDA should set minimum standards for such auditors and audits, with oversight and implementation being assigned to an accreditation and standards body.

REFERENCES

AFDO (Association of Food and Drug Officials). 2009. *Draft State Resource Survey*. York, PA: AFDO.

Albersmeier, F., H. Schulze, G. Jahn, and A. Spiller. 2009. The reliability of third-party certification in the food chain: From checklists to risk-oriented auditing. *Food Control* 20:927–935.

Business Dictionary. 2010. *Definition: "Inspection."* http://www.businessdictionary.com/definition/inspection.html (accessed March 31, 2010).

Busta, F. F. 2009. IFT submitted comments to the Perspectives on FDA's Role in Ensuring Safe Food Meeting, Washington, DC, March 24, 2009.

CFSAN/FDA (Center for Food Safety and Applied Nutrition/U.S. Food and Drug Administration). 2005. *Food CGMP Modernization—A Focus on Food Safety*. Rockville, MD: FDA. http://www.fda.gov/Food/GuidanceComplianceRegulatoryInformation/CurrentGoodManufacturingPracticesCGMPs/ucm207458.htm (accessed May 14, 2010).

DeWaal, C. S., and D. Plunkett. 2007. *Building a Modern Food Safety System: For FDA Regulated Foods*. CSPI White Paper. Washington, DC: Center for Science in the Public Interest.

FDA (U.S. Food and Drug Administration). 2009a. *Investigations Operations Manual 2009*. Rockville, MD: FDA. http://www.fda.gov/ICECI/Inspections/IOM/default.htm (accessed March 2, 2010).

FDA. 2009b. *Establishing a Fully Integrated National Food Safety System with Strengthened Inspection, Laboratory and Response Capacity*. http://www.fda.gov/downloads/ForFederalStateandLocalOfficials/UCM183650.pdf (accessed March 2, 2010).

FDA. 2009c. *Guidance for Industry: Voluntary Third-Party Certification Programs for Foods and Feeds*. http://www.fda.gov/RegulatoryInformation/Guidances/ucm125431.htm (accessed March 2, 2010).

FDA. 2010. *Framework of the FDA Animal Feed Safety System* (Fourth Draft). Washington, DC: FDA.

Fraser, L. M. 2009. *FDA's Regulatory Authority and Division of Responsibility for Food Safety*. Paper presented at Institute of Medicine/National Research Council Committee on Review of the FDA's Role in Ensuring Safe Food Meeting, Washington, DC, March 24, 2009.

GAO (U.S. Government Accountability Office). 2004. *Food Safety: FDA's Imported Seafood Safety Program Shows Some Progress, but Further Improvements Are Needed*. Washington, DC: GAO.

GAO. 2005a. *Overseeing the U.S. Food Supply: Steps Should Be Taken to Reduce Overlapping Inspections and Related Activities*. Washington, DC: GAO.

GAO. 2005b. *Oversight of Food Safety Activities: Federal Agencies Should Pursue Opportunities to Reduce Overlap and Better Leverage Resources*. Washington, DC: GAO.

GAO. 2008. *FDA Has Provided Few Details on the Resources and Strategies Needed to Implement Its Food Protection Plan*. Washington, DC: GAO.

Givens, J. M. 2009. *Review of FDA's Role in Ensuring Safe Food (FDA's Approach to Risk Based Inspections—A Field Perspective)*. Paper presented at Institute of Medicine/National Research Council Committee on Review of the FDA's Role in Ensuring Safe Food Meeting, Washington, DC, March 24, 2009.

Glavin, M. 2008. *Revitalizing ORA: Protecting the Public Health Together in a Changing World: A Report to the Commissioner*. Washington, DC: FDA.

Gombas, D. E. 2009. *FDA's Role in Food Safety A Produce Industry Perspective*. Paper presented at Institute of Medicine/National Research Council Committee on Review of the FDA's Role in Ensuring Safe Food Meeting, Washington, DC, March 24, 2009.

Halloran, J. 2009. *Consumer Perspectives from the Consumers Union*. Paper presented at Institute of Medicine/National Research Council Committee on Review of the FDA's Role in Ensuring Safe Food Meeting, Washington, DC, March 24, 2009.

Hampton, P. 2005. *Reducing Administrative Burdens: Effective Inspection and Enforcement.* London, UK: Her Majesty's Treasury.

Henson, S., and J. Humphrey. 2009. *The Impacts of Private Food Safety Standards on Food Chain and on Public Standard-Setting Processes.* Paper presented at Report to the Codex Alimentarius Commission, 32nd Session, Rome, Italy, June 29–July 4, 2009.

HHS (U.S. Department of Health and Human Services). 2010. *FDA Inspections of Domestic Food Facilities.* http://www.oig.hhs.gov/oei/reports/oei-02-08-00080.pdf (accessed on May 17, 2010).

Kraemer, D. W. 2009. *FDA's Risk Based Prevention.* Paper presented at Institute of Medicine/National Research Council Committee on Review of the FDA's Role in Ensuring Safe Food Meeting, Washington, DC, March 24, 2009.

Kusserow, R. P. 1991. *FDA Food Safety Inspection.* Edited by U.S. Department of Health and Human Services. Washington, DC: Office of the Inspector General.

Mavity, S. 2009. *Safety of Imported Foods: A Perspective from a Company in the Seafood Industry.* Paper presented at Institute of Medicine/National Research Council Committee on Review of the FDA's Role in Ensuring Safe Food Meeting, Washington, DC, May 28, 2009.

Osterholm, M. T. 2009. *Role of Foodborne Disease Surveillance and Food Attribution in Food Safety.* Paper presented at Institute of Medicine/National Research Council Committee on Review of the FDA's Role in Ensuring Safe Food Meeting, Washington, DC, March 24, 2009.

Plunkett, D. 2009. *Perspectives on FDA's Role in Ensuring Safe Food.* Paper presented at Institute of Medicine/National Research Council Committee on Review of the FDA's Role in Ensuring Safe Food Meeting, Washington, DC, March 24, 2009.

Scott, J. 2009. *GMA Perspective on FDA's Role in Ensuring Safe Food.* Paper presented at Institute of Medicine/National Research Council Committee on Review of the FDA's Role in Ensuring Safe Food Meeting, Washington, DC, March 24, 2009.

Solomon, S. 2009. *Regulating in the Global Environment.* Paper presented at Institute of Medicine/National Research Council Committee on Review of the FDA's Role in Ensuring Safe Food Meeting, Washington, DC, March 24, 2009.

Wagner, R. 2009. *FDA'S Current Approach to Risk Based Domestic Inspection Planning.* Paper presented at Institute of Medicine/National Research Council Committee on Review of the FDA's Role in Ensuring Safe Food Meeting, Washington, DC, March 24, 2009.

Yudin, R. C., and K. R. Schneider. 2008. *European Food Safety Certification—The "GlobalGAP" Standard and its Accredited Certification Program.* Gainesville: University of Florida Extension.

9

Improving Food Safety and Risk Communication

According to the National Research Council (NRC) (NRC, 1989), risk communication is "an interactive process of exchange of information and opinion among individuals, groups, and institutions. It involves multiple messages about the nature of risk and other messages, not strictly about risk, that express concerns, opinions, or reactions to risk messages or to legal and institutional arrangements for risk management." Communication with stakeholders is an essential activity of any regulatory agency. In a food safety regulatory agency, the various stakeholders provide different perspectives on factors that enter into the decision-making process of a risk-based food safety management system. Indeed, this type of communication with stakeholders is integral to a risk-based approach and is an important aspect of many of the steps in such an approach as delineated in Chapter 3.

Risk communication can also be viewed more broadly as a policy tool available to the U.S. Food and Drug Administration (FDA) to achieve its food safety–related public health objectives. As such, risk communication encompasses a range of activities, from consulting with the public or professional organizations, to meeting with governmental partners, to designing and delivering recalls or warnings. Preceding chapters have addressed several aspects of risk communication in various contexts, focusing on such topics as identifying the roles of different partners (Chapter 4), sharing data (Chapter 5), and integrating federal activities with those of state and local governments (Chapter 7). This chapter complements those discussions by focusing on risk communication activities at the FDA across contexts, but with emphasis on those contexts in which the FDA provides messages or training to inform and support food safety–related decisions and behaviors.

The Food Protection Plan (FPP) explicitly includes communication as one key step in responding to food safety problems, but it also mentions other FDA actions that entail communication (e.g., risk assessments for prevention, compliance guides, technical advice, training programs or materials for food safety workers and industry) (FDA, 2007). This responsibility is also implied in legislation that directs the FDA to enhance various specific communication functions.[1,2] Accordingly, the agency's website states that: "[t]he FDA is also responsible for helping the public get the accurate, science-based information they need to use medicines and foods to improve their health" (FDA, 2009a).

The FDA's food risk communication activities range from issuing recalls and outbreak notifications, to sharing information about food defense with other countries, to providing guidance and training materials for food safety organizations and individuals. The FDA communicates risks both indirectly, by regulating the labeling and advertising of some products, and directly, by developing and sharing information with all parties in the food system. While the agency's ultimate goal is to protect the public health, the specific objectives, audiences, and methods of its communications differ across tasks and contexts (FDA, 2009a). Communications during crises are a major FDA responsibility[3]; during a recall, for example, the agency is required to ensure efficient and effective communications, reaching people throughout the food system rapidly with actionable messages. In contrast, training and guidance about food safety involve long-term partnerships and collaborations with, for example, professional associations and educational institutions.

Dramatic changes in food production and distribution systems (see Chapter 2) and additional knowledge about the epidemiology and determinants of foodborne illness have resulted in a food safety enterprise that is increasingly complex. For example, worldwide feed production has nearly doubled since 1980—from 370 million tons in 1980 to 614 million tons in 2004 (IFIF, 2009), and the number of food facilities increased by 10 percent from 2003 to 2007 (GAO, 2008a). This complexity adds to the challenges of communicating food safety information to food suppliers, preparers, consumers, and other stakeholders. As populations grow, as food sources globalize, and as production increases in scale, the potential for rapidly

---

[1] *Food and Drug Administration Amendments Act of 2007*, Public Law 110-85, 110th Cong. (September 27, 2007).

[2] *FDA Food Safety Modernization Act of 2009*, 111th Cong., 1st sess., Congressional Record 510 IS. (March 3, 2009).

[3] *Food and Drug Administration Amendments Act of 2007*, Public Law 110-85, 110th Cong. (September 27, 2007).

evolving crises—and the need for effective crisis communication—escalates (GAO, 2004a, 2008b).

Food safety and risk communications are critical at numerous points in the food system, from training field workers and restaurant or institutional food service employees to alerting consumers who may have contaminated products in their kitchens (Taylor and David, 2009). This chapter begins with a general overview of the FDA's risk communication and education activities. In particular, it highlights the FDA's most recent progress in this area, such as the establishment of the Transparency Task Force and the Risk Communication Advisory Committee (RCAC). It examines the communication efforts that are needed during crisis situations, such as recalls. Communication with the food industry is emphasized as an area that warrants increased attention. The chapter also offers recommendations for enhancing food safety and risk communication activities with regard to consumers, public health officials, and other health professionals. Finally, the chapter underscores the importance of conducting social research to design messages and to evaluate risk communication efforts as an essential element of a risk-based approach.

FOOD RISK COMMUNICATION AND EDUCATION AT THE FDA

Risk communication and education is one way the FDA can help ensure food safety. To be effective, risk communication requires an understanding of the needs of those involved, two-way communication, and evaluation (NRC, 1989). As with other interventions, the use of communication and education as policy tools needs to be part of strategic planning in a risk-based approach (see Chapter 3). In addition, decisions to adopt specific communication or education interventions should be based on empirical evidence of effectiveness. In essence, developing a risk-based approach such as that recommended in Chapter 3 is the first step in developing effective risk communication and education activities as policy interventions. An appropriate approach to assessing the level of risk and identifying the possible prevention and mitigation points in food production, processing, distribution, and preparation will also identify the points at which risk communication can reduce risk. This knowledge will enable the FDA to respond consistently and appropriately to stakeholders' needs for information. In addition, such an approach should serve to identify those stakeholders that can collaborate most effectively with the FDA to reduce risk at different points in the system. As discussed in Chapter 3, the strategic planning process should identify the various stakeholders and how they will be consulted and engaged for their contributions. Included in the stakeholder list should be the subgroup of consumers, industry workers, and health professionals that is the focus of this chapter. The committee agrees with the general risk communication steps and actions in the FPP, but it concludes that the necessary details of implementation are lacking. The committee was unable to obtain detailed information about the FDA's communication and education programs specifically related to foods; therefore, the information in this chapter was obtained from public meetings and the FDA website.

As noted, the FDA's risk communication responsibilities are specified in the Food and Drug Administration Amendments Act of 2007 (FDAAA). The act also directs the agency to establish and consult with the RCAC, which is composed of risk communication experts from academia and industry as well as representatives of consumer advocacy groups (FDA, 2009b).

One recent positive development has been the introduction of foodsafety. gov, a website managed by the U.S. Department of Health and Human Services (HHS) as a collaborative effort of the White House, HHS, the U.S. Department of Agriculture (USDA), the FDA, the Centers for Disease Control and Prevention (CDC), and the National Institutes of Health. Its purpose is to consolidate food safety information produced by various federal agencies that have a role in the regulation of the U.S. food supply and to provide the public with current information about food safety. Containing very little technical jargon, the website is designed for consumers and food safety educators and also for vulnerable populations. Much of the website contains information about food safety alerts, prevention, food preparation, causes of food poisoning, and how state and federal governments respond to foodborne illness outbreaks. The website also links to the official websites of the FDA, USDA, and CDC. Written content is supplemented by simple charts, videos, audio podcasts, and social media tools that allow for two-way communication.

Numerous entities within the FDA are engaged in communication (see Table 9-1). The agency's risk communication activities are coordinated by an internal Communication Council. A risk communication director in the Immediate Office of the Assistant Commissioner for Planning leads the agency's strategic planning process and is in charge of coordinating both the internal Communication Council and the external RCAC.[4] The lack of past strategic planning for risk communication and education suggests that prior to these initiatives, risk communication and education efforts at the FDA lacked a cohesive strategy.

Work of the RCAC

The RCAC was established specifically as an FDA advisory body on communications with patients and consumers, recognizing that the agency

---

[4] Personal communication, Nancy M. Ostrove, FDA RCAC, Washington, DC/North Gaithersburg Hilton, February 28, 2008.

TABLE 9-1 Description of Communication-Related Activities at the U.S. Food and Drug Administration (FDA)

Office of the Commissioner	
Office of Foods	• Directs a program of public outreach and communication on food safety, nutrition, and other food-related issues to advance the FDA's public health and consumer protection goals.
Office of Legislation	• Works with members of Congress and staff on legislative proposals that grant new agency authority. • Provides Congress with requested information on FDA programs and policies.
Office of Chief of Staff, Office of Executive Secretariat	• Serves as the FDA's liaison to the U.S. Government Accountability Office and the U.S. Department of Health and Human Services (HHS) Office of the Inspector General on several highly visible studies. • Coordinates numerous high-level briefings for the commissioner and manages the FDA's review and clearance process for executive correspondence, memorandums of understanding, reports to Congress, consumer correspondence, and other items.
Office of External Affairs, Office of External Relations	• Arranges briefings between the commissioner and outside stakeholders on crucial FDA issues. • Manages high-level outreach to various stakeholder groups on all major FDA announcements. Develops a series of innovative "listening sessions" between the commissioner and major stakeholders. • Continues to refine and strengthen the FDA's newly designed home page and its web-based consumer information program, producing articles to support the FDA's public health mission and establishing new distribution channels for this material.
Office of External Affairs, Office of Public Affairs (OPA)	• Provides numerous announcements of agency actions, including food recalls and implementation of requirements under the Food and Drug Administration Amendments Act of 2007. • Conducts crisis communication activities, such as the response to the outbreak of *Salmonella* Saintpaul. • Provides public affairs presence at FDA public meetings, congressional hearings, and advisory committee meetings and responds to inquiries from members of the media.

continued

TABLE 9-1 Continued

Office of External Affairs, Office of Special Health Issues	• Is responsible for engaging, collaborating, and communicating with health professionals, patients, patient advocates, and other special-interest populations about FDA regulatory decisions and policies. • The "FDA Updates for Health Care Professionals" e-list provides recent announcements related in particular to human medical product safety, human medical product approvals, opportunities to comment on proposed rules, upcoming public meetings, and other information of interest to health professionals. • Has a new health professional webpage—MedWatch—to serve as a portal for FDA information, particularly safety-related information of interest to health professionals.
Office of Policy, Planning, and Budget, Office of Policy	• Handles high-priority, cross-cutting, and novel regulatory issues, and coordinates the issuance and publication of all FDA regulations, notices, and guidance documents.
Office of Policy, Planning, and Budget, Office of Planning	• Analyzes risk communication activities and assists agency components in planning to improve the effectiveness of those activities. • Coordinates the Risk Communication Advisory Committee (RCAC). • Sets up internal pilot projects for testing messages prior to issuance. Completed a national survey of physicians concerning their perceptions about emerging and uncertain risks of medical products, the results of which will guide communications directed toward that audience. • Leads the process to develop the FDA's Strategic Plan for Risk Communication, as well as a prioritized research agenda. • Coordinates the presentation of the strategic plan and research agenda to the RCAC for feedback.
Office of the Counselor to the Commissioner, Office of Crisis Management	• Provides coordination and strategic management of the FDA's response to numerous incidents concerning FDA-regulated commodities, including outbreaks, natural disasters, and actual or potential product defects that pose a risk to human or animal health (e.g., melamine-contaminated infant formula, salmonella in imported produce, flooding in the midwest). • Charged with meeting the HHS goal to improve the FDA's ability to respond quickly and efficiently to crises and emergencies that involve FDA-regulated products.
Advisory Committee Oversight and Management Staff	• Works to maintain and improve the transparency, integrity, and consistency of the FDA's advisory committee program. • Published important new draft guidance on when the FDA convenes advisory committee meetings. • Helped improve the FDA webpage on advisory committees, increasing the program's transparency and improving public access to important information.

TABLE 9-1 Continued

FDA Centers and Office of Regulatory Affairs (ORA)	
Center for Food Safety and Applied Nutrition	• Manages the 1-800-SAFEFOOD information line and e-mail inquiries from consumers, industry, and other constituents; this information line averages around 2,100 inquiries monthly. • Develops and implements comprehensive risk communication roll-out strategies to reach all stakeholder groups, domestic and international, including industry, consumers, state and local public health and regulatory agencies, the clinical community, and media, with FDA messages related to emergencies as well as new regulations and guidance and other initiatives. • Directs the development of long-term consumer education campaigns for multiple targeted audiences and messages related to food safety and nutrition best practices. • Maintains a comprehensive stakeholder directory. • Coordinates with other FDA entities and develops major media news releases and social media (Web 2.0) tools related to emergency response communications for foodborne outbreaks and major recalls. • Conducts social research to support communication efforts.
Center for Veterinary Medicine	• Protects human and animal health by regulating animal drugs and feeds for millions of companion animals, poultry, cattle, swine, and other animal species. • Communicates frequently with veterinarians, industry, the public, and other stakeholders about product recalls, new animal drug approvals, guidance for industry, and other animal health issues.
Office of Regulatory Affairs (ORA), Division of Federal State Relations	• Uses a number of mechanisms to provide accurate and timely information to state, local, and tribal partners. • Serves an advisory role to field public affairs specialists.
ORA, Public Affairs Specialists	• Located in ORA field offices, work within their local communities around the country to promote and protect the public health and work closely with OPA to deliver FDA messages. • In addition to serving the general public, work with traditionally underserved populations, such as women, seniors, and ethnic minority communities. • Reach a variety of audiences—including health professionals and students, government and industry representatives, and members of community groups and faith-based organizations—through outreach and educational programs, workshops, conferences, exhibits, and speeches. • Take the pulse of the public, reporting consumer concerns to agency management. This feedback guides future FDA programs so that messages are better targeted to consumer concerns, and agency decisions are responsive to developing public health policy.

needs to communicate more effectively with the public and based on recommendations in the Institute of Medicine (IOM)/NRC report *The Future of Drug Safety: Promoting and Protecting the Health of the Public* (IOM/NRC, 2007). As noted, the FDAAA of 2007 chartered the RCAC, establishing a mandate for the committee to advise the FDA on its risk communication activities in general and on crisis communications during recalls. The RCAC consists of a core of 15 voting members selected by the commissioner for their expertise in such fields as social marketing and health literacy, and for their experience in risk communication and work with patients, consumers, and health professional organizations (FDA, 2009b). Since its inception, the RCAC has held nine public meetings, some of which have addressed food risk communication issues. Meeting agendas have included the review of a draft strategic plan for risk communication at the FDA, research on risk communication, and communication strategies during food recalls and outbreaks (FDA, 2009c,d).

As an example of its advisory role, the RCAC was consulted with regard to communication with the public during food recalls, which remains problematic. Specifically, the RCAC was asked about the appropriateness of a draft press release template for communicating with consumers during Class 1 recalls.[5]

The FDA receives formal and informal recommendations during the RCAC meetings. Informally, for example, the committee chair proposed the different types of expertise needed for effective risk communication. In addition, the chair suggested considering a model recommended by the Canadian Standards Association, and adopted by some government agencies, that requires two-way communication between risk managers and stakeholder representatives throughout the development and implementation of a program (CSA, 1997). Following a more formal process, the RCAC adopted the resolutions in Box 9-1 at its August 2008 meeting. After receiving RCAC recommendations, the FDA reports back to the committee in subsequent meetings on its progress, for example, with regard to risk communication funding in the FDA supplemental budget.[6]

One of the first actions of the RCAC in 2008 was to advise the FDA to engage in strategic planning of its risk communication activities (FDA, 2009d). With this impetus and with attention to aligning its specific strategies with the risk communication–related goals of the FPP (improve risk communications to the public, industry, and other stakeholders [FDA, 2007]), the FDA developed a draft Risk Communication Strategic Plan

---

[5] A Class I recall is a situation in which there is a reasonable probability that the use of or exposure to a violative product will cause serious adverse health consequences or death.

[6] Personal communication, Nancy M. Ostrove, FDA RCAC, Washington, DC/North Gaithersburg Hilton, February 28, 2008.

BOX 9-1
Risk Communication Advisory Committee
Resolutions, August 2008

- The U.S. Food and Drug Administration (FDA) should consider risk communication as a strategic function.
- The FDA should engage in strategic planning of its risk communication activities.
- The FDA should find ways to do risk communication research efficiently, ensuring that communications are designed in a timely fashion to a scientific standard.
- The FDA should routinely present quantitative risk and benefit information, in formats consistent with its regulatory constraints.
- The FDA should develop a participatory design and testing process for FDA consumer communication. The process should include vulnerable groups with barriers to understanding and access.

SOURCE: FDA, 2009d.

(FDA, 2009e). The plan, which was aligned with the goals of the HHS Strategic Plan, presents the FDA's strategies for risk communication and proposes ways to improve the agency's science base, its capacity for action, and its policy processes (see Box 9-2). Also, communication is included in the FPP explicitly as one key step in responding to food safety problems. The three primary goals in the draft Risk Communication Strategic Plan are

(1) expand FDA capacity to generate, disseminate, and oversee risk communication;
(2) optimize FDA policies on communicating risks and benefits; and
(3) strengthen the science that supports effective risk communication (FDA, 2009e).

In this plan, the FDA states its view that risk communication is a two-way process integral to carrying out its mission effectively, that such communication must be adaptable to the various needs of the parties involved, and that it should be evaluated to ensure optimal effectiveness (FDA, 2009e).

BOX 9-2
Summary of U.S. Food and Drug Administration (FDA)
Risk Communication Strategic Plan

Expand the FDA's *capacity* to generate, disseminate, and oversee effective risk communication.

Capacity Strategy 1: Streamline and more effectively coordinate the development of communication messages and activities.

Capacity Strategy 2: Plan for crisis communications.

Capacity Strategy 3: Streamline processes for conducting communication research and testing, including evaluation.

Capacity Strategy 4: Clarify roles and responsibilities of staff involved in drafting, reviewing, testing, and clearing messages.

Capacity Strategy 5: Increase staff with decision and behavioral science expertise and involve them in communication design and message development.

Capacity Strategy 6: Improve the effectiveness of the FDA's website and Web tools as primary mechanisms for communicating with different stakeholders.

Capacity Strategy 7: Improve two-way communication and dissemination through enhanced partnering with government and nongovernment organizations.

The FDA's Transparency Task Force

On January 21, 2009, President Obama issued two memorandums to the heads of executive departments and agencies expressing a commitment to promoting transparency and openness in government (FDA, 2009f; GPO, 2009). These memorandums were followed by the Open Government Directive in December 2009 (OMB, 2009). Executive departments and agencies have been charged with harnessing new technologies to disclose information about operations and decisions online and to make this information readily available to the public. In addition, executive departments and agencies have been instructed to solicit public input and feedback to identify information of greatest use to the public (GPO, 2009).

Accordingly, the FDA has formed a Transparency Task Force (see

Optimize the FDA's *policies* on communicating risks and benefits.

Policy Strategy 1: Develop principles to guide consistent and easily understood FDA communications.
Policy Strategy 2: Identify consistent criteria for when and how to communicate emerging risk information.
Policy Strategy 3: Re-evaluate and optimize policies for engaging with partners to facilitate effective communication about regulated products.
Policy Strategy 4: Assess and improve FDA communication policies in areas of high public health impact.

Strengthen the *science* that supports effective risk communication

Science Strategy 1: Identify gaps in key areas of risk communication knowledge and implementation, and work toward filling those gaps.
Science Strategy 2: Evaluate the effectiveness of FDA's risk communication and related activities, and monitor those of other stakeholders.
Science Strategy 3: Translate and integrate knowledge gained through research/evaluation into practice.

SOURCE: FDA, 2009e.

Box 9-3), which includes the agency's principal deputy commissioner, center directors, associate commissioner for regulatory affairs, chief counsel, and chief scientist (FDA, 2009g). The task force is soliciting public opinion on various communication and transparency matters and has held two public meetings. The first public meeting, held on June 24, 2009 (FDA, 2009h), was meant to solicit input on how the agency can make useful and understandable information about its activities and decision making more transparent and readily available to the public. The second public meeting, on November 3, 2009, was held to receive comments on three specific issues: (1) early communication about emerging safety issues, (2) disclosure of information about product applications that are abandoned or withdrawn by the applicant before approval, and (3) communication of agency decisions about pending product applications (FDA, 2009i). In addi-

---

BOX 9-3
Transparency Task Force Action Items

- Seek public input on issues related to transparency.
- Recommend ways that the agency can better explain its operations, activities, processes, and decision making, compatible with the agency's goal of appropriately protecting confidential information.
- Identify information the U.S. Food and Drug Administration (FDA) should provide about specific agency operations, activities, processes, and decision making, including enforcement actions, recalls, and product approvals.
- Identify problems and barriers, both internal and external, to providing useful and understandable information about FDA activities and decision making to the public, taking into consideration health literacy and the needs of special populations.
- Identify appropriate tools and new technologies for informing the public.
- Recommend changes to FDA's current operations (e.g., internal policies and procedures, standards, information formats, guidance) to improve the agency's ability to provide such information to the public in a timely and effective manner.
- Recommend legislative or regulatory changes, if appropriate, to improve the FDA's ability to provide such information to the public.
- Submit a written report to the Commissioner on the Task Force's findings and recommendations.

SOURCE: FDA, 2009g.

---

tion to these meetings, the FDA has established a Transparency Blog, which also provides opportunities to learn about, and provide feedback on, what the agency is doing, specific topics prompted by the FDA, the basis for its decisions, and the processes used to make those decisions (FDA, 2009j). In response to comments and requests in these forums, the FDA has created a website explaining the basics of its activities.[7]

The task force was to submit a written report to the FDA commissioner approximately 6 months after being convened, and the commissioner was to report back and confer with the Secretary of HHS on the recommendations in the report. The FDA envisions that implementation of the task force's

---

[7] See http://www.fda.gov/AboutFDA/Basics (accessed October 8, 2010).

recommendations will make agency actions, decisions, and underlying processes more transparent to the public while still meeting the agency's goal of appropriately protecting confidential information. Further, implementation of the recommendations should reduce the need for public requests for agency information under the Freedom of Information Act (FDA, 2009g). To date, this transparency initiative has resulted in recommendations that the FDA plans to implement in three different phases: (1) development of a web-based resource that will provide information about commonly misunderstood agency activities; (2) formulation of an approach to making information and decision making more transparent; and (3) transparency specifically to regulated industry. As planned, in December 2009 the task force submitted a written report to the HHS Secretary detailing progress in implementing phase 1, the launching of the FDA basics website.[8]

Although the task force is an admirable effort and intuitively valuable, an evaluation of its activities would be premature since it has been in place for only a few months. The committee encourages its continuation and future evaluation of this new activity.

COMMUNICATING AT A TIME OF CRISIS: FOOD RECALLS AND OUTBREAKS

The number of food recalls issued annually has increased by an order of magnitude in the last two decades and is expected to continue increasing with improved detection technologies (GAO, 2004b). The most common tool the FDA now uses to mitigate emerging outbreaks is public warning.[9] During these recalls, the FDA currently sends an e-mail to all state public health departments and key stakeholders (e.g., the Food Allergy and Anaphylaxis Network in the case of allergens) to post on their websites, and it posts the same information on its own website and on foodsafety.gov. The FDA has also begun using social media and provides Twitter feed about recalls on request.[10] Section 1003 of the FDAAA contains provisions concerning enhancing the quality and speed of the FDA's communication with the public in recall situations.[11,12]

In its 6-month and 1-year FPP progress reports, the FDA reported the development of templates for recalls that it presented to the RCAC in 2008 (FDA, 2008a,b). These templates were tested within the agency's

---

[8] See http://www.fda.gov/AboutFDA/Basics (accessed October 8, 2010).

[9] Personal communication, Nancy M. Ostrove, FDA RCAC, Washington, DC/North Gaithersburg Hilton, February 28, 2008.

[10] Personal communication, Nancy M. Ostrove, FDA RCAC, Washington, DC/North Gaithersburg Hilton, February 28, 2008.

[11] FDAAA, Public Law 110-85, 110th Cong. (September 27, 2007).

[12] *Code of Federal Regulations Food and Drugs* § 7.42 Recall strategy (2003).

own heterogeneous workforce and used as surrogate groups representing public responses. The RCAC provided specific advice on the development of these templates during one of its meetings with the FDA, as noted above. The FDA has also considered partnerships with other organizations as a way of carrying out formative evaluations of communication strategies.

For food recalls, the FDA recognizes that people must be given answers to three key questions: (1) What is the product? (2) What is the concern? and (3) What do I need to do? In a national survey on awareness of and behavioral responses to food recalls, Hallman and colleagues (2009) found that the messaging used during the most recent food recalls had been ineffective in leading consumers to take action. Messages must be delivered quickly with clear criteria for identifying a recalled product and the symptoms caused by consumption of the product. They also need to provide motivational information on the appropriate course of action without frightening consumers, which the survey results suggest is lacking since few respondents had ever looked for recalled food products in their homes. The survey revealed that, while most Americans hear or read about food recalls, they fail to recognize recalled products and feel that food recalls are more relevant to other consumers. Consumers are unaware of the frequency of food recalls and exhibit widespread misconceptions about the division of responsibilities between federal agencies in such situations. Nearly 75 percent named the FDA as responsible for meat and poultry recalls (which are the responsibility of USDA); 48 percent failed to identify any agency as responsible for fruit and vegetable recalls, and just 32 percent identified the FDA as the responsible agency. Thus, despite awareness of recent food recalls, an illusion of invulnerability and a lack of knowledge about the food recall process appear to be widespread among American consumers. These findings signify the need for a clear, coordinated, and centralized communication strategy for food recalls.

This need for information applies to feed as well. Failures in communication during the melamine-associated pet food recall of 2007 spurred the passage of special sections (1002 and 1003) of the FDAAA directed at ensuring the safety of pet food and animal feed. These improvements to the feed safety system include "posting information about a recall in a single location on FDA's Web site" and establishing a Reportable Food Registry for feed in addition to food (Covington and Burling, LLP, 2007; FDA, 2008b,c).

Further, the FDA has been criticized for damaging the food industry by issuing overly general messages (e.g., do not eat raw spinach). It is important to recognize that during the course of a recall, government officials are challenged to be expeditious about communicating with the public while also being accurate and specific about the contaminated product. Protecting the public health without inhibiting sales of safe food requires a delicate balance when the information needs to be provided quickly.

Another challenge in managing recalls is communicating their termination. FDA regulations provide that a recall will be terminated only when "it is reasonable to assume that the product subject to the recall has been removed and proper disposition or correction has been made commensurate with the degree of hazard of the recalled product."[13] The regulations require the FDA to provide written notification of termination to the recalling firm, but they do not address the communication of such information to the public. Risk perception research shows that consumers generally do not know when recalls end and tend to play it safe by avoiding the general category of the recalled product for months thereafter (Cuite et al., 2007). The FDA's procedures regarding recall termination need to be reviewed so that economic losses can be minimized to the extent possible consistent with protecting the public health.

The FDA is working on a set of goals for understanding how to better use food distribution and communication networks to reach consumers. The agency is concerned about being able to reach consumers with timely updates as recall situations evolve.[14] If consumers receive a behavioral cue at an opportune moment—for example, when they are purchasing or preparing food—they can reduce their risk of foodborne illness (e.g., Nauta et al., 2008). Grocery store receipts (Hallman et al., 2009), televised and online recipe and cooking information (Powell, 2000; Mathiasen et al., 2004), newspaper recipe and menu sections, and vending machines are examples of contact points at which recall information could be communicated.

A cursory analysis of online government portals for food recall information shows that the new foodsafety.gov website is prominent, but so, too, are other federal government sites, such as the Joint Institute for Food Safety and Applied Nutrition's foodrisk.org and the USDA National Agricultural Library site foodsafety.nal.usda.gov. These latter sites may confuse consumers, however, because either they do not link to foodsafety.gov for food recalls, or they link to more than one site with information about recalls. The current design of foodsafety.gov includes an immediately visible recall window, as required in Section 1003 of the FDAAA, but other parts of the website link to other websites for core food safety information. The more that linking steps are required, the greater is the potential for communication failures. Consumers, educators, and state and local governments cannot at present find food recall information and report food safety prob-

---

[13] 21 C.F.R. 7.55(a).

[14] Personal communication, Nancy M. Ostrove, FDA Risk Communication Advisory Committee, National Transportation Safety Board Conference Center, Washington, DC, August 13, 2009.

lems and foodborne illnesses on a single authoritative website. Section 1003 states that the FDA website and recall database shall be easily accessed and understood by the public; without an empirical evaluation, it is difficult to demonstrate that these goals have been achieved.[15]

EDUCATING THE FOOD INDUSTRY

As stated above, risk and safety communications are critical at numerous points in the food system. Food producers, processors, and retailers play a vital part in the prevention of foodborne illness and require education tailored to their role in the food safety system. For example, effective training of industry personnel is a critical component of a preventive, risk-based food safety system and is necessary for successful implementation of Hazard Analysis and Critical Control Points (HACCP) (NACMCF, 1997). As the leading food safety oversight agency, the FDA must incorporate the risk and safety communication needs of the food industry and regulators into its risk communication strategy.

Food service workers at institutions, such as schools or nursing homes, that purchase and prepare food for large numbers of potentially sensitive subpopulations are an important control point for risk communication in the food safety system. In fact, the majority of foodborne illnesses in confirmed outbreaks in OutbreakNet for 2007[16] were associated with exposures outside the home, with 30 percent of illnesses attributed to restaurants or delis. Rising trends in eating out, food preparation and service employment, and a high proportion of young (Bureau of Labor Statistics, 2009), foreign-born (ROC-United, 2009; Bureau of Labor Statistics, 2010a), and Hispanic or Latino workers in food service (Bureau of Labor Statistics, 2010a; ROC-United, 2009, 2010) underscore the importance of targeting this sector for food safety training. Food preparation and service workers rely primarily on short-term on-the-job training to prepare for the work (Bureau of Labor Statistics, 2010b). While a lack of health care benefits and illness policies contribute to workers showing up for work when ill (ROC-United, 2009),

---

[15] Section 1003 reads: "(1) work with companies, relevant professional associations, and other organizations to collect and aggregate information pertaining to the recall; (2) use existing networks of communication, including electronic forms of information dissemination, to enhance the quality and speed of communication with the public; and (3) post information regarding recalled human and pet foods on the Internet Web site of the Food and Drug Administration in a single location, which shall include a searchable database of recalled human foods and a searchable database of recalled pet foods, that is easily accessed and understood by the public" (FDAAA, Section 1003, Public Law 110-85. 110th Cong. [September 27, 2007]).

[16] OutbreakNet. Foodborne Outbreak Online Database. See http://wwwn.cdc.gov/foodborneoutbreaks/Default.aspx (accessed October 8, 2010).

studies of food service employees suggest that targeted training in the positive outcomes of specific behaviors (e.g., hand washing making it less likely that people will get sick), in combination with reducing barriers to such behaviors (e.g., convenient facilities, available time), can contribute to needed improvements in food safety behaviors (Howells et al., 2008; Pilling et al., 2008, 2009; see also Green and Selman, 2005).

Numerous sources of information and training materials currently exist for the food industry. The Center for Food Safety and Applied Nutrition (CFSAN) posts training materials and notices on its website under the Retail Food Protection's Industry and Regulatory Assistance and Training Resources page, as well as under Food Defense (FDA, 2009k,l). In addition, industry associations provide comprehensive and standardized training materials for the food industry. For example, ServSafe is well recognized as the leading training program for food retailers (ServSafe, 2009). Grocery Manufacturers of America has developed a HACCP guide for the food industry that is frequently modified by others to suit their needs (GMA, 2009). Other groups, such as the National Environmental Health Association, also provide training materials for the food industry (NEHA, 2008).

The feed industry relies heavily on trade associations such as the American Feed Industry Association, the National Grain and Feed Association, and specific food animal associations (e.g., the National Pork Producers Council, National Turkey Federation, U.S. Poultry and Egg Association) for information and training. Further, many land grant universities have developed feed safety bulletins and other educational materials and have those materials available on their websites. Not unlike conferences addressing specialty crops, nearly every conference targeting livestock production includes topics on safe feed/safe food. While all of these mechanisms are excellent sources for the industry, however, some may be expensive for small processors and retailers (Behnke, 2009).

The Cooperative Extension System provides a broad range of educational programs and serves as a resource for food safety training and information for the food industry. Regulatory agencies frequently refer food producers, particularly small establishments, to Cooperative Extension Services for training and information on food safety and the implementation of new regulations. Cooperative Extension Services often advertise their programs through their websites and by mailing risk communication and training notifications to the food industry. They frequently set their training schedules months in advance but get little, if any, advance notice of the implementation of new regulations. As a result, they can be overwhelmed when new regulations are issued. In addition, funding shortfalls compound the problem as state and federal agencies cut their budgets. Therefore, while Cooperative Extension Services are a good resource for meeting the food industry's educational needs, their ability to serve the large number of food processors and retailers in the United States is limited. Also, few Land Grant institutions have spent the time and effort to develop significant expertise in feed production and safety, although, based on the experience of committee members, this situation is slowly beginning to change (Behnke, 2009).

One particular subgroup of the food industry that may not have the resources to update its workforce on the latest policy developments and may need more targeted attention is small producers, processors, and retailers. Hirsch and Cutter (2006) used several methods to examine the training and support available to small and very small meat and poultry establishments. They also conducted a mail survey and later organized a workshop to learn from small and very small meat and poultry producers in the Northeast about their sources of information and the value and quality of training available to them. The results point to the inadequacies of, and barriers to, training and the need for standardization (Hirsch and Cutter, 2006).

The committee is unaware of similar studies for the portion of the food industry regulated by the FDA. Yet while the study by Hirsch and Cutter focuses on USDA-regulated establishments, it clearly demonstrates the need for a comprehensive, standardized education and training program for the food industry, and the industry training needs it identifies could impact producers of FDA-regulated products as well. The committee concluded that a similar study should be conducted to identify training needs in the FDA-regulated portion of the food industry.

OTHER TARGETED POPULATIONS

In addition to information for industry, the FDA creates and collates on its website important information for targeted populations, such as consumers, industry, and health professionals. This section addresses the importance of enhancing communications with these populations.

Consumers

While the food industry—from the farm to the retailer—plays an essential part in mitigating the risks from foods, consumers also play a role in reducing their risks from food through appropriate food purchases and handling (Nauta et al., 2008). Understanding what consumers know, value, and do is an essential first step in providing them with relevant information in a form they can understand and use; risk communication research can bridge the gap between what experts say and consumers hear, or need to hear, about handling food safely (Fischhoff and Downs, 1997; Morgan et al., 2001; Bruhn, 2005; Fischhoff, 2009). If consumers are to make informed food consumption decisions, they also need information with which to weigh benefits and risks—for example, to understand when the nutritional benefits of foods may outweigh the risks from potential trace contaminants (IOM, 2007).

While in some cases consumers may be unaware of food risks, in others they may be unnecessarily worried because they lack specifics on what they can do to protect themselves effectively. Although estimates of the percentage of Americans that have confidence in the safety of the food supply vary considerably because of methodological differences across surveys, in general confidence appears lower today than it has been since 2001 (Gallup, 2010). Public opinions about, and confidence in, food safety are highly responsive to specific food safety incidents (Cuite et al., 2007; Blendon et al., 2009), although, as with other risks (Weinstein, 1989; Rothman et al., 1996), consumers generally tend to be optimistic and, as noted above, to believe that foodborne illnesses and food recalls are more relevant to the general public than to themselves (Miles and Scaife, 2003; Hallman et al., 2009). Kinsey and colleagues (2009) analyzed the influence of media attention on consumer confidence and concluded that media coverage has a significantly negative effect on consumer confidence in the safety of the food system. Overall, favorable attitudes toward the FDA declined from 1997/1998 to 2010 (from 75 percent to 58 percent) (The Pew Research Center, 2010). This general trend toward lower confidence in the FDA, however, may be due not only to food safety incidents and coverage by the media but also to increasing general distrust in the U.S. government (and in the FDA in particular) since the late 1990s (The Pew Research Center, 2010). Kinsey and collaborators' most recent data[17] show that confidence in food safety has neither decreased further nor increased much in the last year.

According to FDA research (Levy et al., 2008), several safe food practices have increased in the United States over the last decade. Consumer knowledge about foodborne pathogens, high-risk foods, vulnerable populations, and safe food-handling practices has also increased in recent years, although this knowledge is sometimes incomplete or wrong (FSIS, 2002). On the other hand, despite increased self-reported use of safe food-handling practices, food preparers do not always follow these practices (Redmond and Griffith, 2003; Anderson et al., 2004; Howells et al., 2008; Abbot et al., 2009). The International Food Information Council found that for some practices, such as washing hands, the majority of those surveyed reported using them as a precaution. For other practices, the percentages of use reported were lower—for example, 50 and 25 percent, respectively, for using a different or freshly cleaned cutting board for each type of food and for using a food thermometer to check the doneness of meat and poultry

---

[17] Personal communication, Jean Kinsey, Director, The Food Industry Center, University of Minnesota, May 21, 2010.

items (IFIC, 2009). Other research shows that younger people in particular are increasingly ignorant of safe food-handling practices and foodborne illness (Byrd-Bredbenner et al., 2007a,b); young adults (aged 18–25) are the age group most likely to engage in risky food handling (Byrd-Bredbenner et al., 2007a,b).

Although these findings about precautionary behaviors are disappointing, they may reflect consumers' difficulty in understanding what to do. Once consumers become aware of the risk associated with particular food-handling and consumption behaviors (e.g., consuming certain raw foods), they may become concerned; however, they are unlikely to take protective action unless they see the risk as personal, know what to do to reduce the risk, and are confident that they can do it (Prochaska and Velicer, 1997; Prochaska et al., 2002; Brewer et al., 2004, 2007; Weinstein et al., 2007; Cuite et al., 2008). Social pressures and practices can also influence consumer behaviors (Cialdini and Goldstein, 2004; Cialdini, 2005, 2007; Abroms and Maibach, 2008).

Risk communications that build on empirical evidence of, and interactive exchanges about, consumer understanding and food risks and benefits can help consumers make informed decisions (Morgan et al., 2001; Bruhn, 2005; Fischhoff, 2009). In the United States, people currently learn about food safety from a variety of sources, ranging from social networks and television to specific government programs (Cuite et al., 2008; Hallman et al., 2009). Use of these sources varies by consumer circumstances. For example, in a 2008 study (Kwon et al., 2008), Special Supplemental Nutrition Program for Women, Infants, and Children (WIC) recipients surveyed reported receiving food safety information from WIC (78.7 percent), family (63.1 percent), and television (60.7 percent). In a 2003 survey conducted in Lubbock, Texas (Whatley et al., 2005), family and friends were cited overwhelmingly as sources of food safety information. With respect to young adults, home economics classes are becoming increasingly rare (Beard, 1991); instead, young adults learn about food safety primarily from their parents, with very few (5 percent) reporting never learning about it (Byrd-Bredbenner et al., 2007a,b).

Certain groups—infants and children, pregnant women, and older persons—are deemed biologically and clinically more susceptible to food safety risks. This susceptibility stems in part from altered or adversely affected immune systems or chemical kinetics, the sensitivity of developing organ systems to toxicological insult, or the effects of age-related diseases, treatments, and declining physiological function (Kendall et al., 2006; Hayashi, 2009).

In addition, the United States is becoming increasingly diverse both culturally and ethnically, adding complexity to the food safety messages provided to the public. This increased diversity will likely have an important impact on the risk of food safety incidents for several reasons. First, ethnic and cultural food preferences may affect the distribution of domestic food consumption, altering risks to consumers. For example, diets high or low in processed meats or raw vegetables may affect the general risks of foodborne illness associated with these food categories. Second, various groups may differ in socioeconomic status or access to different types of foods (French, 2003; Zenk et al., 2009), again altering food safety risks. Also, various ethnic groups may have special dietary traditions and recipes associated with altered risk because of either food content or special methods of preparation. For example, *Yersiniosis* infections associated with unsafe preparation of chitterlings in Georgia have been documented and addressed through communications (Georgia Division of Public Health, 1998). Likewise, the consumption of Mexican-style soft cheese resulted in *Listeriosis* infections among pregnant Hispanic women (MMWR, 2001). There have also been documented problems with contaminated food products in retail ethnic food establishments (Rudder, 2006). The special food safety issues associated with diverse ethnic and cultural food acquisition, preparation, and dietary practices have been only partially evaluated and deserve additional attention.

Health Professionals

From the FDA's perspective, both the public and clinical health professional communities are important audiences for food safety education and risk communication. This is especially true for specific subgroups, such as doctors, educators, media specialists, and others who either work with food safety or mediate risk communications with the public or other stakeholders. In addition to guidance for producers to minimize food contamination,[18,19] the FDA's website includes information for health professionals and educators on the latest advisories regarding pathogens and diagnoses of foodborne illness.[20] It also offers information designed to assist the states in laboratory analysis and inspectional procedures.[21] While state and local public health agencies conduct important food safety–related work, such as surveillance and testing, they often require information from other states

---

[18] See http://www.fda.gov/Food/GuidanceComplianceRegulatoryInformation/GuidanceDocuments/ProduceandPlanProducts/ucm064574.htm (accessed October 8, 2010).

[19] See http://www.fda.gov/Food/GuidanceComplianceRegulatoryInformation/GuidanceDocuments/Seafood/FishandFisheriesProductsHazardsandControlsGuide/default.htm (accessed October 8, 2010).

[20] See http://www.fda.gov/Food/ResourcesForYou/HealthCareProfessionals/default.htm (accessed October 8, 2010).

[21] See http://www.fda.gov/Food/GuidanceComplianceRegulatoryInformation/ComplianceEnforcement/default.htm (accessed October 8, 2010).

and the federal government to carry out this work, generating an important set of multidirectional communication needs (see Chapter 5). In addition, food safety–related programs and surveillance findings from state and local public health agencies—as well as those from federal agencies such as the FDA, USDA, and CDC—must be communicated clearly to the public.

Communicating with the clinical health community is also critical to maintaining food safety. Severe food-related adverse clinical events are almost always detected in the clinical care system. Such patients need to be identified, treated, and reported to public health agencies, again necessitating effective communication channels. In addition to this detection and surveillance role, the clinical care system plays a critical preventive role in food safety. Health professionals manage many patients with conditions that place them at increased risk of harm from tainted or contaminated foods, as well as patients who use special diets to control various chronic illnesses. In both of these cases, the FDA and other federal agencies have an important role in communicating about food-related risks to primary care, specialty, and dietetic professionals who specify diets for such patients.

MECHANISMS FOR EFFECTIVE INFORMATION EXCHANGE AND TRANSPARENCY

The FDA has available a number of mechanisms to enhance its food risk communication and education efforts. They include stakeholder involvement through formal partnerships, ad hoc public forums and consultations, and innovative interactive web tools.

An example of a formal partnership is the Partnership for Food Safety Education (PFSE), a nonprofit collaboration of industry, government, and consumer groups. PFSE launched its food safety initiative, Fight BAC!, under the Clinton Administration, but is no longer funded solely by the government. Its goal is to educate consumers about safe food-handling practices (PFSE, 2006). Another example of such a partnership is the International Food Protection Training Institute, which has the FDA as a partner and was established to deliver career-spanning training for state and local food protection professionals.

The FDA also has many partnerships with academic, domestic, and international organizations and governments through formal agreements (FDA, 2009m). As of 2004, there were more than 50 interagency agreements governing food safety (GAO, 2004a); in 2005, 71 such agreements were identified (GAO, 2005). The U.S. Government Accountability Office recommends that the FDA use these agreements to reduce spending on duplicate efforts and to share resources so as to stretch limited funds. Memorandums of understanding (MOUs) also exist between the FDA and universities for collaboration in the areas of education, research, and outreach. There are currently 12 such MOUs in effect, most of them between the FDA and one university.

In addition to those formal partnerships to facilitate communication, other means of collaborating would enhance the FDA's risk communication activities. Tabletop discussions,[22] public forums, and consultations with scientists and advocacy groups on critical decisions would enable the agency to anticipate new needs and reactions to new activities and adapt appropriately. The media, advocacy groups, and scientists should be essential partners in the agency's efforts to communicate with the public. However, the FDA's activities have been less than transparent to many parties over the last decade. Advocacy groups and others have been surprised by FDA actions that have at times been taken without consultation or communication with stakeholders, nor have they been full participants at media briefings.[23] One concern raised during an RCAC public meeting was the difficulty of obtaining timely information from the FDA. During the same meeting, according to journalist Kathryn Foxhall, the FDA was identified as among the most stringent agencies in applying permission-to-speak systems, which were implemented across the federal government more than a dozen years ago. All communications with reporters go through a public relations officer and may be subject to additional clearances. This process has been characterized as effectively destroying the relationship between the media and the agency. In Ms. Foxhall's words, "Agencies track, monitor, control, and chill our conversations with staff."[24] One way of learning about diverse needs is to talk to those in the mass media with special interests in food safety on a regular basis. Lacking good relationships with the press, the FDA is unlikely to gain the scientific and authoritative profile it needs to communicate effectively with the public.

As noted above, mechanisms for two-way communication with the public can lead to improved foodborne illness surveillance. Interactive websites can be used to collect information from the public as well as to present information, and they are increasingly used in government to gather both general and program- or product-specific feedback and suggestions. Communications with less conventional sources of information on food safety may be possible as part of an effective FDA-based communication program. For example, allowing members of the public to report putative outbreaks through a health professional (e.g., their primary physician) could serve as an early warning system for local, state, and federal agencies. Similar

---

[22] A tabletop discussion is a focused practice activity that places the participants in a simulated situation requiring them to function in the capacity that would be expected of them in a real event.

[23] Personal communication, Tony Corbo, Food and Water Watch, September 2009.

[24] Personal communication, Katherine Foxhall, FDA RCAC, Washington, DC/North Gaithersburg Hilton, February 28, 2008.

mechanisms, such as the Vaccine Adverse Event Reporting System (Chen et al., 1994) or the Consumer Complaint Monitoring System in USDA's Food Safety and Inspection Service (Dubrawski et al., 2006), have already been implemented in other venues. Such data cannot be taken at face value, but methods are being developed to take advantage of the information they provide (Dubrawski et al., 2006). Mechanisms for ongoing surveillance in health systems can be built into electronic health records (EHRs) so that suspected foodborne illnesses are reported. For example, it may be possible for EHRs to generate surveillance messages automatically based on specific clinical text, as well as to generate educational messages relevant to food safety for patients and clinicians when certain clinical situations arise. Communications with drug manufacturers could be another important source of surveillance through automated monitoring of prescriptions or sales of medications, such as antidiarrheal drugs. All of these approaches would require thorough research and demonstration, and in some cases legislative change, but their potential for enhancing food risk communications warrants the effort.

RESEARCH, EVALUATION, AND CONTINUOUS IMPROVEMENT

Given the importance of communications with stakeholders as one of the interventions in the FDA's tool kit of interventions, decisions about how to best provide these communications should be based on data collected (see also Chapters 3 and 5). Through research, the FDA estimates consumers' awareness, understanding, and reported behaviors related to food contaminants, such as methyl mercury, *Salmonella*, pathogenic *Escherichia coli*, and *Listeria monocytogenes*. These results are used to inform and evaluate the FDA's policies and rules as well as its public information and educational outreach on safe food handling and preparation. The FDA's typical research methods are both quantitative (surveys, experiments) and qualitative (focus groups, interviews, mental modeling).

Research can also help target messages that are more effective at reaching different cultural and ethnic groups, people with varying levels of education or language skills, and other subpopulations. Media segmentation and multimodal strategies may help reach more people than conventional methods. New social media marketing and viral marketing approaches may enhance the value of the FDA's communication efforts (Gosselin and Poitras, 2008). The Consumer Studies Team at CFSAN helps set program priorities and informs communications within CFSAN and across the FDA and other agencies (e.g., the Federal Trade Commission, the U.S. Environmental Protection Agency, USDA, and CDC). As of February 2008, the team included eight social scientists from a variety of disciplines conducting both survey and experimental research.[25] The team members typically design all of their own research protocols, perform their own data analyses, and use an extramural contractor for field service.

Recognizing that the FDA is not a research institution, there is nevertheless a need to reorient its activities so that empirical evidence from research constitutes the basis for its interventions (see Chapter 6). While the deficiencies of the FDA's risk communication research have been noted (e.g., IOM, 2007), the creation and recent activities of the RCAC and the internal Communications Committee are promising developments that may enhance the agency's research efforts in this critical area. In its May 6–7, 2010, meeting with the RCAC, which focused on research, the FDA reported that a research priority list was being developed with previous input from the RCAC.

An effective food safety system requires dedicated funding for behavioral and social science research on food safety risk communication and education, as well as a capacity to conduct this research. As noted in Chapter 3, academic programs generally do not offer adequate training and education in risk analysis disciplines, including risk communication. In particular, there is value in evaluating the role of past communication techniques in crisis situations, such as during the outbreaks related to peppers and peanuts (Cuite et al., 2005). Retrospective review using both formative and summative approaches can make subsequent communication programs more effective. Moreover, social and behavioral science research on the food safety knowledge and patient advice practices of public health professions should drive the FDA's educational activities targeted to those groups. Surveillance of food industry knowledge and practices can also identify the educational needs of those stakeholders. The committee did not receive sufficient information from the FDA to evaluate the research capacity in social and behavioral sciences pertaining to risk communication in the food safety area.

One potential avenue for educating consumers and promoting safe food handling, for which further research on effectiveness is needed, is labeling of food products with respect to safety. In the United States, some laws or regulations mandate safety information on food labels. For example, raw or partially cooked meat and poultry products must contain information on cooking, storage, and handling. Also, U.S. law requires that eight food allergens be identified in plain English on all food labels, although it does not require any advisories. Otherwise, food producers and retailers are under no obligation to use food labels that contain food safety advice, and they are often reluctant to do so. There are likely many reasons for this, including the large amount of information that might be placed in the lim-

---

[25] Personal communication, Steven Bradbard, FDA RCAC, Washington DC/North Gaithersburg Hilton, February 28, 2008.

ited space on labels (e.g., nutritional content, source content, traceability of sources, eco-friendly procedures, techniques of manufacture, suggested recipes) and the difficulty of communicating risk in such a small space, including warnings about special high-risk groups (e.g., *Listeriosis* among pregnant women) (Caswell, 2006). It is also likely that food manufacturers do not want to deter food purchasers by implying that their product is categorically unsafe.

Current food safety–related label messages that appear to be simple and straightforward are actually unregulated by the FDA and may be subject to varied interpretation; an example is "sell by" or "best if used by" on date labels. In focus groups, messages such as the product contains "antilisterial" agents were not well received (Lenhart et al., 2008) and perhaps not fully understood. Similar issues may exist in labeling for potential food allergens, where different messages ("may contain," "shared equipment," "same plant") may be correct but do not convey information that is helpful in interpreting risk and promoting appropriate behavior (Pieretti et al., 2009). It is likely that underlying some of these problems of effective labeling is the challenge of communicating risk and appropriate responses in a way that effectively guides healthful attitudes and behaviors. The FDA should develop and sustain a label research program to inform the design of safety labels that effectively communicate and enhance safe food-handling behaviors among consumers. When a suitable body of evidence is available, regulations for mandatory safety messages on food products should be considered.

A Slow Process for Research Approval and Funding

Information sharing is a critical policy tool (OTA, 1995) that, to be effective, can require audience-based assessments and product evaluations (e.g., Schriver, 1989, 1996; Roth et al., 1990). Implementation of the FDA's social science research agenda can be slowed by many factors, some of which are common to any research agenda, such as the sensitive nature of new research and emerging topics, collaboration with others, funding cycles and budgets, and standard operating procedures for review and clearance at the level of the center, agency, and department. Another factor recognized by the RCAC to be a barrier to the FDA's ability to conduct communication-related research in a timely and scientifically sound manner is the current interpretation of the Paperwork Reduction Act (PRA) of 1990.[26] The act stipulates that agencies must seek public comment (through 60-day notices in the *Federal Register*) on proposed research involving the

---

[26] *Paperwork Reduction and Federal Information Resources Management Act of 1990*, 101st Cong.

collection of information and receive clearance from the Office of Management and Budget (OMB) if ten or more subjects are involved in such research. The agency publishes its response to public comments in a 30-day *Federal Register* notice, which reopens the docket for an additional public comment period. When this comment period closes, the agency again reviews comments, provides OMB with written responses, and addresses any remaining OMB concerns. Negotiations between OMB and the FDA, possibly including changes in the research plan and/or the instruments, may take as long as 7 or 8 months before OMB approval. Exceptions to standard PRA requirements are made for focus groups and interviews, rapid response surveys, and 30-day emergency OMB approval. In an effort to find a solution to these delays, the RCAC recommended that the FDA identify the public welfare implications of *not* testing its communications. The RCAC also recommended that the FDA submit a proposal to OMB for a protocol for evaluating food safety communication research that would balance the public welfare needs associated with the FDA's mandate and the requirements of PRA (FDA, 2009e).

Concurrently with this review by OMB, the Research Involving Human Subjects Committee (RIHSC) (the FDA's Institutional Review Board [IRB]) is tasked with reviewing all studies using human subjects. Every FDA center has an RIHSC liaison who reviews materials submitted in support of such research. Most social science research involving adults is considered exempt from full review unless it uses high-risk populations and/or studies highly sensitive topics. Nevertheless, even partial reviews, required under 45 Code of Federal Regulations (CFR) 46.101, can delay research projects.

Nationally, social and behavioral research conducted in pursuit of better communication, education, or policies continues to be impeded, and in some cases discouraged, by unnecessarily restrictive and intrusive human subjects review procedures developed for biomedical research (Schrag, 2009). In a 2006 study of the effectiveness of IRBs, "removing or reducing scrutiny of many fields within the social sciences and humanities that pose minimal risk" is a key recommendation (Gunsalus et al., 2007, p. 3). While OMB review may be the more onerous of the reviews to which FDA consumer studies are subjected, there is evidence that IRB reviews hamper and discourage such research as well. As an example, the FDA often uses its own workforce as surrogate groups representing public responses, which is a less than ideal subject sample. Given that such research does not collect sensitive personal information, is not overly intrusive, and likely contributes to more effective communications and warnings and therefore to public protection, consideration should be given to reducing or eliminating human subjects–related review requirements under 45 CFR 46.101 for social science research—in particular, research on perceptions and communications that meets appropriate confidentiality standards. A recent study at the University of Michigan characterizes "the tenor of the national conversation regarding the system for protecting human subjects from harm" as follows: "Regulations and policies are often narrowly and conservatively interpreted; terms and definitions are not clearly defined; the system is burdened with documentation requirements; and there is a paucity of empirical evidence to guide ethical decision making" (Pennell et al., 2008, p. vii). The need for OMB and IRB reviews may also be discouraging the FDA from conducting surveys or other data collection efforts that are more representative than focus groups.

Risk Communication Capacity

Effective risk communication programs require understanding public responses to messages, targeting the correct audiences, developing technologies and partnerships to reach targeted groups, and being familiar with information networks (NIH, 2008). As is the case for any federal agency with a public health mandate, the FDA cannot communicate successfully without interaction and advice, and it needs to build its internal capacity to design and evaluate risk communications. Capacity for effective communication is a function of organizational structure as well as human and technological resources. While the Consumer Studies Team at the FDA focuses on consumer studies, its emphasis with regard to food-related research is primarily on nutrition labeling, and its ability to conduct research is currently limited.[27]

With a small social science research group, significant research clearance requirements, and resource barriers to conducting empirical evaluations and research studies, the FDA has faced an uphill battle in developing its food safety education and risk communication efforts. Recent regulatory and organizational changes have improved the prospects for addressing these barriers, but much remains to be done to make the FDA a trusted and authoritative resource for food safety information so it can meet its food safety communication responsibilities effectively.

KEY CONCLUSIONS AND RECOMMENDATIONS

The RCAC, established in 2008, and the 2009 risk communication strategic planning are positive initiatives that will help the FDA improve its risk communication efforts. Although the FDA is on a path toward developing critical risk communication capacity, effective implementation of its risk communication strategic plan will require integrating such communication

---

[27] Personal communication, Donald Zink, Senior Science Advisor, FDA/CFSAN, September 25, 2009.

into an overarching risk-based management strategy. For example, elements of the strategic plan, such as determining criteria for communicating risk information in areas of high public health impact, require a clearly articulated approach that is embraced throughout the agency. In an era of instantaneous communications and multiple media, transparency in communications about food safety issues is essential.

Many partners, including regulatory agencies, provide food safety education to the public in various formats; that is, there is no single, authoritative voice on food safety in the United States. This is of concern especially for communications in times of crises, such as national outbreaks, which demand a coordinated and centrally controlled plan. While the FDA, with other federal agencies, has established foodsafety.gov, a website intended to better provide food safety information to the public, enhancements to this gateway are needed. Likewise, many partners (e.g., trade organizations, Cooperative Extension Services at universities) are engaged in training industry in food safety, but coordination, research, and evaluation of these efforts are essential and appear to be lacking. Standardized food safety training and education for public health officials in state and local (including territorial and tribal) governments do not exist and are currently not being investigated or evaluated. While the FDA has many communication-related partnering arrangements in place, there is room for creative progress to take advantage of new information and communication technologies.

For the FDA to improve its food safety messages, scientific evaluation of risk communication as part of an overall social science research portfolio is essential. The results of such research make it possible to understand consumers' knowledge, perceptions, and behaviors, including those of populations with heightened vulnerability to food hazards. Whether the research is extramural or intramural, obtaining approval and funding for a human subjects study currently requires a long, stringent process. Because risk communication studies are often time sensitive, this lengthy approval process deters investigators from conducting valuable research on food safety messages. Surveillance of those who may contribute to providing protection from foodborne illness, such as public health professionals and industry personnel, can also help in the FDA's selection of communication interventions.

The committee recommends that the FDA continue to respond to the advice of the RCAC and offers the following recommendations to enhance the FDA's risk communication and education functions.

Recommendation 9-1: In its effort to integrate risk communication into the recommended risk-based food safety management system, the FDA should play a leadership role in coordinating the education of the food industry, the public, clinical health professionals, and public

health officials at all government levels. The FDA could carry out its leadership role in educating industry personnel, health professionals, and public health officials by seeking authority to mandate the setting of training standards, preparing training materials, certifying trainers, and providing technical support for the interpretation of policies and for the implementation of the risk-based approach.

Recommendation 9-2: In collaboration with other federal agencies, the FDA should continue efforts to develop a single source of authoritative information on food safety practices, foodborne illness and risks, and crisis communications. The FDA, with other federal agencies, should develop a coordinated plan for communicating in one voice with all affected parties during crises so that stakeholders receive timely, clear, and accurate information from a single recognizable source.

To enhance these communication efforts, reducing barriers to and conducting more consumer research will be essential. To this end, the committee makes the following recommendation.

Recommendation 9-3: The FDA should improve its understanding of the knowledge and behavior of industry, health professions personnel, and consumers with respect to food safety, paying specific attention to knowledge about demographic groups that are particularly susceptible to food risks.

In making critical decisions about risk communication to implement recommendations 9-1, 9-2, and 9-3, the FDA should explore new mechanisms (e.g., tabletop discussions, public forums, consultations) for expanding its use of strategic partnerships and collaborations.

REFERENCES

Abbot, J. M., C. Byrd-Bredbenner, D. Schaffner, C. M. Bruhn, and L. Blalock. 2009. Comparison of food safety cognitions and self-reported food-handling behaviors with observed food safety behaviors of young adults. *European Journal of Clinical Nutrition* 63(4):572–579.

Abroms, L. C., and E. W. Maibach. 2008. The effectiveness of mass communication to change public behavior. *Annual Review of Public Health* 29:219–234.

Anderson, J. B., T. A. Shuster, K. E. Hansen, A. S. Levy, and A. Volk. 2004. A camera's view of consumer food-handling behaviors. *Journal of the American Dietetic Association* 104(2):186–191.

Beard, T. D. 1991. HACCP and the home: The need for consumer education. *Food Technology* 45:123–124.

Behnke, K. 2009. *Feed Manufacturing and the Connection to Human Health.* Paper presented at Institute of Medicine/National Research Council Committee on Review of the FDA's Role in Ensuring Safe Food Meeting, Washington, DC, March 25, 2009.

Blendon, R. J., K. J. Weldon, J. M. Benson, and M. J. Herrmann. 2009. *Peanut Product Recall Survey.* Harvard Opinion Research Program. Harvard School of Public Health. http://www.hsph.harvard.edu/news/press-releases/2009-releases/peanut-product-recall-survey-americans-reduce-risk-sick.html. (accessed May 23, 2010)

Brewer, N. T., N. D. Weinstein, C. L. Cuite, and J. E. Herrington, Jr. 2004. Risk perceptions and their relation to risk behavior. *Annals of Behavioral Medicine* 27(2):125–130.

Brewer, N. T., G. B. Chapman, F. X. Gibbons, M. Gerrard, K. D. McCaul, and N. D. Weinstein. 2007. Meta-analysis of the relationship between risk perception and health behavior: The example of vaccination. *Health Psychology* 26(2):136–145.

Bruhn, C. M. 2005. Explaining the concept of health risk versus hazards to consumers. *Food Control* 16:487–490.

Bureau of Labor Statistics, U.S. Department of Labor. 2009. *Occupational Outlook Handbook, 2010–11 Edition, Food and Beverage Serving and Related Workers.* http://www.bls.gov/oco/ocos162.htm (accessed May 11, 2010).

Bureau of Labor Statistics, U.S. Department of Labor. 2010a. *Table 11: Employed Persons by Detailed Occupation, Sex, Race, and Hispanic or Latino Ethnicity.* http://www.bls.gov/cps/cpsaat11.pdf (accessed May 11, 2010).

Bureau of Labor Statistics, U.S. Department of Labor. 2010b. *Table 1.4: Occupations with the Largest Job Growth.* http://www.bls.gov/emp/ep_table_104.htm (accessed May 11, 2010).

Byrd-Bredbenner, C., J. Maurer, V. Wheatley, D. Schaffner, C. Bruhn, and L. Blalock. 2007a. Food safety self-reported behaviors and cognitions of young adults: Results of a national study. *Journal of Food Protection* 70(8):1917–1926.

Byrd-Bredbenner, C., J. Maurer, V. Wheatley, E. Cottone, and M. Clancy. 2007b. Food safety hazards lurk in the kitchens of young adults. *Journal of Food Protection* 70(4):991–996.

Caswell, J. 2006. Quality assurance, information tracking, and consumer labeling. *Marine Pollution Bulletin* 53:650–656.

Chen, R. T., S. C. Rastogi, J. R. Mullen, S. W. Hayes, S. L. Cochi, J. A. Donlon, and S. G. Wassilak. 1994. The Vaccine Adverse Event Reporting System (VAERS). *Vaccine* 12(6):542–550.

Cialdini, R. B. 2005. Basic social influence is underestimated. *Psychological Inquiry* 16(4):158–161.

Cialdini, R. B. 2007. Descriptive social norms as underappreciated sources of social control. *Psychometrika* 72(2):263–268.

Cialdini, R. B., and N. J. Goldstein. 2004. Social influence: Compliance and conformity. *Annual Review of Psychology* 55:591–621.

Covington and Burling, LLP. 2007. New legislation regulating pet food and other animal feed. In *Food and Drug E-Alert.* Washington, DC: Covington and Burling, LLP.

CSA (Canadian Standards Association). 1997. *Risk Management: Guidelines for Decision-Makers.* Toronto, Canada: CSA.

Cuite, C. L., H. L. Aquino, and W. K. Hallman. 2005. An empirical investigation of the role of knowledge in public opinion about GM food. *International Journal of Biotechnology* 7(1-3):178–194.

Cuite, C. L., S. C. Condry, M. L. Nucci, and W. K. Hallman. 2007. *Public Response to the Contaminated Spinach Recall of 2006.* Rutgers University, NJ: Food Policy Institute.

Cuite, C. L., N. D. Weinstein, K. Emmons, and G. Colditz. 2008. A test of numeric formats for communicating risk probabilities. *Medical Decision Making* 28(3):377–384.

Dubrawski, A., K. Elenberg, A. Moore, and M. Sabhnani. 2006. *Monitoring Food Safety by Detecting Patterns in Consumer Complaints.* Paper presented at Proceedings of the National Conference on Artificial Intelligence, American Association for Artificial Intelligence/Innovative Applications of Artificial Intelligence, Boston, MA.

FDA (U.S. Food and Drug Administration). 2007. *Food Protection Plan: An Integrated Strategy for Protecting the Nation's Food Supply.* Rockville, MD: FDA.

FDA. 2008a. *FDA Food Protection Plan: Six-Month Progress Summary.* Rockville, MD: FDA.

FDA. 2008b. *Food Protection Plan: One-Year Progress Summary.* Rockville, MD: FDA.

FDA. 2008c. *Third Edition: Draft Framework of the FDA Animal Feed Safety System,* FDA. Rockville, MD: FDA.

FDA. 2009a. *About FDA: What We Do.* http://www.fda.gov/AboutFDA/WhatWeDo/default. htm (accessed December 10, 2009).

FDA. 2009b. *Risk Communication Advisory Committee 2008.* http://www.fda.gov/ohrms/dockets/ac/oc08.html#RCAC (accessed December 10, 2009).

FDA. 2009c. *2009 Meeting Materials, Risk Communication Advisory Committee to the Food and Drug Administration.* http://www.fda.gov/AdvisoryCommittees/CommitteesMeetingMaterials/RiskCommunicationAdvisoryCommittee/ucm116558.htm (accessed December 10, 2009).

FDA. 2009d. *Risk Communication Advisory Committee 2008.* http://www.fda.gov/ohrms/dockets/ac/oc08.html#RCAC (accessed December 10, 2009).

FDA. 2009e. *Strategic Plan for Risk Communication at the Food and Drug Administration* (Draft April 15, 2009). Rockville, MD: FDA.

FDA. 2009f. *Memorandum of January 21, 2009 Freedom of Information Act.* http://fdatransparencyblog.fda.gov/ (accessed January 13, 2010).

FDA. 2009g. *Transparency Task Force Mission.* http://www.fda.gov/AboutFDA/WhatWeDo/FDATransparencyTaskForce/ucm163781.htm (accessed March 12, 2010).

FDA. 2009h. *June 24, 2009 Public Meeting on Transparency: Meeting Materials.* http://www.fda.gov/AboutFDA/WhatWeDo/FDATransparencyTaskForce/ucm170422.htm (accessed March 12, 2010).

FDA. 2009i. *FDA Transparency Task Force.* http://www.fda.gov/AboutFDA/WhatWeDo/FDA-TransparencyTaskForce/default.htm (accessed December 10, 2009).

FDA. 2009j. *FDA Transparency Blog.* http://fdatransparencyblog.fda.gov/ (accessed December 10, 2009).

FDA. 2009k. *Industry and Regulatory Assistance and Training Resources for Retail Food.* http://www.fda.gov/Food/FoodSafety/RetailFoodProtection/IndustryandRegulatoryAssistanceandTrainingResources/default.htm (accessed December 10, 2009).

FDA. 2009l. *Food Defense & Emergency Response: Training.* http://www.fda.gov/Food/FoodDefense/Training/default.htm (accessed December 10, 2009).

FDA. 2009m. *FDA Memoranda of Understanding.* http://www.fda.gov/AboutFDA/PartnershipsCollaborations/MemorandaofUnderstandingMOUs/default.htm (accessed December 10, 2009).

Fischhoff, B. 2009. Risk perception and communication. In *Oxford Textbook of Public Health,* 5th ed., edited by R. Detel, M. Beaglehole, M. A. Lansang, and M. Gulliford. Oxford, UK: Oxford University Press. Pp. 940–952.

Fischhoff, B., and J. S. Downs. 1997. Communicating foodborne disease risk. *Emerging Infectious Diseases* 3(4):489–495.

French, S. A. 2003. Pricing effects on food choices. *Journal of Nutrition* 133(3):841S–843S.

FSIS (Food Safety and Inspection Service). 2002. *Changes in Consumer Knowledge, Behavior, and Confidence Since the 1996 PR/HACCP Final Rule.* PR/HACCP Rule Evaluation Report. Washington, DC: USDA.

Gallup. 2010. *Nutrition and Food.* http://www.gallup.com/poll/6424/Nutrition-Food.aspx (accessed May 12, 2010).

GAO (U.S. Government Accountability Office). 2004a. *Federal Food Safety and Security System: Fundamental Restructuring Is Needed to Address Fragmentation and Overlap.* Washington, DC: GAO.

GAO. 2004b. *Food Safety: USDA and FDA Need to Better Ensure Prompt and Complete Recalls of Potentially Unsafe Food.* Washington, DC: GAO.

GAO. 2005. *Oversight of Food Safety Activities: Federal Agencies Should Pursue Opportunities to Reduce Overlap and Better Leverage Resources.* Washington, DC: GAO.

GAO. 2008a. *Federal Oversight of Food Safety: FDA Has Provided Few Details on the Resources and Strategies Needed to Implement Its Food Protection Plan.* Washington, DC: GAO.

GAO. 2008b. *Federal Oversight of Food Safety: FDA's Food Protection Plan Proposes Positive First Steps, but Capacity to Carry Them Out Is Critical.* Washington, DC: GAO.

Georgia Division of Public Health. 1998. Healthcare providers: Be alert for yersiniosis. *Georgia Epidemiology Report* 14(9).

GMA (Grocery Manufacturers Association). 2009. *Grocery Manufacturers Association Offers Online HACCP Training.* http://www.gmatraining.com/ (accessed December 10, 2009).

Gosselin, P., and P. Poitras. 2008. Use of an Internet "viral" marketing software platform in health promotion. *Journal of Medical Internet Research* 10(4):e47.

GPO (U.S. Government Printing Office). 2009. Presidential documents. *Federal Register* 74(15):4683–4684. http://www.gpo.gov/fdsys/pkg/FR-2009-01-26/pdf/E9-1773.pdf (accessed January 13, 2010).

Green, L. R., and Selman, C. 2005. Factors impacting food workers' and managers' safe food preparation practices: A qualitative study. *Food Protection Trends* 25(12):981–990.

Gunsalus, C. K., E. Bruner, N. Burbules, L. D. Dash, M. W. Finkin, and J. Goldberg. 2007. Improving the system for protecting human subjects: Counteracting IRB Mission Creep. University of Illinois Law & Economics Research Paper No. LE06-016. *Qualitative Inquiry* 13(5):617–649.

Hallman, W. K., C. L. Cuite, and N. H. Hooker. 2009. *Consumer Responses to Food Recalls: 2008 National Survey Report.* New Brunswick: Rutgers, The State University of New Jersey.

Hayashi, Y. 2009. Scientific basis for risk analysis of food-related substances with particular reference to health effects on children. *Journal of Toxicological Sciences* 34(2): SP201–SP207.

Hirsch, D. W., and C. N. Cutter. 2006. *Preparing Small and Very Small Meat and Poultry Establishments for the Future of HACCP: A Cooperative Approach.* Storrs, CT: The University of Connecticut and the Pennsylvania State University.

Howells, A. D., K. R. Roberts, C. W. Shanklin, V. K. Pilling, L. A. Brannon, and B. B. Barrett. 2008. Restaurant employees' perceptions of barriers to three food safety practices. *Journal of the American Dietetic Association* 108(8):1345–1349.

IFIC (International Food Information Council Foundation). 2009. *2009 Food & Health Survey.* Washington, DC: IFIC.

IFIF (International Feed Industry Federation). 2009. *Welcome to the World of Feed!* http://www.ifif.org/global_stats1.php (accessed December 21, 2009).

IOM (Institute of Medicine). 2007. *Seafood Choices: Balancing Benefits and Risks.* Washington, DC: The National Academies Press.

IOM/NRC (National Research Council). 2007. *The Future of Drug Safety: Promoting and Protecting the Health of the Public.* Washington, DC: The National Academies Press.

Kendall, P. A., Hillers, V. V., and L. C. Medeiros. 2006. Food safety guidance for older adults. *Clinical Infectious Diseases* 42(9):1289–1304.

Kinsey J., R.W. Harrison, D. Degeneffe, and G. Ferreira. 2009. Index of consumer confidence in the safety of the United States food system. *American Journal of Agricultural Economics* 91(5):1470–1476.

Kwon, J., A. N. S. Wilson, C. Bednar, and L. Kennon. 2008. Food safety knowledge and behaviors of Women, Infant, and Children (WIC) program participants in the United States. *Journal of Food Protection* 71(8):1651–1658.

Lenhart, J., P. Kendall, L. Medeiros, J. Doorn, M. Schroeder, and J. Sofos. 2008. Consumer assessment of safety and date labeling statements on ready-to-eat meat and poultry products designed to minimize risk of listeriosis. *Journal of Food Protection* 71(1):70–76.

Levy, A. S., C. J. Choiniere, and S. B. Fein. 2008. Practice-specific risk perceptions and self-reported food safety practices. *Risk Analysis* 28(3):749–761.

Mathiasen, L. A., B. J. Chapman, B. J. Lacroix, and D. A. Powell. 2004. Spot the mistake: Television cooking shows as a source of food safety information. *Food Protection Trends* 24(5):328–334.

Miles, S., and V. Scaife. 2003. Optimistic bias and food. *Nutrition Research Reviews* 16(1):3–19.

MMWR (Morbidity and Mortality Weekly Report). 2001. Outbreak of *Listeriosis* associated with homemade Mexican-style cheese—North Carolina, October 2000–January 2001. *Morbidity and Mortality Weekly Report* 50(26):560–562.

Morgan, M. G., B. Fischhoff, A. Bostrom, and C. Atman. 2001. *Risk Communication: The Mental Models-Approach*. New York: Cambridge University Press.

NACMCF (National Advisory Committee on Microbiological Criteria for Foods). 1997. *Hazard Analysis and Critical Control Point Principles and Application Guidelines*. Washington, DC: NACMCF. http://www.fda.gov/Food/FoodSafety/HazardAnalysisCriticalControlPointsHACCP/ucm114868.htm (accessed April 22, 2010).

Nauta, M. J., A. R. H. Fischer, E. D. van Asselt, A. E. I. de Jong, L. J. Frewer, and R. de Jonge. 2008. Food safety in the domestic environment: The effect of consumer risk information on human disease risks. *Risk Analysis* 28(1):179–192.

NEHA (National Environmental Health Association). 2008. *NEHA Food Safety Training: Protecting Environmental Health Through Education*. http://www.nehatraining.org/ (accessed December 10, 2009).

NIH (National Institutes of Health). 2008. *Making Health Communication Programs Work*. Bethesda, MD: U.S. Department of Health and Human Services.

NRC (National Research Council). 1989. *Improving Risk Communication*. Washington, DC: National Academy Press.

OMB (Office of Management and Budget). 2009. *Open Government Directive*. Presidential Memorandum M-10-06, December 8, 2009. http://www.whitehouse.gov/omb/assets/memoranda_2010/m10-06.pdf (accessed January 13, 2010).

OTA (Office of Technology Assessment). 1995. *Environmental Policy Tools*. www.fas.org/ota/reports/9517.pdf (accessed March 16, 2010).

Pennell, S., S. Ziniel, and Z. Lepkowski. 2008. *Survey of Investigator Experiences in Human Research. The Institute for Social Research, University of Michigan*. www.ohrcr.umich.edu/news/surveyexperiences.pdf (accessed January 13, 2010).

The Pew Research Center. 2010. *People and Their Government: Distrust, Discontent, Anger and Partisan Rancor*. Washington, DC: The Pew Research Center.

PFSE (Partnership for Food Safety Education). 2006. *About PFSE*. http://www.fightbac.org/content/view/1/16/ (accessed December 10, 2009).

Pieretti, M. M., D. Chung, R. Pacenza, T. Slotkin, and S. H. Sicherer. 2009. Audit of manufactured products: Use of allergen advisory labels and identification of labeling ambiguities. *Journal of Allergy and Clinical Immunology* 124(2):337–341.

Pilling, V. K., L. A. Brannon, C. W. Shanklin, A. D. Howells, and K. R. Roberts. 2008. Identifying specific beliefs to target to improve restaurant employees' intentions for performing three important food safety behaviors. *Journal of the American Dietetic Association* 108(6):991–997.

Pilling, V. K., L. A. Brannon, C. W. Shanklin, W. Carol, K. R. Roberts, B. B. Barrett, and A. D. Howells. 2009. Intervention improves restaurant employees' food safety compliance rates. *International Journal of Contemporary Hospitality Management* 21(4):459–478.

Powell, D. A. 2000. Food safety and the consumer—perils of poor risk communication. *Canadian Journal of Animal Science* 80(3):393–404.

Prochaska, J. O., and W. F. Velicer. 1997. The transtheoretical model of health behavior change. *American Journal of Health Promotion* 12(1):38–48.

Prochaska, J. O., C. A. Redding, and K. E. Evers. 2002. The transtheoretical model and stages of change. In *Health Behavior and Health Education: Theory, Research, and Practice*, edited by K. Glanz, B. K. Rimer and F. M. Lewis. San Francisco, CA: Jossey-Bass. Pp. 99–120

Redmond, E. C., and C. J. Griffith. 2003. Consumer food handling in the home: A review of food safety studies. *Journal of Food Protection* 66(1):130–161

ROC-United (Restaurant Opportunities Centers United). 2009. *Burned: High risks and low benefits for workers in the New York City restaurant industry.* A joint publication of ROC-United and ROC-NY. http://www.rocunited.org/what-we-know (accessed May 11, 2010).

ROC-United. 2010. *Behind the Kitchen Door. The Hidden Cost of Low Road Jobs in Chicagoland's Thriving Restaurant Industry.* http://www.rocunited.org/what-we-know (accessed May 11, 2010).

Roth, E., M. G. Morgan, B. Fischhoff, L. Lave, and A. Bostrom. 1990. What do we know about making risk comparisons? *Risk Analysis* 10(3):375–387.

Rothman, A. J., W. M. Klein, , and N. D. Weinstein. 1996. Absolute and relative biases in estimations of personal risk. *Journal of Applied Social Psychology* 26(14):1213–1236.

Rudder, A. 2006. Food safety and the risk assessment of ethnic minority food retail businesses. *Food Control* 17(3):189–196.

Schrag, Z. M. 2009. How talking became human subjects research: The federal regulation of the social sciences, 1965–1991. *Journal of Policy History* 21(1):3–37.

Schriver, K. A. 1989. Evaluating text quality: The continuum from text-focused to reader-focused methods. *IEEE Transactions in Professional Communication* 32(4):238–255.

Schriver, K. A. 1996. *Dynamics in Document Design: Creating Text for Readers.* New York: John Wiley & Sons.

ServSafe. 2009. *ServSafe.* http://www.servsafe.com/ (accessed December 10, 2009).

Taylor, M. R., and S. D. David. 2009. *Stronger Partnerships for Safer Food: An Agenda for Strengthening State and Local Roles in the Nation's Food Safety System: Final Report.* San Francisco, CA: School of Public Health and Health Services, The George Washington University.

Weinstein, N. D. 1989. Optimistic biases about personal risks. *Science* 4935:1232–1233.

Weinstein, N. D., A. Kwitel, K. D. McCaul, R. E. Magnan, M. Gerrard, and F. X. Gibbons. 2007. Risk perceptions: Assessment and relationship to influenza vaccination. *Health Psychology* 26(2):146–151.

Whatley, K. W., D. L. Doerfert, M. Kistler, and L. Thompson. 2005. An examination of the food safety information sources and channels utilized and trusted by residents of Lubbock, Texas. *Journal of Agricultural Education* 46(3):70–81.

Zenk, S. N., L. L. Lachance, A. J. Schulz, G. Mentz, S. Kannan, and W. Ridella. 2009. Health promoting community design/nutrition: Neighborhood retail food environment and fruit and vegetable intake in a multiethnic urban population. *American Journal of Health Promotion* 23(4):255–264.

10

Modernizing Legislation to Enhance the U.S. Food Safety System

In the 1906 Pure Food and Drugs Act, for the first time Congress prohibited interstate commerce in "adulterated" food, which included, among other things, food "contain[ing] any added poisonous or other added deleterious ingredient which may render such article injurious to health" and food "consist[ing] in whole or in part of a filthy, decomposed, or putrid animal or vegetable substance."[1] The government could enforce these and all other provisions of the 1906 act through the collection and examination of specimens, criminal prosecution, the seizure and condemnation of violative articles, and the sampling and exclusion of imported goods.[2]

In 1938, Congress repealed the 1906 act and replaced it with the Federal Food, Drug, and Cosmetic Act (FDCA), which, as amended, is still in effect today.[3] While preserving, with a few minor changes, the 1906 adulteration provisions quoted above,[4] the 1938 act enhanced the U.S. Food and Drug Administration's (FDA's) food safety authority in various significant ways, including (1) a provision defining a food as adulterated "if it has been prepared, packed, or held under insanitary conditions whereby it may have become contaminated with filth, or whereby it may have been rendered injurious to health"; (2) a section empowering the FDA to establish an emergency permit system for food contaminated with microorganisms; and (3) a section providing for the establishment of tolerances for unavoid-

---

[1] *Federal Food and Drugs Act of 1906*, Sec. 7.
[2] *Federal Food and Drugs Act of 1906*, Sec. 2, 3, 10, 11.
[3] *Federal Food, Drug, and Cosmetic Act (FDCA)*, 21 U.S.C. §§ 301 et seq., 1938.
[4] FDCA 402(a)(1), (3).

293

able poisonous and deleterious substances.[5] In addition, for food and all other regulated products, the 1938 FDCA added injunction proceedings and mandatory establishment inspection to the enforcement tools included in the 1906 act.[6]

Since 1938, Congress has occasionally amended the FDCA to further enhance the FDA's power to accomplish its food safety mission. Notable examples of these amendments include the Food Additives Amendments of 1958, creating a premarket approval system for food additives; the Color Additives Amendments of 1960, creating a premarket approval system for color additives; and the Animal Drugs Amendments of 1968, creating a unified scheme for all aspects of animal drug regulation, including ensuring the safety of animal drug residues in food.[7] More recently, the Public Health Security and Bioterrorism Preparedness and Response Act of 2002 (Bioterrorism Act)[8] strengthened the food safety provisions of the FDCA by, among other things, (1) authorizing the FDA to administratively detain food for which there is "credible evidence or information indicating that such article presents a threat of serious adverse health consequences or death to humans or animals,"[9] (2) mandating the registration of food facilities,[10] (3) giving the FDA access to industry records related to food that "presents a threat of serious adverse health consequences or death to humans or animals,"[11] (4) empowering the FDA to require the maintenance of records needed by the agency "to identify the immediate previous sources and the immediate subsequent recipients of food,"[12] and (5) requiring prior notice of imported food shipments. Finally, in 2007 Congress added a new section to the FDCA (the Food and Drug Administration Amendments Act of 2007) requiring the FDA to establish a Reportable Food Registry for the reporting of instances in which there is a "reasonable probability that the use of, or exposure to, [a] food will cause serious adverse health consequences or death to humans or animals."[13]

Nevertheless, in some other fundamental respects, the law under which

---

[5] FDCA 402(a)(4), 404, 406.

[6] FDCA 302, 704.

[7] *Food Additives Amendment*, 72 Stat. 1784 (1958); *Color Additive Amendments*, 74 Stat. 397 (1960); *Animal Drug Amendments*, 82 Stat. 342 (1968).

[8] *Public Health Security and Bioterrorism Preparedness and Response Act of 2002 (Bioterrorism Act)*, HR 3448, 107th Cong, 2nd sess. (FDCA 801(m)).

[9] FDCA 304(h).

[10] FDCA 415.

[11] FDCA 414(a).

[12] FDCA 414(b).

[13] FDCA 417.

the FDA must ensure the safety of 80 percent of Americans' food supply[14] remains unchanged since 1938, despite the dramatic changes in food production and distribution patterns that have taken place since (see Chapter 2). For example, the provisions of the FDCA that the agency invokes most often in attempting to prevent and address the pathogenic infection of food read exactly the same as they did 72 years ago.[15]

The FDA needs to have the power to fulfill its food safety mission in the face of an increasingly complex and global food supply. In this chapter, the committee recommends some important legislative changes to this end. As shown by the length of the food safety bills currently under consideration in Congress, this chapter cannot address every area in which statutory amendments may be warranted; instead, it highlights those the committee deems most critical. For example, this chapter does not address authorities, such as embargo power[16] and civil monetary penalties, that might be helpful but less essential to ensure public health than the ones discussed below. Furthermore, this chapter does not consider how much money Congress should appropriate for the FDA's food safety activities or what funding mechanisms the agency should use. Although the committee supports increasing funding for the FDA to the extent necessary to implement the recommendations contained in this report, it is also firmly convinced that simply putting more money into the food safety system as it is currently constituted, without essential reforms, would be insufficient from a public health perspective and an inefficient expenditure of resources.

Finally, the legislative recommendations in this chapter are not intended to suggest that the FDA does not already have the authority in question under current law. Various existing statutory provisions give the agency broad discretion and flexibility that might encompass the powers discussed herein. There are instances in which a specific authority has not been explicitly given to the FDA, so that legal interpretations might result in differences in opinion that would raise controversy among stakeholders. In these cases, the committee concluded that it would be helpful to provide such authorities to the FDA explicitly. For example, the committee recommends giving the FDA explicit authority to mandate that food facilities establish preventive process controls, maintain records, and provide the agency with access to these records during inspections. Yet even without such explicit statutory authority, the FDA has promulgated Hazard Analysis and Criti-

---

[14] The term "food," as defined in the FDCA, includes "all articles used for food or drink for man or other animals" and thus encompasses what is commonly known animal "feed." Throughout this chapter, therefore, as throughout the rest of the report, the word "food" includes animal feed unless otherwise noted.

[15] See FDCA 402(a)(1), (3), (4) (*Adulterated Food*); 404 (*Emergency Permit Control*).

[16] As discussed later in the chapter, the committee does recommend that the FDA be given the power to issue cease distribution orders as part of a broader mandatory recall authority.

cal Control Points (HACCP) regulations that impose such requirements on seafood and juice processors. The agency issued both of these rules pursuant to section 701(a) of the FDCA (21 U.S.C. 371(a)), which gives the FDA broad "authority to promulgate regulations for the efficient enforcement of this Act." For the juice HACCP rule, the agency also relied in part on section 361 of the Public Health Service Act (42 U.S.C. 264), under which the FDA commissioner has been delegated power to "make and enforce such regulations as in [her] judgment are necessary to prevent the introduction, transmission, or spread of communicable diseases from foreign countries into the States or possessions, or from one State or possession into any other State or possession" (HHS/FDA, 1995, 2001).[17]

The seafood and juice HACCP rules have not been challenged in court as unreasonable interpretations of the statutes, and the rules might well survive such challenges if they arose. Nonetheless, the FDA should be able to impose preventive controls based on hazard analysis and risk, as defined in Chapter 3, on all food facilities—and to exercise the other powers enumerated below—free of any doubt that it has the authority do so. The agency is prone to hesitate before pursuing measures based on broad delegations of authority rather than detailed statutory provisions, and agency actions taken pursuant to such broad delegations are more vulnerable to court challenge. Hence, the committee believes it is important to revise the FDCA to expressly provide the FDA with explicit authorities in the areas of facility registration, preventive controls, performance standards, risk-based inspection, access to records, traceability, mandatory recall, reporting of adulteration, and banning of all food imports from a country if a review of its food safety system indicates that the public health is at risk.

FACILITY REGISTRATION

The FDA cannot have an adequate food safety program unless it knows exactly where food is being produced, processed, packed, and held. Section 415 of the FDCA, "Registration of Food Facilities," currently requires food facilities, both domestic and foreign, to register with the FDA. Although the act requires registrants to notify the agency of changes in the submitted information, it does not mandate regular reregistration in the absence of such changes. Moreover, it does not provide for the suspension of the registration of a facility that has committed violations that threaten the public health. The act needs to be amended to include mandatory periodic reregistration and, with adequate procedural protections, FDA authority to suspend registrations.

The FDCA's definition of a "facility" subject to the registration require-

---

[17] 42 U.S.C. 264 sec. 361.

ment is limited to "any factory, warehouse, or establishment (including a factory, warehouse, or establishment of an importer) that manufactures, processes, packs, or holds food."[18] Many food importers, however, never physically possess the food they import and thus fall outside this definition. To enhance the FDA's ability to trace and apply the act to imported foods, the definition of "facility" should be amended to embrace entities in the business of importing foods from foreign countries even if these entities do not "manufacture, process, pack, or hold" the foods (see Appendix E).

Section 415 of the act also explicitly exempts farms, restaurants, and other retail food establishments from the definition of "facility" and thus from the current registration requirement. The committee believes that, to enhance the agency's ability to trace food along its entire production and distribution chain, all domestic farms, restaurants, and other food service and retail food establishments ought to be required to register with the FDA. This is not to say that such establishments should be subject to the same panoply of requirements as, for example, food factories and warehouses. Congress might sensibly decide to exempt farms, restaurants, and other food service and retail food establishments from requirements other than registration imposed on all "food facilities." Therefore, the goal of universal registration should probably not be achieved by simply amending the definition of "facility" in section 415(b)(1) to delete the exception for farms, restaurants, and retail establishments.

PREVENTIVE CONTROLS

As demonstrated by its promulgation of the seafood and juice HACCP rules, the FDA has found authority under current law to impose preventive process control regimes on food facilities. Nonetheless, the FDCA needs to be amended not only to make this authority explicit, but also to mandate that all registered food facilities have such controls in place. Every food facility ought to be required to conduct a hazard evaluation, identify potential hazards, implement preventive controls, monitor the controls, establish corrective actions, and maintain comprehensive records of the system's implementation. Each facility should also be required to prepare a food safety plan that sets forth the hazard evaluation results, the identified preventive controls, and the facility's program for monitoring the preventive controls, validating them, taking corrective action, and keeping records. In addition, the act needs to specify that the food safety plan and the implementation records must be made available to FDA inspectors. Finally, the act should state that if a facility fails to satisfy these requirements for preventive controls based on hazard analysis and risk, any food produced,

---

[18] FDCA 415(b)(1).

processed, packed, or held in that facility is considered adulterated under section 402 of the act.

The committee discussed the possibility of recommending mandatory testing for pathogens. However, it concluded that the FDA should address this complex issue on a case-by-case basis, pursuant to the overall risk-based food safety management approach proposed in this report.

PERFORMANCE STANDARDS

The FDCA needs to be amended to require the FDA to periodically issue enforceable, risk- and science-based performance standards for pathogens and other contaminants significant to public health. The agency should be required to use a risk-ranking approach to prioritize the development and issuance of those standards.

RISK-BASED INSPECTION

A process for making decisions about what, when, and how to inspect is essential for an efficient food safety system. In Chapter 3, the committee recommends that the FDA use a risk-based approach to make decisions and allocate resources. In Chapter 8, the committee specifically calls for a review and update of FDA inspection processes so they are consistent with a risk-based approach. Although the FDA is already thinking through its decision-making process for the conduct of inspectional activities, the committee concluded that this is one key area that requires a congressional mandate.

The FDCA needs to be amended to require the FDA to adopt a risk-based approach to both the frequency and intensity of inspections. The committee also believes, however, that the law should establish minimum standards for the frequency and intensity of inspection of all food facilities, regardless of their risk ranking. Moreover, the committee believes it is important to maintain some element of randomness in the scheduling and targeting of inspections.

ACCESS TO RECORDS

The FDCA as currently written expressly authorizes the FDA to demand access to only four categories of records relating to food: (1) those showing the movement of food in interstate commerce kept by shippers/carriers and by recipients of interstate shipments,[19] (2) those kept pursuant to FDA regulations by shippers/carriers regarding sanitary transportation practices,[20] (3) those relating to infant formula,[21] and (4) those needed to determine whether a food is adulterated and presents a threat of serious adverse health consequences or death.[22] The agency has access to documents under the fourth provision, added by the Bioterrorism Act of 2002, only if it has a "reasonable belief" that the food is adulterated and presents a threat of serious health consequences or death.[23]

In contrast, with respect to prescription drugs, nonprescription drugs intended for human use, and restricted devices, the FDCA provides the FDA with broad access to records bearing on whether the products are adulterated, misbranded, or otherwise in violation of the act. The committee believes that Congress needs to give the FDA similarly broad access to records in food facilities. As explained above, the effective enforcement of a food safety system based on preventive controls depends on the FDA's having access to each facility's food safety plan and implementation records. But in light of the fact that other categories of documents may also bear on food safety, the FDA's access should not be limited to preventive control documents.

TRACEABILITY

Section 414(b) of the FDCA, added by the Bioterrorism Act of 2002, authorizes the FDA to issue regulations requiring food facilities, excluding farms and restaurants, to establish and maintain "records . . . needed by the Secretary for inspection to allow the Secretary to identify the immediate previous sources and the immediate subsequent recipients of food . . . in order to address credible threats of serious adverse health consequences or death to humans or animals."[23] Such regulations cannot require that facilities maintain those records for longer than 2 years. The agency issued such regulations in 2004.[24] These regulations, in accordance with the statute, exempt farms and restaurants from all the requirements, and they also exempt entities that sell directly to consumers from the requirement to identify subsequent recipients. The FDA has access to these records under the same standard applicable to all records sought under

---

[19] FDCA 703(a).

[20] FDCA 703(b).

[21] FDCA 704(a)(3).

[22] FDCA 414(a). This category was added by the *Bioterrorism Act of 2002.*

[23] *Public Health Security and Bioterrorism Preparedness and Response Act of 2002 (Bioterrorism Act).*

[24] 21 CFR 1.326-1.368.

the Bioterrorism Act; the agency must have a "reasonable belief that an article of food is adulterated and presents a threat of serious adverse health consequences or death to humans or animals."[25] The committee believes that the FDCA needs to be amended to require farms to maintain records identifying immediate subsequent recipients, other than individual consumers, and restaurants to maintain records identifying immediate previous sources.

MANDATORY RECALL

When confronting a food safety emergency, the FDA can often depend on state governments to use their embargo authority to stop the distribution and sale of the adulterated food. Moreover, section 304(h)(1)(A) of the FDCA gives the FDA itself the power to administratively detain any article of food if an officer or qualified employee of the agency "has credible evidence or information indicating that such article presents a threat of serious adverse health consequences or death to humans or animals."[26] However, the FDA does not currently have explicit authority to mandate a recall of the products it regulates, with the exception of infant formula, medical devices, and biological products.

In communications with the committee, the FDA maintained that it should be given the power to order a company to recall an adulterated food when necessary to protect the public health. The bills currently under consideration in Congress give the FDA the power, subject to specified procedures, to issue a cease distribution order and a subsequent recall order when there is a reasonable probability that a food will cause serious adverse health consequences or death.[27]

In most instances, the FDA does not need mandatory recall authority to fulfill its food safety mission. The agency has developed a sophisticated and highly successful "voluntary recall" process with respect to food as well as all other products it regulates (Title 21 CFR—"Food and Drugs," Subpart J, "Establishment, Maintenance, and Availability of Records," 2004; Degnan, 2006, pp. 107–113). Food companies almost always cooperate with FDA-requested recalls, and even when companies resist, the agency

---

[25] 21 CFR 1.361.

[26] A detention order may be issued by an "officer or qualified employee" of the FDA, but such order must be approved by the commissioner or by an official designated by the commissioner who ranks no lower than district director (FDCA 304(h)(1)). A claimant for a detained article may appeal the detention order, and the commissioner must, after providing an opportunity for an informal hearing, confirm or terminate the order within 5 days of when the appeal is filed (FDCA 304(h)(4)(A)).

[27] HR759, *Food and Drug Administration Globalization Act of 2009*; S510 IS, *FDA Food Safety Modernization Act of 2009*.

can usually induce cooperation through the threat of negative publicity. Indeed, the voluntary recall process is normally so efficacious that the FDA rarely uses its mandatory authority even in those areas in which it possesses such authority. For example, although the FDA has had mandatory recall authority over medical devices since 1990, the committee learned that the agency has invoked this power only ten times, and never since 1994.[28]

Nonetheless, the committee concludes that there may be rare circumstances, involving uncooperative food distributors, in which the FDA needs the power to formally order a party to cease distribution of an article of food and recall it. Congress thus needs to amend the statute to provide the FDA with such authority with respect to foods that are adulterated under section 402 of the FDCA and may cause serious health consequences or death. To ensure that the existence of mandatory recall authority does not undermine the carefully honed and highly effective voluntary system already in place, Congress should require the FDA to always provide the party in question an opportunity to cease distribution and recall an article voluntarily (according to terms prescribed by the agency) before it issues an order. If the party refuses to proceed voluntarily, the FDA should then have the power to order the party to cease distribution immediately, but the party should, except in instances of imminent danger, be given an opportunity for an expeditious informal hearing before the FDA modifies the order to mandate recall.

REPORTING OF ADULTERATION

In 2007, Congress amended the FDCA to require all registered food facilities to report to the FDA, through an electronic portal into a Reportable Food Registry, any "article of food . . . for which there is a reasonable probability that the use of, or exposure to, such article of food will cause serious adverse health consequences or death to humans or animals."[29] While the committee supports the concept of this registry, it is concerned that the mandatory reporting requirement may lead to a reduction in testing by food facilities reluctant to report any problems they may find. Section 417(d)(2) exempts from the reporting requirement any party that detects the adulteration prior to the transfer of the food to another party and corrects the adulteration or destroys the food. The committee believes this safe harbor ought to be extended to parties that detect adulteration even after transfer of the food to an immediately subsequent party as long

---

[28] Personal communication, Joanna Weitershausen, Center for Devices and Radiological Health, FDA, September 30, 2009.
[29] FDCA 417.

as the responsible party corrects the adulteration (or causes it to be corrected) or destroys the food (or causes it to be destroyed).

AUTHORITY TO BAN ALL FOOD IMPORTS FROM A COUNTRY

The U.S. Department of Agriculture's Food Safety and Inspection Service (FSIS) administers the Federal Meat Inspection Act, the Poultry Products Inspection Act, and the Egg Products Inspection Act (FSIS/USDA, 2009a). Pursuant to these statutes and implementing regulations, FSIS permits imports of meat, poultry, and egg products only from countries it has certified as having inspection systems that ensure that exported food products meet American food safety standards.[30] FSIS makes the determination that a country's food regulatory system provides food safety protections equivalent to those provided by U.S. domestic regulatory programs (and thus that the country is eligible to export meat, poultry, or egg products) based on document reviews, on-site audits, and port-of-entry reinspection (FSIS/USDA, 2009b).

The FDCA does not require the FDA to make a similar country-by-country equivalence determination, and the committee does not believe that such an approach would be practicable for the agency, which has jurisdiction over a much more global and diverse imported food supply relative to FSIS. Nonetheless, in administering a risk-based food safety system, the FDA might decide to review the regulatory systems of some or all of the nations that export food to the United States. In addition, the agency might conclude, based on a comprehensive risk assessment, that a particular country's food safety regulatory system is so inadequate that all food imports from that country should be banned. The FDCA needs to be amended to empower the FDA to ban all food imports from a country if the agency concludes, in light of a review of that country's food safety regulatory system, that such a measure is necessary to protect the public health. The committee also concluded that, rather than dramatically increasing inspectors in foreign countries, the FDA should use a risk-based approach to prioritize inspections at the border (see Chapter 3).

KEY CONCLUSIONS AND RECOMMENDATIONS

The FDA bears responsibility for ensuring the safety of 80 percent of the nation's food supply. Despite the dramatic developments in food production and distribution that have occurred since the 1938 enactment of the FDCA, the main statutory provisions under which the agency carries out its food safety mission remain largely unchanged. These provisions are broad

---

[30] See Title 9 CFR 327.2 (meat), 381.196 (poultry), 590.910 (egg products).

delegations of power rather than detailed grants of authority. The agency is often reluctant to take action without an explicit mandate to do so, and those actions it does take in the absence of express statutory authorization are vulnerable to court challenge. Therefore, the committee believes the FDCA needs to be revised to detail the FDA's authorities in the areas of facility registration, preventive controls, performance standards, risk-based inspection, access to records, traceability, mandatory recall, reporting of adulteration, and banning of all food imports from a country if a review of its food safety system indicates that the public health is at risk.

Recommendation 10-1: Congress should consider amending the FDCA to provide explicitly and in detail the authorities the FDA needs to fulfill its food safety mission. The following are the most critical areas in which Congress should enact amendments: mandatory reregistration of food facilities and FDA authority to suspend registrations for violations that threaten the public health, mandatory preventive controls for all food facilities, FDA authority to issue enforceable performance standards, mandatory adoption by the FDA of a risk-based approach to inspection frequency and intensity, expansion of the FDA's access to records, FDA authority to mandate recalls, and FDA authority to identify countries with inadequate food safety systems and to ban all imports from such countries.

REFERENCES

Degnan, F. H. 2006. *FDA's Creative Application of the Law: Not Merely a Collection of Words* (2nd edition). Washington, DC: Food and Drug Law Institute.

FSIS/USDA (Food Safety and Inspection Service/U.S. Department of Agriculture). 2009a. *Regulations, Directives & Notices: Acts & Authorizing Statutes.* http://www.fsis.usda.gov/regulations_&_policies/acts_&_authorizing_statutes/index.asp (accessed December 9, 2009).

FSIS/USDA. 2009b. *Regulations & Policies/International Affairs/Import Information/Equivalence Process.* http://www.fsis.usda.gov/regulations_&_policies/Equivalence_Process/index.asp (accessed December 9, 2009).

HHS/FDA (U.S. Department of Health and Human Services/U.S. Food and Drug Administration). 1995. Procedures for the safe and sanitary processing and importing of fish and fishery products. Final rule. *Federal Register* 60(242):665905–65202.

HHS/FDA. 2001. Hazard Analysis and Critical Control Point (HAACP): Procedures for the safe and sanitary processing and importing of juice. Final rule. *Federal Register* 66(13):6138–6202.

11

Achieving the Vision of an Efficient Risk-Based Food Safety System

Preceding chapters have presented a variety of recommendations aimed at improving the U.S. Food and Drug Administration's (FDA's) food safety–related activities. Box 11-1 lists some of the areas in which the committee found that significant improvements are warranted. In formulating its recommendations, the committee emphasized the need for the FDA to move toward a risk-based approach to food safety. Recognizing that many enhancements (e.g., leadership commitment, staff retention, strategic planning) can be realized without structural changes, the committee initially formulated its recommendations in the context of the FDA's current food safety management structure. Subsequently, however, the committee concluded that while some recommendations pertain only to the FDA's functions and operations, success in implementing many others will be achieved only through cooperation with partners that play important roles in maintaining food safety. As the study progressed and the committee's ideas matured, it became clear that the effectiveness of the FDA's food safety programs will not be fully realized without organizational changes both in the structure of the agency itself and across the multiple government agencies and departments with food safety responsibilities.

Such changes will not occur without strong leadership with a clear vision for reform and the capacity (i.e., resources) and authority to implement the changes effectively. Leadership should direct change and be authorized to redirect resources and bring in new personnel with the appropriate expertise. The agency leaders with responsibility for implementing the changes must also have the appropriate support at high levels of governmental oversight. At the same time, not just high-level management but also

---

BOX 11-1
Selected Proposed Improvements in the U.S. Food and Drug Administration's (FDA's) Food Safety Management Highlighted Throughout This Report

- Apply the recommended risk-based approach to the management of all domestic and imported foods and hazards, whether derived from food or animal feed or from intentional (i.e., with the intent to harm) or inadvertent contamination (Chapter 3).
- Address the lack of resources (e.g., data infrastructure, human capacity) and organization for the implementation of a risk-based food safety management system. Access to appropriate resources (personnel, data, models) in support of this effort is central to the success of the FDA's future food safety risk management activities (Chapter 3).
- Identify metrics with which to measure the effectiveness of intervention strategies and the food safety system as a whole (Chapter 3).
- Define the roles of the various parties sharing responsibility for food safety, and develop a road map with defined criteria for food safety governance, that is, the level and intensity of policy interventions and plans to evaluate them (Chapter 4).
- Develop a strategic plan to identify data needs for a risk-based approach, and establish mechanisms to coordinate, capture, and integrate the data (Chapter 5). This includes data collected by state and local (including tribal and territorial) governments (Chapter 7), field personnel (Chapter 5), and the food industry (Chapter 5).
- Remove barriers to the practical utilization of data to support a risk-based system, including problems with data sharing and gaps in analytical expertise within the FDA (Chapter 5).

---

the entire team tasked with facilitating agency changes must have the necessary vision, understanding, and experience to implement those changes. Further, since many FDA food safety activities are inextricably linked to those of other agencies with food safety jurisdiction (federal, state, and local) (see Table 2-1 in Chapter 2), coordination and collaboration with these agencies will be essential. As discussed in Chapter 3, moreover, change cannot occur without careful prior planning and substantial investments in physical, human, and financial resources. Finally, the need for strong leadership implies that appropriate legislative authority must be given to the agency (see Chapter 10).

- Conduct strategic planning and coordination of the FDA's food safety research portfolio, keeping in mind the need to partner with other groups in carrying out the agency's research function, including the value of funding mechanisms to facilitate cooperative research between the FDA and external entities (Chapter 6).
- Integrate state and local food safety programs with the ultimate goal of making these food surveillance, inspectional, and analytical systems full partners in the national food safety program (Chapter 7).
- Address the existence of barriers to improving the efficiency of inspections, such as the fact that the FDA's food programs do not have direct authority over the work of inspectors, resulting in substantial delays in policy implementation in the field, the inefficiency of inspection procedures, and underutilization of other sources of information, such as state inspections (Chapter 8).
- Continue development of a single source of authoritative government information on food safety, safe food practices, foodborne illnesses and risks, and crisis communications (Chapter 9).
- Create a coordinated and centrally controlled plan for communicating with one voice with all affected parties during food safety crises, including coordination of recalls, so that all constituents (producers, distributors, retailers, and consumers) receive timely and reliable information (Chapter 9).
- Modernize the legislative framework to give the FDA the necessary legal authority to perform its role in ensuring and enhancing the safety of FDA-regulated foods (Chapter 10).

For more than a decade, various organizations, consumer groups, and individuals have recommended organizational changes in the U.S. food safety system, with the goal of increasing its efficiency and enhancing the public health (IOM/NRC, 1998; GAO, 2004, 2005a, 2007, 2008; Gombas, 2009; Halloran, 2009; IOM, 2009; Plunkett, 2009; Scott, 2009; Waldrop, 2009).[1] Furthermore, governments in other countries

---

[1] Gaps in Food Safety Illustrated by the Peanut Products Outbreak, Testimony before the Senate Committee on Agriculture, Nutrition, and Forestry, Washington, DC, February 5, 2009.

have reorganized and adapted their food safety systems to reflect current circumstances (GAO, 2005b). More recently, in congressional testimony on federal oversight of food safety and the FDA's Food Protection Plan (FPP), Lisa Shames, the U.S. Government Accountability Office's director of natural resources and environment (GAO, 2008), stated that:

> it is important to note that FDA is one of 15 federal agencies that collectively administer at least 30 laws related to food safety. This fragmentation is a key reason we designated federal oversight of food safety as a high-risk area. Two agencies have primary responsibility—FDA is responsible for the safety of virtually all foods except for meat, poultry, and processed egg products, which are the responsibility of the United States Department of Agriculture (USDA). In addition, among other agencies, the National Marine Fisheries Service in the Department of Commerce conducts voluntary, fee-for-service inspections of seafood safety and quality; the Environmental Protection Agency regulates the use of pesticides and maximum allowable residue levels on food commodities and animal feed; and the Department of Homeland Security is responsible for coordinating agencies' food security activities. This federal regulatory system for food safety, like many other federal programs and policies, evolved piecemeal, typically in response to particular health threats or economic crises. (GAO, 2008, p. 3)

As of this writing, change is already under way, as evidenced by the creation of the White House Food Safety Working Group (FSWG) in March 2009. The FSWG was formed by the Obama Administration to address the critical need for cooperation across the spectrum of federal food safety agencies (FSWG, 2009a). Chaired by the Secretaries of the U.S. Department of Health and Human Services and USDA, the FSWG "will coordinate with other agencies and senior officials to advise the President on improving coordination throughout the government, examining and upgrading food safety laws, and enforcing laws that will keep the American people safe" (FSWG, 2009a). According to Agriculture Secretary Thomas J. Vilsack:

> The Working Group will be an important tool for gathering ideas as to how we can strengthen the food safety system to be more accountable and accessible to the public it protects, flexible enough to quickly resolve new safety challenges that emerge, and able to meet the robust needs of our rapidly changing world. (HHS, 2009)

In an effort to foster transparency and openness, the FSWG has invited public participation and is focusing on five basic principles similar to those in the FDA's FPP:

(1) Respond rapidly to outbreaks and facilitate recovery.

(2) Expand risk-based inspection and enforcement.
(3) Focus on prevention.
(4) Target resources effectively.
(5) Strengthen surveillance and risk analysis. (FSWG, 2009b)

The FSWG proposes to strengthen federal coordination by clarifying responsibilities, improving accountability, and modernizing current statutes. Thus its establishment is, at the time of this writing, a critical first step toward a comprehensive overhaul of the U.S. food safety management system, with the FDA as a key player (FSWG, 2009b).

The committee strongly supports the direction being taken by the FSWG. It is concerned, however, that these efforts remain piecemeal. A review of the FSWG website reveals little activity since the group's inception, and its membership is unclear. To be effective, the FSWG must include experts with the depth of background in food safety needed to understand the multitude of issues facing those agencies charged with food safety oversight. Increased transparency and stakeholder participation would strengthen and enhance the role of the FSWG as the leader in planning and implementing the comprehensive overhaul needed to optimize the U.S. food safety management system. The remainder of this chapter addresses issues relevant to reorganization and resource allocation within the FDA and approaches to the unification of food safety activities across the multiple agencies and departments with food safety responsibilities.

ISSUES RELEVANT TO REORGANIZATION AND RESOURCE ALLOCATION

Barriers to Change Within the FDA

As outlined in Chapter 2, FDA responsibilities relative to the nation's food supply lie within multiple centers and units. As it currently stands, there are deep-seated and fundamental differences in the cultures within the various FDA units. Historical differences in mission, financing, legal authorities and responsibilities, and institutional traditions have led to disparate perspectives on food safety issues among these units (Bell, 2009; Osterholm, 2009). A good example is the differing visions for the Center for Food Safety and Applied Nutrition (CFSAN) and the Office of Regulatory Affairs (ORA). Past studies (Glavin, 2008) have also noted the conflicts inherent in the FDA's dual roles of law enforcement and protection of the public health. Policy setting for FDA food and feed regulation has historically resided with CFSAN (formerly the Bureau of Foods) and the Center for Veterinary Medicine (CVM), respectively, which are headed by a director. On the other hand, enforcement of policies and regulations is carried out by ORA, which is headed by an associate commissioner. Much of ORA's organizational culture is focused on its law enforcement role. CFSAN and CVM employees, on the other hand, are not law enforcement officers (Givens, 2009). Thus, ORA investigators can request data while they conduct an inspection, and these data may be helpful in guiding regulatory decisions that affect the public health. On the other hand, if these data reveal policy violations, they can also become the basis for regulatory action against a food facility. This possibility could contribute to hesitancy on the part of industry to share potentially important data with the FDA (see Chapter 5).

Historically, ORA district offices sought approval from CFSAN (or the Bureau of Foods) for legal action when sufficient evidence existed, in the opinion of CFSAN scientists/administrators, to support such action. Over time, more authority was ceded to the ORA regions/districts to take action on specific findings without center approval or concurrence. Establishing field research centers and strengthening support for ORA laboratories as part of ORA's "revitalization strategies" were perceived by some as usurping what was traditionally a function of CFSAN scientists (Swann, 1993; Glavin, 2008). The relationship between the two centers has reportedly varied over time with changes in personnel and personal relationships among leaders within the offices of the director at CFSAN and the associate commissioner for regulatory affairs, as well as at lower echelons within each organization.

A related problem that derives from this division of roles at the FDA is that inspectors under the jurisdiction of ORA have responsibilities for more than one type of FDA-regulated product. As a result, the agency has imprecise data on the proportion of field resources dedicated to food safety (Givens, 2009; Solomon, 2009). This situation appears to be due to the policy that individual inspectors are not assigned to specific types of facilities (foods, drugs, devices, cosmetics) but handle a variety of establishments in their jurisdictions (Givens, 2009). Although maintaining a workforce with diverse training in foods, drugs, devices, and cosmetics purportedly provides the agency with flexibility, the committee argues that it results in an inspection force that may not have sufficient expertise in food safety (see Chapter 8) (Givens, 2009; Wagner, 2009).

In summary, the separation of the public health and enforcement roles within the FDA and the lack of clarity about their overlap have resulted in a situation in which CFSAN and CVM, the agency's food and feed policy arms, have little direct authority over the FDA's activities in the field. This lack of direct authority hampers the FDA's ability to prioritize such activities as inspections, the collection of data necessary to drive a risk-based food safety management system, and even the implementation of new or updated CFSAN policies. These are essential activities that are central to the

FDA's success in managing food safety with a risk-based approach; implementing many of the recommendations in this report will not be feasible if these problems persist.

Efficient Use of Resources

Among other factors, the organizational structure at the FDA contributes to a setting in which the utilization of available resources is often less than ideal. This report has pointed to various areas in which such operational inefficiencies exist at the FDA; two particularly important areas are discussed below.

One area of concern for the committee that has also been highlighted by others (GUIRR/NAS, 2009) is the lack of coordination of the nation's food safety and defense research portfolios. Within the FDA, in the absence of a strong organizational focus with a well-defined strategic plan, food safety–related research has evolved into a poorly integrated network of research centers, institutes, and laboratories (see Chapter 6). The ORA laboratories play into this issue; their work is focused on enforcement, but with appropriate agency restructuring, they could well be a critical source of data to support risk-based food safety management. As part of any organizational restructuring, changes to the agency's research portfolio (and laboratory functions) will be necessary, including reallocation of irrelevant or poorly performing initiatives and identification of future resources needed to support risk-based efforts.

Data infrastructure issues are a second area of critical importance with respect to resource allocation and internal reorganization. Underlying virtually all of the recommendations made in this report is the fundamental need for reliable data to guide the decision-making process. Reliable data must be appropriate (fit-for-purpose), complete, available, and representative of all sectors and stakeholders (Bell, 2009; Osterholm, 2009; Plunkett, 2009; Scott, 2009). As described in Chapter 5, there are many technical, cultural, and perhaps even legal barriers to meeting such data needs, including inadequate information technology (IT) infrastructure, cultures that discourage the sharing of data, and delays or lack of collaboration in sharing data due to misunderstandings about legal constraints. Also, the lack of high-quality personnel to carry out the collection, analysis, and management of data has been highlighted in this report as a barrier to good data infrastructure and management (Chapter 5). At the most basic level, the FDA must give top priority to the development of robust IT systems that can accommodate the data available from multiple partners; such systems must be designed to collect the right data in the right format to facilitate risk-based decision making. In any internal FDA reorganization, an applied statistician and an IT/data manager with experience in developing and maintaining large databases must be included in the top management group, and their respective divisions must have access to the necessary resources and work collaboratively to create a modern data management system.

Current Approaches to Internal FDA Reorganization

As this report is being written, the FDA has initiated internal reorganization plans that would integrate the food safety functions of, CFSAN and CVM. The committee is encouraged by, and strongly supportive, of the creation of the Office of Foods with authority over CFSAN and CVM (see Chapter 2). However, this consolidation will not resolve concerns associated with the separation of the enforcement and public health roles of ORA and the centers, respectively. In fact, based on the problems discussed above, the committee concluded that if the FDA is to accomplish its food safety mission efficiently, its food programs should have complete authority over field activities related to the foods it regulates. The committee is also concerned about how the plans currently being developed will deal with structuring the agency's research mission and with addressing the IT and data management deficiencies highlighted in this report.

UNIFICATION OF FOOD SAFETY ACTIVITES ACROSS MULTIPLE AGENCIES AND DEPARTMENTS

In keeping with its statement of task, the committee did not conduct an in-depth review of the whole food safety system and responsible government agencies. Nor has the committee considered or evaluated the pros and cons of all potential organizational changes that might address the current challenges reviewed in this report. The committee does believe, however, that certain key organizational changes described below would enhance the ability of the FDA, and the federal government in general, to ensure food safety.

The committee concludes that focusing attention on risk-based priorities, workforce development, and the integration of activities currently scattered among many poorly coordinated agencies would result in a marked increase in efficiency throughout the system. While the resource and organizational issues to be addressed may appear to be daunting in the short term, it is highly likely that well-designed components of an integrated food safety system would, in the long run, save money and improve the public health.

Similar sentiments have been expressed by government officials in other countries that have recently reorganized their food safety systems (see Appendix C). Although evaluations of the outcomes of these reorganizations are still in progress, officials in each country believe that the final balance will be a positive one. In addition to improvements in efficiency, such as less overlap in inspections and more consistent and timely enforcement of laws and regulations, some countries cite areas that should result in savings, such as reduced duplication of inspections and lower costs associated with administrative personnel (GAO, 2005b).

There are well-documented difficulties inherent in any internal restructuring of government agencies, difficulties that are magnified when such efforts involve reorganizing across agencies and departments that have traditionally operated independently. The committee is aware that any reorganization efforts directed at the food safety system will require careful planning and may require stepwise implementation. Regardless of the final structure of the food safety system, it must include data management and analytical functions that will ensure that the data needs of a risk-based food safety system are met. The approaches described below reflect what could be an evolutionary process in which the first step—creation of a centralized risk-based analysis and data management center—leads toward accomplishing the more challenging goal of a unified food safety agency.

Creation of a Centralized Risk-Based Analysis and Data Management Center

A risk-based food safety system requires the analytical capacity to assess food safety risks and policy interventions and the ability to access data from a broad array of sources. To meet these needs, the committee envisions the establishment of a centralized center with risk-based analysis and data management functions. The need for data to support a scientific basis for decision making has been articulated by the White House FSWG as well as a variety of other public and private groups (Taylor and Hoffman, 2001; GAO, 2004, 2005a; Taylor and Batz, 2008). The proposed center would serve as an information hub or broker that would streamline data collection from a variety of sources to support a risk-based approach. Such data might include epidemiological and farm-to fork surveillance data collected at the national level; inspectional, laboratory, and epidemiological data collected at the state and local levels; supporting food safety data, such as industry surveillance and academic research findings; and other relevant data related to food safety and food defense.

Establishment of a centralized food safety data management function would be an important step toward the implementation of a risk-based approach to food safety management. However, the act of collating and organizing data does not necessarily mean that the right data have been collected or that the data will be used appropriately. Therefore, this center also needs to house the analytic capacity, including the appropriate scientific and technical expertise, to identify (in consultation with the relevant agencies) specific data needs, ensure that data are collected in an appropriate manner, and analyze the data with the clear goal of supporting risk-based food safety decision making.

The committee envisions several advantages to the establishment of such a centralized risk-based analysis and data management center. On the analytical side, having such a center responsible for all food safety data, irrespective of agency, would go a long way toward developing the much-needed capacity that is currently lacking. The center's independence from a specific regulatory agency would not preempt any agency's prerogative to develop its own approach to food safety management, but would eliminate the need for each agency to develop its own comprehensive expertise in risk and decision analysis. This in turn would reduce interagency competition for available scientific resources (including personnel), reduce redundancy, harmonize analytical methods, and increase efficiency. Specifically, because the agencies involved would not have competing analytic groups, the center concept would ensure a consistent technical approach to surveillance, data analysis, and modeling. On the data management side, the centralized nature of this body would help overcome some of the current barriers to data acquisition and transfer, keeping in mind that additional actions needed to overcome the data sharing barriers identified in Chapter 5 would have to be considered during the center's establishment. The ability of such a center to promote communication, collaboration, and sharing of data among government agencies is central to its value.

Positioning the risk-based analysis and data management center as a free-standing (independent) entity that is not directly answerable to any one regulatory agency would also result in a scientifically credible source of unbiased data and analytic capacity. This model is consistent with the need for separation of the risk management and assessment functions, which is central to the assurance that risk-based decision making is objective and not influenced to support a predetermined policy or political agenda (NRC, 1983, 1996). Further, within such a structure, it may be easier to recruit and retain scientists and maintain the interactive and multidisciplinary scientific base essential to the functioning of such an organization. Although it is important to stress that this center should be independent from political influence, it is also essential that the strategic plan for the center be developed to address the needs of the regulatory food safety agencies. The term "independent" in this context means free from political influence but accountable to the public health needs and mission of the regulatory agencies. In Europe, quasi-governmental research institutes (such as the National Institute for Public Health and the Environment in the Netherlands or the European Food Safety Authority) serve the dual purposes of functioning as a hub for national data collection and providing the independent scientific and analytical expertise necessary to support policy decision making. The proposed center could be established as an entity in its own right or as a step toward the ultimate establishment of a single, unified food safety agency.

Creation of a Single, Unified Food Safety Agency

For well over a decade, many responsible suggestions have been made that the major elements of the U.S. food safety system would be more effective and efficient if many of the core activities of multiple agencies were consolidated into a single food agency (IOM/NRC, 1998; National Commission on the Public Service, 2003; GAO, 2005b; IOM, 2009). The committee concluded that, to effect the risk-based approach and actions proposed in this report, a unified food safety agency will ultimately be essential. Such an agency would have overall authority for all aspects of the risk-based food safety system outlined in Chapter 3, from planning and data collection to policy and regulatory development, including oversight of all food safety inspections. Its functions would be supported by the centralized risk-based analysis and data management center described above; in fact, the unified entity would be responsible for this center.

Establishment of a single food safety agency would certainly be challenging. It would require reorganization of various federal agencies and buy-in from several congressional committees to facilitate changes to many food safety–related laws and regulations (IOM/NRC, 1998; GAO, 2004). Given the jurisdictional and political ramifications, an immediate and total reorganization of this magnitude probably is not feasible. Nonetheless, it is the consensus of this committee that core federal food safety responsibilities should ultimately reside within a single entity having a unified administrative structure, a clear mandate, a dedicated budget, and above all, full responsibility for oversight of the entirety of the safety of the nation's food supply.

KEY CONCLUSIONS AND RECOMMENDATIONS

The committee is confident that the recommendations offered in this report constitute a series of actions that would enhance the FDA's food programs and their ability to ensure food safety now and in the future. The committee is encouraged by changes already occurring in the FDA's food programs, such as the establishment of the Office of Foods in 2009. However, the committee has not been persuaded that the consolidation of responsibility represented by the establishment of this office will resolve issues associated with the current separation of the FDA's food safety–related enforcement and public health roles and the lack of authority of CFSAN and CVM over inspection and enforcement. In addition, food safety in the

United States today is managed by multiple government agencies, hampering the efficiency and effectiveness of the overall food safety system.

Efficiency in working toward the common goal of ensuring food safety and the public health will be greatly enhanced if the recommendations in this report are implemented in the context of the organizational changes outlined in this chapter. The committee realizes that there are many potential avenues to the evolution and implementation of those organizational changes and that there are serious barriers to overcome. Hence, the importance of in-depth analysis and planning of the implementation process cannot be overemphasized. With regard to the overall organization and functioning of the FDA, the committee makes the following recommendations.

> **Recommendation 11-1:** The committee recommends that the FDA's Office of Foods have complete authority over and responsibility for all field activities for FDA-regulated foods, including inspection, sampling, and testing of foods. Implementing this recommendation would resolve issues associated with the separation between the agency's enforcement functions and larger public health roles and responsibilities, and ensure a well-trained field workforce with specialized expertise in food safety and risk-based principles of food safety management.

> **Recommendation 11-2:** There is a compelling need to elevate and unify the nation's food safety enterprise so that the FDA and relevant sister agencies can better ensure a safe food supply. The committee recognizes that organizational change to enhance the effectiveness and efficiency of the nation's food safety system as a whole is an evolutionary process that would require careful analysis, planning, and execution. With this in mind, the committee recommends that the federal government move toward the establishment of a single food safety agency to unify the efforts of all agencies and departments with major responsibility for the safety of the U.S. food supply.

> **Recommendation 11-3:** Regardless of the evolution of the food safety system, an integrated, unimpeded, and centralized approach to risk-based analysis and data management is required to enhance the FDA's and the broader federal government's ability to ensure a safe food supply. To achieve this goal, and as a potential intermediate step toward the creation of a single food safety agency, the committee recommends the establishment of a centralized risk-based analysis and data management center. This center should be provided with the staff and supporting resources necessary to conduct rapid and sophisticated assessments of short- and long-term food safety risks and of policy interventions, and to ensure that the comprehensive data needs of the recommended

risk-based food safety management system are met. This center should be as free from external political forces and influence as possible and accountable to the public health needs and mission of the regulatory agencies.

REFERENCES

Bell, J. W. 2009. *The USFDA & Ensuring Food Safety: Perspective of a Seafood Scientist.* Paper presented at the Institute of Medicine/National Research Council Committee on Review of the FDA's Role in Ensuring Safe Food Meeting, Washington, DC, March 24, 2009.

FSWG (Food Safety Working Group). 2009a. *About FSWG.* http://www.foodsafetyworkinggroup. gov/ContentAboutFSWG/HomeAbout.htm (accessed December 07, 2009).

FSWG. 2009b. *Food Safety Working Group: Key Findings.* http://www.foodsafetyworkinggroup. gov/FSWG_Key_Findings.pdf (accessed February 18, 2010).

GAO (U.S. Government Accountability Office). 2004. *Federal Food Safety and Security System: Fundamental Restructuring Is Needed to Address Fragmentation and Overlap.* Washington, DC: GAO.

GAO. 2005a. *Oversight of Food Safety Activities: Federal Agencies Should Pursue Opportunities to Reduce Overlap and Better Leverage Resources.* Washington, DC: GAO.

GAO. 2005b. *Food Safety: Experiences of Seven Countries in Consolidating Their Food Safety Systems.* Washington, DC: GAO.

GAO. 2007. *Long-Term Fiscal Challenge: Comments on the Bipartisan Task Force for Responsible Fiscal Action Act.* Washington, DC: GAO.

GAO. 2008. *Federal Oversight of Food Safety: FDA's Food Protection Plan Proposes Positive First Steps, but Capacity to Carry Them Out Is Critical.* Washington, DC: GAO.

Givens, J. M. 2009. *Review of FDA's Role in Ensuring Safe Food (FDA's Approach to Risk Based Inspections—A Field Perspective).* Paper presented at Institute of Medicine/National Research Council Committee on Review of the FDA's Role in Ensuring Safe Food Meeting, Washington, DC, March 24, 2009.

Glavin, M. 2008. *Revitalizing ORA: Protecting the Public Health Together in a Changing World, a Report to the Commissioner.* Rockville, MD: U.S. Food and Drug Administration.

Gombas, D. E. 2009. *FDA's Role in Food Safety: A Produce Industry Perspective.* Paper presented at Institute of Medicine/National Research Council Committee on Review of the FDA's Role in Ensuring Safe Food Meeting, Washington, DC, March 24, 2009.

GUIRR/NAS (Government-University-Industry Research Roundtable of the National Academy of Sciences). 2009. *Technology Workshop on Food Safety and National Defense, September 29–30, 2009.* http://sites.nationalacademies.org/PGA/guirr/PGA_053569 (accessed April 7, 2010).

Halloran, J. 2009. *Consumer Perspectives from the Consumers Union.* Paper presented at Institute of Medicine/National Research Council Committee on Review of the FDA's Role in Ensuring Safe Food Meeting, Washington, DC, March 24, 2009.

HHS (U.S. Department of Health and Human Services). 2009. *News Release: Obama Administration Launches Food Safety Working Group.* www.hhs.gov/news, http://www.hhs. gov/news/press/2009pres/05/20090521a.html (accessed March 29, 2010).

IOM (Institute of Medicine). 2009. *HHS in the 21st Century: Charting a New Course for a Healthier America.* Washington, DC: The National Academies Press.

IOM/NRC (National Research Council). 1998. *Ensuring Safe Food: From Production to Consumption.* Washington, DC: National Academy Press.

National Commission on the Public Service. 2003. *Urgent Business for America: Revitalizing the Federal Government for the 21st Century*. Washington, DC: National Academy of Public Administration. www.uscourts.gov/newsroom/VolckerRpt.pdf (accessed March 29, 2010).

NRC (National Research Council). 1983. *Risk Assessment in the Federal Government: Managing the Process*. Washington, DC: National Academy Press.

NRC. 1996. *Understanding Risk: Informing Decisions in a Democratic Society*. Washington, DC: National Academy Press.

Osterholm, M. T. 2009. *Role of Foodborne Disease Surveillance and Food Attribution in Food Safety*. Paper presented at Institute of Medicine/National Research Council Committee on Review of the FDA's Role in Ensuring Safe Food Meeting, Washington, DC, March 24, 2009.

Plunkett, D. 2009. *Perspectives on FDA's Role in Ensuring Safe Food*. Paper presented at Institute of Medicine/National Research Council Committee on Review of the FDA's Role in Ensuring Safe Food Meeting, Washington, DC, March 24, 2009.

Scott, J. 2009. *GMA Perspective on FDA's Role in Ensuring Safe Food*. Paper presented at Institute of Medicine/National Research Council Committee on Review of the FDA's Role in Ensuring Safe Food Meeting, Washington, DC, March 24, 2009.

Solomon, S. 2009. *Regulating in the Global Environment*. Paper presented at Institute of Medicine/National Research Council Committee on Review of the FDA's Role in Ensuring Safe Food Meeting, Washington, DC, March 24, 2009.

Swann, J. P. 1993. The development of research as a recognized function of the field. In *Highlights in the History of Field Science in the FDA*. Rockville, MD: FDA History Office.

Taylor, M. R., and M. B Batz. 2008. *Harnessing Knowledge to Ensure Food Safety: Opportunities to Improve the Nation's Food Safety Information Infrastructure*. Gainesville, FL: Food Safety Research Consortium.

Taylor, M. R., and S. A. Hoffman. 2001. *Redesigning Food Safety: Using Risk Analysis to Build a Better Food Safety System*. Washington, DC: Resources for the Future.

Wagner, R. 2009. *FDA'S Current Approach to Risk Based Domestic Inspection Planning*. Paper presented at Institute of Medicine/National Research Council Committee on Review of the FDA's Role in Ensuring Safe Food Meeting, Washington, DC, March 24, 2009.

Waldrop, C. 2009. *Consumer Federation of America Perspectives on FDA's Role in Ensuring Safe Food*. Verbal testimony at Institute of Medicine/National Research Council Committee on Review of the FDA's Role in Ensuring Safe Food Meeting, Washington, DC, March 24, 2009.

Appendix A

Workshop Agendas

**Review of U.S. Food and Drug Administration's (FDA's)
Role in Ensuring Safe Food**

The Keck Center of the National Academies
Room 100
500 Fifth Street, NW
Washington, DC 20001
January 29, 2009

AGENDA

Open Session—Meeting with Sponsor—11:00 a.m. to 2:30 p.m.

11:00 a.m.	**Welcome and Introductions** *Robert Wallace, Committee Chair*
11:15 a.m.	**FDA's Perspective on the Statement of Task** *David Acheson, Associate Commissioner for Foods*
1:00 p.m.	**FDA's Perspective on the Statement of Task (continued)** *David Acheson, Associate Commissioner for Foods*

Perspectives on FDA's Role in Ensuring Safe Food

Venable LLP Conference Center
8th floor Capitol Room
575 7th Street, NW
Washington, DC 20004
March 24–25, 2009

AGENDA

March 24

8:45 a.m.   **Welcome and Purpose of Workshop**
               Robert Wallace, Committee Chair

               Session 1: FDA Organization and Responsibilities
               Moderator: Robert Wallace

8:50 a.m.   **FDA's Organization and Responsibilities**
               *Leslye Fraser, Office of Regulations, Policy, and Social
               Sciences, FDA/Center for Food Safety and Applied
               Nutrition (CFSAN)*

9:30 a.m.   **FDA's Legal Authority**
               Lars Noah, University of Florida

9:50 a.m.   **FDA's Resources**
               Joseph Levitt, Hogan & Hartson

10:10 a.m.   **Break**

10:30 a.m.   **Role of Foodborne Disease Surveillance and Food
               Attribution in Food Safety**
               *Dale Morse, Office of Science, New York State Department
               of Health*
               *Mike Osterholm, Center for Infectious Disease Research
               and Policy, University of Minnesota*
               *David Warnock, Division of Foodborne, Bacterial and
               Mycotic Diseases, Centers for Disease Control and
               Prevention*

Session 2: Approaches to Food Safety Prevention, Inspection, and Research
Moderator: Lee-Ann Jaykus

11:30 a.m.   **FDA's Approach to Risk-Based Inspections**
Steven Solomon, FDA/ORA
Roberta Wagner, Office of Compliance, FDA/CFSAN
Steven Kendall, FDA/ORA

12:30 p.m.   Lunch

1:30 p.m.   **FDA's Risk-Based Prevention**
Donald Kraemer, Office of Food Safety, FDA/CFSAN

2:00 p.m.   **Research Priorities**
Steven Musser, Office of Regulatory Science, FDA/CFSAN

2:30 p.m.   **Panel Discussion with Session 2 Speakers**

3:15 p.m.   **Break**

Session 3: Perspectives from Stakeholders
Moderator: Martha R. Roberts

3:35 p.m.   **Consumer Perspectives**
David Plunkett, Center for Science in the Public Interest
Jean Halloran, Consumers Union
Christopher Waldrop, Consumer Federation of America

4:20 p.m.   **Industry Perspectives**
Jenny Scott, Grocery Manufacturers Association
David Gombas, United Fresh Produce Association
Jon Bell, National Fisheries Institute

5:05 p.m.   **Public Comments (3-5 min each)**

5:30 p.m.   **Adjourn**

March 25

The National Academy of Sciences Building
Room 150
2101 Constitution Avenue, NW
Washington, DC 20418

1:00 p.m.   **Effective Risk-Based Approaches for Food Safety**
Bob Buchanan, University of Maryland

FDA's Role in Ensuring Safe Food

The Keck Center of the National Academies
Room K201
500 Fifth Street, NW
Washington, DC 20001
May 28, 2009

AGENDA

Open Session—8:00 a.m.–5:30 p.m.

8:00 a.m.   **Welcome and Purpose of Workshop**
Robert Wallace, Committee Chair

Session 1: Coordination of Food Defense Activities
Moderator: Robert Wallace

8:10 a.m.   **Food Defense Initiatives at FDA**
*LeeAnne Jackson, Office of Food Defense, Communication,
and Emergency Response, FDA/CFSAN*

8:30 a.m.   **Questions from Committee Members**

Session 2: FDA's Risk-Based Activities
Moderator: Lewis Grossman

9:00 a.m.   **Discussion Panel: FDA and State Inspections of Food**
FDA District Office Directors

10:00 a.m.   Break

10:15 a.m.   Anthropogenic and Natural Chemical Contaminants in
Food—Detection and Control
Philip M. Bolger, Office of Food Safety, FDA/CFSAN

10:45 a.m.   Feed and Pet Food Safety at the Center for Veterinary
Medicine
*Martine Hartogensis, Office of Surveillance and
Compliance, FDA/Center for Veterinary Medicine*

11:15 a.m.   Questions from Committee Members

12:15 p.m.   Lunch

Session 3: U.S. Department of Agriculture's (USDA's) Approach to Ensuring Food Safety
Moderator: Joseph Rodricks

1:15 p.m.   General Overview of Food Safety at Food Safety and
Insepction Service (FSIS)
*Dan Engeljohn, Office of Policy and Program
Development, USDA/FSIS*

1:50 p.m.   Proposed Risk-Based Inspection System at FSIS
*Carol Maczka, Office of Data Integration and Food
Protection, USDA/FSIS*

2:15 p.m.   Questions from Committee Members

Session 4: Safety of Imported Foods
Moderator: Tim Jones

2:45 p.m.   USDA Model to Ensure Safety of Imported Foods
*Phil Derfler, Office of Policy and Program Development,
USDA/FSIS*

3:05 p.m.   Break

3:25 p.m.   **European Union Model and Third-Party Certifications for Food Safety**
              Wolf Maier, European Commission

3:45 p.m.   **Ensuring Food Safety of Food Imports**
              Caroline Smith DeWaal, Center for Science in the Public Interest

4:05 p.m.   **Ensuring Food Safety at the Border**
              Cathy Sauceda, U.S. Department of Homeland Security/ Customs and Border Protection

4:25 p.m.   **Perspective from the Industry**
              Steve Mavity, Bumble Bee Foods, LLC

4:45 p.m.   **Questions from Committee Members**

5:30 p.m.   **Meeting Adjourned**

Appendixes B–G are not printed in this book.
They are available on the CD in the back of this book.

Appendix H

Glossary

Agreement on Sanitary and Phytosanitary Measures (SPS Agreement) Agreement concerning the application of food safety and animal and plant health regulations as established by the World Trade Organization in 1995. Under these agreements, countries can set their own standards for safety as long as they are based on science.

Appropriate level of protection A way to express, on a population level, what level of risk a society is prepared to tolerate or considers to be achievable to protect human, animal, or plant life or health within its territory.

Biologics/biological products A wide range of products including vaccines, blood and blood components, allergenics, somatic cells, gene therapy, tissues, and recombinant therapeutic proteins. These products are regulated by the U.S. Food and Drug Administration (FDA).

Biomolecule Any molecule that is involved in the maintenance and metabolic processes of living organisms. Biomolecules include carbohydrate, lipid, protein, nucleic acid, and water molecules.

Biosecurity A strategic and integrated approach that encompasses the policy and regulatory frameworks (including instruments and activities) used in analyzing and managing risks in the sectors of food safety, animal life and health, and plant life and health, including associated environmental risk. Biosecurity covers the introduction of plant pests, animal pests and diseases, and zoonoses; the introduction and release of genetically modified organisms and their products; and the introduction and management of invasive alien species and genotypes.

Bioterrorism The intentional release of viruses, bacteria, or other agents used to cause illness or death in people, animals, or plants.

Bottom-up data Data that model the path of pathogens from their source through the food supply chain to health outcomes.

CARVER+Shock A risk assessment tool that enables users to conduct assessments of the risks of, and vulnerabilities to, intentional contamination of a food production and distribution process. Its use by the food and agriculture sector and government agencies originates in its use by military special operations forces. The acronym stands for Criticality, Accessibility, Recuperability, Vulnerability, Effect, and Recognizability, which are the factors considered in assessing risk and vulnerability.

Class I recall A situation in which there is a reasonable probability that the use of, or exposure to, a violative product will cause serious adverse health consequences or death.

Classified information According to U.S. Code Title 18, any information or material that has been determined by the U.S. Government—pursuant to an executive order, statute, or regulation—to require protection against unauthorized disclosure for reasons of national security, and any restricted data, as defined in the Atomic Energy Act of 1954.

Cooperative Extension System A network of nationwide offices staffed by one or more experts who provide useful, practical, and research-based information to agricultural producers, small business owners, youth, consumers, and others in rural areas and communities of all sizes.

Decision analysis An applied branch of decision theory that offers individuals and organizations a methodology for making decisions; it also offers techniques for modeling decision problems mathematically and determining optimal decisions numerically. Decision models have the capacity for accepting and quantifying human subjective inputs, including judgments of experts and preferences of decision makers. Implementation of these models can take various forms ranging from simple paper-and-pencil procedures to sophisticated computer programs known as decision aids or decision systems.

Detention without physical examination (DWPE) An enforcement mechanism by which the FDA can detain shipments of imported products without having to actually analyze those shipments.

Electronic Foodborne Outbreak Reporting System (eFORS) A web-based reporting system used by the U.S. Centers for Disease Control and Prevention (CDC) to collect basic summary data from states on all reported foodborne illness outbreaks.

Electronic Laboratory Exchange Network (eLEXNET) A web-based information network that allows comparison of laboratory analysis findings and serves as a warning system for potentially hazardous foods.

Embargo authority When referring to food, the authority to issue and enforce a stop sale, stop use, removal, or hold for a food or processing equipment when there is probable cause to believe that it is dangerous, unwholesome, fraudulent, or insanitary.

Enterprise architecture A blueprint for organizational change and a foundation for information technology management, describing the current operation of an organization, how it intends to operate in the future, and how it plans to reach these goals.

Entry line Each portion of an import shipment that is listed as a separate item on an entry document. Items in an import entry having different tariff descriptions must be listed separately.

Epidemiology The study of the occurrence, distribution, and determining factors associated with the health and diseases of a population; the study of how often health events or diseases occur in different groups and why.

Etiology The cause or origin of a disease.

Food contaminant A substance that may be present in foods as a result of environmental contamination, cultivation practices, or production processes. If present above certain levels, these substances can pose a threat to human health. Some contaminants are formed naturally; carried over to food from water, air, or soil; or created as a by-product of the food production process itself.

Food defense A collective term used by agencies including the FDA, the U.S. Department of Agriculture (USDA), and the U.S. Department of Homeland Security to denote activities associated with protecting the nation's food supply from deliberate or intentional acts of contamination or tampering. The term encompasses other similar verbiage, such as counterterrorism.

Food Protection Plan A plan issued by the FDA in 2007 to lay out the agency's integrated strategy for food safety and food defense. The three core elements of the plan are prevention, intervention, and response.

Food safety risk The likelihood of harm to health resulting from exposure to hazardous agents in the food supply.

Food Safety Working Group (FSWG) A group created by President Obama in 2009 to advise him on how to upgrade the U.S. food safety system. It is chaired by the Secretaries of the U.S. Department of Health and Human Services and USDA.

Foodborne illness An illness, usually either infectious or toxic in nature, caused by an agent that enters the body through the ingestion of food.

FoodNet A collaborative project of CDC, USDA, the FDA, and 10 Emerging Infections Program sites. It consists of active surveillance for foodborne illnesses and related epidemiologic studies designed to help public health officials better understand the epidemiology of foodborne illnesses in the United States.

FoodSHIELD A web-based platform whose mission is to support federal, state, and local regulatory agencies and laboratories in defending the food supply through web-based tools that enhance threat prevention and response, risk management, communication and asset coordination, and public education.

Functional genomics The study of genes, their resulting proteins, and the role played by the proteins in the body's biochemical processes.

Hazard A biological, chemical, or physical agent in or condition of food with the potential to cause an adverse health effect.

Hazard Analysis and Critical Control Points (HACCP) A production control system for the food industry. It is a process that identifies where potential contamination can occur (the critical control points) and strictly manages and monitors these points as a way of ensuring that the process is under control and that the safest possible product is being produced. HACCP is designed to prevent rather than detect potential hazards.

Information science The collection, organization, storage, retrieval, exchange, interpretation, and use of information.

iRISK A web-based risk-ranking prototype used to compare microbial and chemical hazards to support risk management decisions.

Iterative approach The repetition of a numerical or non-numerical process whereby the results from one or more stages are used to form the input to the next stage. Generally the recycling of the process continues until some preset goal is achieved, or the process result is constantly repeated.

Melamine A synthetic chemical with a variety of industrial uses, including the production of resins and foams, cleaning products, fertilizers, and pesticides. If ingested in sufficient amounts, melamine can result in kidney failure and death.

Memorandum of understanding (MOU) A document outlining the terms and details of an agreement between parties, including each party's requirements and responsibilities.

Metabolomics The science of measurement and analysis of metabolites, such as sugars and fats, in the cells of organisms at specific times and under specific conditions. The field of metabolomics overlaps with biology, chemistry, mathematics, and computer science.

Molecular surveillance Combines the methods of molecular biology with those of epidemiology in an effort to identify exposure to foodborne pathogens and subsequent disease. The use of molecular biology makes it possible to conduct pathogen surveillance at a genetic level and to determine the associations between contamination and disease when they are separated in space or time. PulseNet and VetNet are examples of molecular surveillance systems.

Multiple criteria decision analysis (MCDA) An approach used to systematically structure and model decision problems in multiple dimensions, with the goal of achieving a well-considered and -justified decision, and to provide a transparent explanation of the decision's basis.

Operational risk management A management approach used by the Departments of Defense and Transportation to identify risks and reduce them to an appropriate level, ensuring that benefits outweigh any risks.

OutbreakNet A network of foodborne disease epidemiologists from all states and CDC that works to improve communication among these partners.

Pathogen An agent causing disease or illness to its host, such as an organism or infectious particle capable of producing disease in another organism.

Phototoxicology Assessment of the toxic and/or carcinogenic potential of chemicals and agents when exposed to light or when applied to photo-treated skin.

Postmarket enforcement A process by which a regulatory agency determines the safety of a product only after it has entered into commerce. For example, manufacturers of foods and cosmetics in the United States generally do not have to submit evidence of safety to the FDA or obtain approval from the agency before putting their products on the market. If the FDA determines that a product is unsafe after it is on the market, the agency may take enforcement action against the product, but in any formal enforcement action, the burden is on the FDA to establish that the product in question is unsafe.

PREDICT (Predictive Risk-Based Evaluation for Dynamic Import Compliance Targeting) A screening tool that will automate decisions currently made by import entry reviewers by utilizing intelligence information from numerous sources. PREDICT will target higher-risk shipments for examination and will expedite the clearance of lower-risk cargo if accurate and complete data are provided by importers and entry filers.

Premarket Approval A process by which a regulatory agency determines whether a product is safe for the public before permitting it to enter into commerce. For example, manufacturers of food and color additives may put a product into commerce in the United States only if the FDA has already determined that the product in question is safe and has approved it for sale. In any formal enforcement action against an unapproved product, the FDA does not have to establish that the product in question is unsafe; rather, the agency will prevail simply by showing that the product has not received the requisite premarket approval.

Prior notice A requirement of the Bioterrorism Act of 2002 that the FDA receive advance notice of food to be imported into the United States before the food arrives.

Protected Critical Infrastructure Information (PCII) program A program established pursuant to the Critical Infrastructure Information Act of 2002 that provides a means for sharing private-sector information with the government while providing assurance that the information will be exempt from public disclosure and will be properly safeguarded.

Proteomics The large-scale study of proteins, particularly their structures and functions.

PulseNet A national network of federal, state, and local laboratories coordinated by CDC that uses standardized collection and sharing of pulsed-field gel electrophoresis (PFGE) molecular subtyping data to link isolates obtained from diverse sources. PulseNet allows scientists at public health laboratories throughout the country to rapidly compare the PFGE patterns of bacteria isolated from ill persons and determine whether those bacteria are similar.

Risk The possibility or probability of loss, injury, disadvantage, or destruction.

Risk analysis A transparent means by which to link the nature and extent of public health protection (risk reduction) achieved as a result of different risk management actions (or interventions). Risk analysis is composed of three activities: (1) risk assessment, (2) risk management, and (3) risk communication.

Risk assessment A process that provides information on the extent and characteristics of the risk attributed to a hazard.

Risk communication The exchange of information and opinions concerning risk and risk-related factors among risk assessors, risk managers, and other interested parties, stakeholders, and the public. In this report, risk communication is applicable when the message is directly related to specific risks (or benefits) of certain behaviors.

Risk management The activities undertaken to control risk.

Risk prioritization A multifactorial approach to ranking risks that considers a wide range of factors (in addition to public health) that might influence prioritization or decision making. Risk prioritization uses tools of both risk assessment and decision analysis to determine the importance of one risk over another, usually in relationship to mitigation. Risk prioritization is inherently used as a risk management tool.

Risk ranking A special form of risk assessment whose purpose is to compare hazards, commodities, or hazard–commodity pairs with respect to their degree of risk relative to one another.

Risk-based food safety system A systematic means by which to facilitate decision making to reduce public health risk in light of limited resources and additional factors that may be considered.

Sunshine laws State and federal statutes requiring that government meetings, decisions, and records be made available to the public.

Surveillance A key component of epidemiology, it can be defined as the ongoing collection, analysis, interpretation, and dissemination of health-related data. Surveillance is one of a number of methods used by epidemiologists to gather information on a disease.

Top-down data Surveillance-based data, such as epidemiological data on illnesses and deaths.

Toxicoinformatics Analysis and integration of genomic, transcriptomic, proteomic, and metabolomic databases with the objective of knowledge discovery and the elucidation of mechanisms of toxicity.

Traceability In the food arena, the ability to trace the history, application, or location of a food under consideration.

Trace-back/trace-forward activities In the food arena, activities performed to determine the origin (trace-back) or distribution (trace-forward) of a product, usually to identify contaminated food. The activities are conducted jointly with local health departments and appropriate federal agencies. They entail the review and analysis of records such as harvesting dates, specific field and product locations, number of packages within a lot, and packing and shipping dates.

User fee A charge for the use of a particular good or service, for example, an entrance fee to a state park or the rental of equipment at a pubic facility. Many government-operated facilities are financed by both tax revenues and user fees.

Viral communications/marketing Use of social networking to rapidly diffuse ideas, marketing campaigns, or other messages.

Zoonotic disease A disease of animals that may be transmitted to humans under natural conditions (e.g., brucellosis, rabies).

Appendix I

Acronyms and Abbreviations

ABI	Automated Broker Interface
ACS	Automated Commercial System
AF	acidified food
AFDO	Association of Food and Drug Officials
AFSS	Animal Feed Safety System
AIDS	acquired immune deficiency syndrome
ALERT	Assure, Look, Employees, Report, Threat
AMS	Agricultural Marketing Service (USDA)
APEC	Asia-Pacific Economic Cooperation
APFSL	Agricultural Products Food Safety Laboratory
APHIS	Animal and Plant Health Inspection Service (USDA)
APHL	Association of Public Health Laboratories
AQIS	Australian Quarantine and Inspection Service
ARS	Agricultural Research Service (USDA)
ASTHO	Association of State and Territorial Health Officials
AVMA	American Veterinary Medical Association
BATF	Bureau of Alcohol, Tobacco, and Firearms (USDOT)
BRC	British Research Consortium
BSE	bovine spongiform encephalopathy
BSL	biosafety level
CAERS	CFSAN Adverse Events Reporting System
CBP	U.S. Customs and Border Protection (DHS)
CDC	U.S. Centers for Disease Control and Prevention

CFI	Center for Foodborne Illness Research and Prevention
CFIA	Canadian Food Inspection Agency
CFR	Code of Federal Regulations
CFSAN	Center for Food Safety and Applied Nutrition (FDA)
CFU	colony forming units
CGMP	current good manufacturing practice
CHB	Customs House Broke
CIA	Central Intelligence Agency
CIFOR	Council to Improve Foodborne Outbreak Response
CIKR	Critical infrastructure and key resources
CRC	CFSAN Review Committee
CSPI	Center for Science in the Public Interest
CU	Consumers Union
CVM	Center for Veterinary Medicine (FDA)
DG SANCO	Directorate General for Health and Consumers (European Commission)
DHS	U.S. Department of Homeland Security
DLC	dioxin-like compound
DNA	deoxyribonucleic acid
DoC	U.S. Department of Commerce
DoD	U.S. Department of Defense
DoI	U.S. Department of the Interior
DOJ	U.S. Department of Justice
DVFA	Danish Veterinary and Food Administration
EFSA	European Food Safety Authority
EHR	electronic health record
EHS-NET	Environmental Health Specialists Network
eLEXNET	electronic Laboratory Exchange Network (FDA)
EPA	U.S. Environmental Protection Agency
Epi-X	Epidemic Information Exchange
ERS	Economic Research Service (USDA)
EU	European Union
FAO	Food and Agriculture Organization
FASCAT	Food and Agriculture Sector Criticality Assessment Tool
FASCC	Food and Agriculture Sector Coordinating Council
FBI	Federal Bureau of Investigation
FDA	U.S. Food and Drug Administration
FDAAA	Food and Drug Administration Amendments Act of 2007
FDCA	Federal Food, Drug, and Cosmetic Act
FEMA	Federal Emergency Management Agency (DHS)

FERN	Food Emergency Response Network
FMI	Food Marketing Institute
FMIA	Federal Meat Inspection Act
FNB	Food and Nutrition Board
FOIA	Freedom of Information Act
FoodNet	Foodborne Diseases Active Surveillance Network
FOUO	For Official Use Only
FPP	Food Protection Plan
FSA	Food Standards Agency (United Kingdom)
FSANZ	Food Standards Australia New Zealand
FSIC	Food Safety Information Council
FSII	Food Safety Information Infrastructure
FSIS	Food Safety and Inspection Service (USDA)
FSLC	Food Safety Leadership Council
FSQS	Food Safety and Quality Service
FSWG	Food Safety Working Group
FTC	Federal Trade Commission
FTE	full-time equivalent/employee
FVO	Food and Veterinary Office (European Union)
FWS	Fish and Wildlife Service (DoI)
FY	fiscal year
GAO	U.S. Government Accountability Office (previously U.S. General Accounting Office)
GAP	Good Agricultural Practice
GAqP	Good Aquacultural Practice
GATT	General Agreement on Tariffs and Trade
GCC	Government Coordinating Council
GC-MS	Gas chromatography-mass spectrometry
GFSI	Global Food Safety Initiative
GIP	Good Importer Practice
GIPSA	Grain Inspection, Packers, and Stockyards Administration (USDA)
GMA	Grocery Manufacturers Association
GMP	Good Manufacturing Practice
GPRA	Government Performance and Results Act
GRAS	generally recognized as safe
HACCP	Hazard Analysis and Critical Control Points
HC	Health Canada
HHS	U.S. Department of Health and Human Services
HIPAA	Health Insurance Portability and Accountability Act
HIV	human immunodeficiency virus

HSIN	Homeland Security Information Network
HSPD	Homeland Security Presidential Directive
IAC	Intertribal Agriculture Council
IEC	International Electrotechnical Commission
IFSS	Integrated Food Safety System
IFT	Institute of Food Technologists
IIT	Illinois Institute of Technology
IOM	Institute of Medicine
IRAC	Interagency Risk Assessment Consortium
IRB	Institutional Review Board
ISO	International Organization for Standardization
IT	information technology
JIFSAN	Joint Institute for Food Safety and Applied Nutrition
LACF	low-acid canned foods
LM	*Listeria monocytogenes*
MARCS	Mission Activity Reporting Compliance System
MCDA	multiple criteria decision analysis
MDP	Microbiological Data Program
MDVP	Methods Development and Validation Program
MHS	Meat Hygiene Service (United Kingdom Food Standards Agency)
MID	Manufacturer Identification
MOU	memorandum of understanding
NACCHO	National Association of County and City Health Officials
NAL	National Agricultural Library (USDA)
NARMS	National Antimicrobial Resistance Monitoring System
NASS	National Agricultural Statistics Service (USDA)
NCFPD	National Center for Food Protection and Defense (DHS)
NCFST	National Center for Food Safety and Technology
NCNPR	National Center for Natural Products Research
NCTR	National Center for Toxicological Research (FDA)
NEHA	National Environmental Health Association
NGO	nongovernmental organization
NIFA	National Institute of Food and Agriculture (USDA)
NIH	National Institutes of Health
NIMS	National Incident Management System
NIPP	National Infrastructure Protection Plan
NLEA	Nutrition Labeling and Education Act

NMFS	National Marine Fisheries Service (DoC)
NOAA	National Oceanic and Atmospheric Administration (DoC)
NORS	National Outbreak Reporting System
NRC	National Research Council or Nuclear Regulatory Commission
NRP	National Response Plan
NZFSA	New Zealand Food Safety Authority
OASIS	Operational and Administrative System for Import Support
OCI	Office of Criminal Investigations (FDA)
OCM	Office of Crisis Management (FDA)
OECA	Office of Enforcement and Compliance Assistance (EPA)
OHA	Office of Health Affairs (DHS)
OMB	Office of Management and Budget
OPA	Office of Public Affairs (FDA)
OPHEP	Office of Public Health Emergency Preparedness
OPPTS	Office of Prevention, Pesticides and Toxic Substances (EPA)
OR	Office of Research (CVM)
ORA	Office of Regulatory Affairs (FDA)
ORACBA	Office of Risk Assessment and Cost-Benefit Analysis (USDA)
ORAU	Office of Regulatory Affairs University
ORD	Office of Research and Development (EPA)
ORM	operational risk management
PART	Program Assessment Rating Tool
PCII	Protected Critical Infrastructure Information
PCR	polymerase chain reaction
PCT	Pesticide Coordination Team
PDP	Pesticide Data Program (USDA)
PFGE	pulsed-field gel electrophoresis
PFSE	Partnership for Food Safety Education
PN	prior notice
PNC	Prior Notice Center
PRA	Paperwork Reduction Act
PREDICT	Predictive Risk-Based Evaluation for Dynamic Import Compliance Targeting
PulseNet	National Molecular Subtyping Network for Foodborne Disease Surveillance
RACT	Risk Assessment Coordination Team
RCAC	Risk Communication Advisory Committee (FDA)

RIHSC	Research Involving Human Subjects Committee
RMF	risk management framework
SAHCDHA	serious adverse health consequences or death to humans or animals
SCC	Sector Coordinating Council
SEB	*Staphylococcal enterotoxin B*
SPPA	Strategic Partnership Program Agroterrorism
SPS	Sanitary and Phytosanitary
SQF	Safe Quality Food
SSA	Sector-Specific Agency
SSP	Sector-Specific Plan
TBT	Technical Barriers to Trade
TDS	Total Diet Study
UF	University of Florida
UK	United Kingdom
UMB	University of Maryland, Baltimore
USDA	U.S. Department of Agriculture
USDOT	U.S. Department of Treasury
WCFS	Western Center for Food Safety
WCL	Washington College of Law
WHO	World Health Organization
WIC	Special Supplemental Nutrition Program for Women, Infants, and Children
WIFSS	Western Institute for Food Safety and Security
WTO	World Trade Organization

Appendix J

Committee Member
Biographical Sketches

ROBERT B. WALLACE, M.D. (*Chair*), is Irene Ensminger Stecher Professor of Epidemiology and Internal Medicine at the University of Iowa Colleges of Public Health and Medicine and Director of the University's Center on Aging. He has been a member of the U.S. Preventive Services Task Force and the National Advisory Council on Aging of the National Institutes of Health. He is a Member of the Institute of Medicine (IOM), past Chair of the IOM's Board on Health Promotion and Disease Prevention, and current Chair of the IOM's Board on the Health of Select Populations. His research interests are in clinical and population epidemiology and focus on the causes and prevention of disabling conditions of older persons. Dr. Wallace has had substantial experience in the conduct of both observational cohort studies of older persons and clinical trials, including preventive interventions related to fracture, cancer, coronary disease, and women's health. He is the site principal investigator for the Women's Health Initiative, a national intervention trial exploring the prevention of breast and colon cancer and coronary disease, and a co-principal investigator of the Health and Retirement Study, a national cohort study of the health and economic status of older Americans. He has been a collaborator in several international studies of the causes and prevention of chronic illness in older persons. Dr. Wallace received his B.S. and M.D. from Northwestern University and M.Sc. in epidemiology from the State University of New York at Buffalo.

DOUGLAS L. ARCHER, Ph.D., is Associate Dean for Research at the Institute of Food and Agricultural Sciences and a Professor in the Food Science and Human Nutrition Department at the University of Florida (UF). He served as Chair of the department until 2001, when he stepped down to return to the faculty. Prior to his arrival at UF, Dr. Archer served as Deputy Director of the U.S. Food and Drug Administration's (FDA's) Center for Food Safety and Applied Nutrition (CFSAN), where he was charged with oversight of the research, regulatory, and policy activities of all food and cosmetic programs, including food additives, food labeling, special nutritionals, seafood, and cosmetics and colors. During his career with the FDA, Dr. Archer was a Commissioned Officer in the United States Public Health Service. He was appointed Assistant Surgeon General in 1990. He has received numerous awards, including three Meritorious Service Medals and the Distinguished Service Medal. His nongovernment awards include the J.C. Frazier Memorial Award from the University of Wisconsin in 1992 and the Ivan Parkin Lectureship in 2005 from the International Association for Food Protection. From 1984 until 1994, Dr. Archer served as Chairman of the Food and Agriculture Organization (FAO)/World Health Organization (WHO) Codex Alimentarius Committee on Food Hygiene, and since 1990, has been a member of the WHO Expert Advisory Panel on Food Safety. He is past U.S. Associate Editor for *Food Control* (and is currently an Editorial Board member) and member of the Advisory Board of the Academic Press Nutrition and Food Science Publications. He is a professional member of the Institute of Food Technologists (IFT) and serves on the Board of Directors of that organization. Dr. Archer is currently a member of the IFT Global Policy and Regulations Committee and is the subject expert for that committee on food hygiene. He has authored or co-authored more than 80 peer-reviewed scientific publications and given hundreds of presentations to scientific organizations, trade organizations, and consumer groups. Dr. Archer received a B.A. in zoology, an M.S. in bacteriology from the University of Maine, and a Ph.D. in microbiology from the University of Maryland.

KEITH C. BEHNKE, Ph.D., is Professor and Feed Technology Research Scientist in the Department of Grain Science and Industry at Kansas State University, where he has been a member of the faculty since 1977. He currently coordinates all feed-processing research and the production of all research feeds manufactured by the Department of Grain Science at Kansas State University. Dr. Behnke's research areas of interest are the effect of feed processing on animal and feed performance, the incorporation of feed additives into livestock feeds, and the utilization of food and nonfood coproducts in livestock feeds. Prior to his position at Kansas State University, he was Group Leader in Processing Research of the Food Division of Far Mar, Co., in Hutchison, Kansas. In 2007, Dr. Behnke was 1 of 15 invited attendees from around the world to the FAO/WHO Expert Meeting on Animal

Feed Impact on Food Safety. He is currently a member of several professional societies and associations, including the American Society of Animal Science, the Poultry Science Association, the American Feed Industry Association, and the Chinese Feed Manufacturing Association, of which he is an honorary member. Dr. Behnke served on the National Research Council's (NRC's) Committee on the Nutrient Requirements of Dogs and Cats. He received his B.S. in feed technology (1968), his M.S. in grain science (1973), and his Ph.D. in grain science (1975) from Kansas State University.

ANN BOSTROM, Ph.D., is Professor and Associate Dean of Research at the Evans School of the University of Washington, where she has been a member of the faculty since 2007. Her research focuses on risk perception, communication, and management and on environmental policy and decision making under uncertainty. Dr. Bostrom previously served on the faculty at the Georgia Institute of Technology from 1992 to 2007, serving most recently as Associate Dean for Research at the Ivan Allen College of Liberal Arts and Professor in the School of Public Policy. She co-directed the Decision Risk and Management Science Program at the National Science Foundation from 1999 to 2001. Dr. Bostrom is currently Associate Editor or Risk Communication Area Editor for *Risk Analysis*, the *Journal of Risk Research*, and *Human and Ecological Risk Assessment*. She has served on various science advisory and NRC and IOM committees, including the IOM Committee on Nutrient Relationships in Seafood: Selections to Balance Benefits and Risks and the NRC Committee on Review of the Tsunami Warning and Forecast System and Overview of the Nation's Tsunami Preparedness. She is a Fellow of the Society for Risk Analysis and the recipient of several awards and fellowships, including an American Statistical Association/National Science Foundation/Bureau of Labor Statistics Research Associateship for the 1991–1992 academic year and the 1997 Chauncey Starr award for a young risk analyst from the Society for Risk Analysis for her work on mental models of hazardous processes. Dr. Bostrom completed postdoctoral studies in engineering and public policy and her Ph.D. in public policy analysis at Carnegie Mellon University, and she holds an M.B.A. from Western Washington University and a B.A. in English from the University of Washington.

ROBERT E. BRACKETT, Ph.D., is Director and Vice President of National Center for Food Safety and Technology at Illinois Institute of Technology (IIT). Prior to his position at IIT, he was Senior Vice President and Chief Scientific and Regulatory Affairs Officer at the Grocery Manufacturers Association (GMA). As Chief Scientific and Regulatory Affairs Officer, Dr. Brackett oversaw all of the association's scientific and regulatory activity, including the operation of its in-house food safety laboratory. Prior to

GMA, he was Director of CFSAN. Dr. Brackett has served elected leadership positions in several professional associations and is a Fellow of the American Academy of Microbiology and the International Association for Food Protection. He serves on the Advisory Boards of the National Center for Food Protection and Defense, the National Center for Food Safety and Technology, Association of Analytical Comunities International, and the Food and Drug Law Institute. Dr. Brackett has won numerous awards, among them the CFSAN Leadership Award for his exceptional contribution in ensuring a "real world" perspective on the risk assessment of *Listeria monocytogenes* and the President's Appreciation Award, International Association for Food Protection, in July 2007. He has been a member of the IOM/Food and Nutrition Board (FNB) Food Forum. Dr. Brackett received his B.S. in bacteriology and his M.S. and Ph.D. in food microbiology, all from the University of Wisconsin.

JULIE A. CASWELL, Ph.D., is Professor and Chair of the Department of Resource Economics at the University of Massachusetts, Amherst. Her research interests include the operation of domestic and international food systems, analysis of food system efficiency, and evaluation of government policy as it affects systems operation and performance, with a particular focus on the economics of food quality, safety, and nutrition. Dr. Caswell has provided her expertise on food safety and labeling issues to the Organization for Economic Cooperation and Development and to FAO. She has held numerous senior positions with the Agricultural and Applied Economics Association and the Northeastern Agricultural and Resource Economics Association. Dr. Caswell has served on IOM committees including the Planning Committee on Future Trends in Food Safety: Changing Market Forces, Emerging Safety Issues, and Economic Impact (a workshop); the Committee on Implications of Dioxin in the Food Supply; and the Committee on Nutrient Relationships in Seafood: Selections to Balance Benefits and Risks. She is currently a member of the Food Forum. She held a Fulbright Distinguished Lectureship at the University of Tuscia in Viterbo, Italy, from April–June 2009. She received her Ph.D. in agricultural economics from the University of Wisconsin.

LEWIS A. GROSSMAN, Ph.D., J.D., is Professor of Law and Associate Dean for Scholarship at American University. He joined the faculty of Washington College of Law (WCL) at American University in 1997. He became Professor of Law in 2003 and Associate Dean for Scholarship in 2008. He teaches and specializes in food and drug law, civil procedure, and American legal history. Prior to joining the faculty of WCL, Dr. Grossman was an associate at the DC firm of Covington and Burling, where he is still employed on an "of counsel" basis and is a member of the food and drug law practice group. Previously, he was clerk for Chief Judge Abner Mikva, U.S. Court of Appeals, D.C. Circuit. Dr. Grossman is co-author (with Peter Barton Hutt and Richard A. Merrill) of *Food and Drug Law: Cases and Materials*, 3rd ed. (Foundation Press, 2007). He is a member of the Food and Drug Law Institute, the American Society for Legal History, and the Supreme Court Historical Society. He has volunteered as a legal consultant for the IOM and NRC Committee on the Framework for Evaluating the Safety of Dietary Supplements. He earned his Ph.D. in history at Yale University, his J.D. at Harvard Law School, and his B.A. at Yale University.

LEE-ANN JAYKUS, Ph.D., is Professor in the Department of Food, Bioprocessing, and Nutritional Sciences and the Department of Microbiology at North Carolina State University. Her current research efforts are varied and include the following: development of molecular methods to detect foodborne pathogens (noroviruses, hepatitis A virus, and bacterial agents such as *Campylobacter* and *Salmonella*) in foods, including pre-analytical sample processing; investigation of persistence and transfer of pathogens in the food preparation environment; and the application of quantitative microbial risk assessment methods to food safety. Dr. Jaykus has collaborated on large, multi-institutional projects to investigate the prevalence and association of pathogens with domestic and imported fresh produce and to study the ecology of the pathogenic *Vibrio* species in molluscan shellfish originating from the Gulf of Mexico. Her professional memberships include the International Association for Food Protection (currently serving as President-Elect), the American Society for Microbiology, the IFT, the Council for Agricultural Science and Technology, and the Society for Risk Analysis. Dr. Jaykus recently completed a 6-year term as a member of the National Advisory Committee on Microbiological Criteria for Foods, and currently is a member of the NRC/IOM Standing Committee for the Review of Food Safety and Defense Risk Assessments, Analyses, and Data and the Committee for Review of the Food Safety and Inspection Service (FSIS) Risk-Based Approach to Public Health Attribution. She earned a Ph.D. in Environmental Sciences and Engineering from the University of North Carolina at Chapel Hill School of Public Health.

TIMOTHY F. JONES, M.D., is State Epidemiologist and Director of the FoodNet Program at the Tennessee Department of Health. In this position, he has been intimately involved in investigating foodborne disease outbreaks. Dr. Jones is nationally active in leading the FoodNet Outbreak Working Group, co-chairing the multiagency Council to Improve Foodborne Disease Outbreak Response, and serving as the liaison between the FDA and the Council of State and Territorial Epidemiologists. Formerly, he practiced medicine in Utah and then joined the U.S. Centers for Disease Control and Prevention's (CDC's) Epidemic Intelligence Service in Tennessee. Dr. Jones has served as a consultant for WHO on foodborne disease issues. He has also been the Council of State and Territorial Epidemiologists's representative to the Association of State and Territorial Health Officials's Food Safety Committee and a participant in Trust for America's Health and Food Safety Research Consortium projects. Dr. Jones is an Associate Editor for the journal *Foodborne Pathogens and Disease*, and has produced over 100 publications and 110 posters and professional presentations. He obtained his M.D. from Stanford University and completed a residency in family medicine at Brown University.

BARBARA KOWALCYK, M.S., is Director of Food Safety at the Center for Foodborne Illness Research and Prevention (CFI). A biostatistician, she became involved in foodborne illness prevention in 2001 following the death of her 2½ year old son, Kevin, from complications due to an *E. coli* O157:H7 infection. Ms. Kowalcyk has volunteered extensively as a consumer advocate for food safety and co-founded CFI in 2006. In addition, she served on the U.S. Department of Agriculture's (USDA's) National Advisory Committee on Microbiological Criteria for Foods from 2005 to 2009 and serves on the Advisory Board for the Georgetown University Health Policy Institute's Produce Safety Project. Ms. Kowalcyk has given numerous presentations on food safety. In addition to her extensive experience in food safety advocacy, she has more than 10 years of experience as a biostatistician conducting clinical research in the pharmaceutical industry. She serves on the NRC Standing Committee on the Use of Public Health Data in FSIS Food Safety Programs. Ms. Kowalcyk earned her B.S. in mathematics from the University of Dayton and her M.S. in applied statistics from the University of Pittsburgh. She is currently pursuing a doctorate in environmental health with a focus in epidemiology/biostatistics at the University of Cincinnati and is a fellow in the Molecular Epidemiology in Children's Environmental Health Training Program.

J. GLENN MORRIS, Jr., M.D., M.P.H.&T.M., is Director of the Emerging Pathogens Institute at the University of Florida, Gainesville, and Professor of Medicine in the College of Medicine. Prior to assuming his current position, he served as Chairman of the Department of Epidemiology and Preventive Medicine at the University of Maryland School of Medicine, Baltimore (UMB), and interim Dean of the UMB School of Public Health. Dr. Morris was an Epidemic Intelligence Service officer at CDC, with responsibility for national foodborne disease surveillance. He played a key role in the development of the Pathogen Reduction/Hazard Analysis and Critical Control Points regulations at USDA/FSIS, where he also created and served as Director of the FSIS Epidemiology and Emergency Response Program. He was instrumental in the creation of FoodNet while at USDA, and subsequently served as co-principal investigator of the Maryland FoodNet site. Dr. Morris maintains an active research program in the area of emerging pathogens and enteric diseases. He also has extensive experience in work with antimicrobial resistance and has served as a member of the National Advisory Committee on Microbiological Criteria for Food. Dr. Morris has authored more than 60 textbook chapters and symposium proceedings and more than 180 articles in peer-reviewed journals. His scholarly contributions were recognized by his election to the American Society for Clinical Investigation in 1996. He has served as a member or consultant on a series of National Academies expert committees dealing with food safety, including the Committee on the Public Health Risk Assessment of Poultry Inspection Programs (member), Committee on the Evaluation of Safety of Fishery Products (member), Committee on Evaluation of USDA Streamlined Inspection System for Cattle (consultant), Committee on Review of the Use of Scientific Criteria and Performance Standards for Safe Food (consultant), and Planning Committee on Foodborne Diseases and Public Health: An Iranian-American Workshop (member). He was also an advisor to the Subcommittee for the Review of FDA Science, FDA Science Board. Dr. Morris is currently a member of the FNB. He received his B.A. from Rice University in Houston and his M.D. and master's in public health and tropical medicine from Tulane University. His residency training in internal medicine was at the University of Texas Southwestern in Dallas and Emory University in Atlanta, with subspecialty training in infectious diseases at the University of Maryland.

MARTHA RHODES ROBERTS, Ph.D., is Special Assistant to the Director of the Florida Experiment Station and Dean for Research, UF, Institute of Food and Agricultural Sciences. She was formerly Deputy Commissioner of Agriculture at the Florida Department of Agriculture and Consumer Services and Assistant Commissioner of Agriculture (she was the first woman in the United States to hold this position). Dr. Roberts is a recipient of numerous awards, including the FDA Commissioner's Special Citation in May 2003 for outstanding leadership and cooperative support of joint regulatory responsibilities in advancing food safety and enhancing the public health mandate and the USDA Animal and Plant Health Inspection Service Administrator of the Year Award in 2003. She has received numerous awards from government and industry and serves on many committees regarding produce safety and agricultural and food policy. She was inducted into the Florida Agricultural Hall of Fame in 2003. Dr. Roberts' previous positions include Chairman of the 48-party Suwannee River Partnership; Co-chair of the Agriculture, Fisheries and Forestry Committee for the Mexico/U.S. Gulf of Mexico States Accord; President of the Association of Food and Drug Officials; Chairman of the Conference for Food Protection, and Chair of Government Relations for IFT and Chair of the IFT Foundation. She served on advisory groups for the FDA (Microbiological Criteria for Foods, Food Advisory Committee), USDA, and other state and industry groups. Currently, Dr. Roberts also works as a private consultant in the food safety, government relations, and agricultural environmental areas and serves on the Farm Foundation Roundtable, Food Foresight food trend analysis group, and the Center for Produce Safety Executive Committee. She received her B.S. in Biology from North Georgia College and her M.S. and Ph.D. in microbiology from the University of Georgia, where she also completed postdoctoral studies in public health.

JOSEPH V. RODRICKS, Ph.D., is a founding principal of ENVIRON International, a technical consulting firm founded in 1982, and a Visiting Professor at the Johns Hopkins University School of Public Health. He is an internationally recognized expert in toxicology and risk analysis and in their uses in regulation, and he has consulted for hundreds of manufacturers, government agencies, and WHO. Dr. Rodricks has authored more than 150 publications on toxicology and risk analysis and has lectured nationally and internationally on these topics. From 1965 to 1980, he was Deputy Associate Commissioner for Health Affairs and Toxicologist for the FDA. Dr. Rodricks has served as a member of a number of NRC and IOM committees, including the Committee on Public Health Risk Assessment of Poultry Inspection Programs, the Committee on Institutional Means for Assessment of Risks to Public Health, the Committee on Scientific Evaluation of Dietary Reference Intakes, and currently the Committee on Decision Making Under Uncertainty; he also serves on the Board on Environmental Studies and Toxicology. He has been certified as a Diplomate of the American Board of Toxicology since 1982. Dr. Rodricks holds a Ph.D. in biochemistry and an M.S. in organic chemistry from the University of Maryland. He was a postdoctoral scholar at the University of California, Berkeley.